Optimizing Health Literacy for Improved Clinical Practices

Vassilios E. Papalois
Imperial College, UK

Maria Theodosopoulou
Imperial College, UK

A volume in the Advances in Medical Technologies and Clinical Practice (AMTCP) Book Series

IGI Global
DISSEMINATOR OF KNOWLEDGE

Published in the United States of America by
IGI Global
Medical Information Science Reference (an imprint of IGI Global)
701 E. Chocolate Avenue
Hershey PA, USA 17033
Tel: 717-533-8845
Fax: 717-533-8661
E-mail: cust@igi-global.com
Web site: http://www.igi-global.com

Library of Congress Cataloging-in-Publication Data

Names: Papalois, Vassilios E., editor. | Theodosopoulou, Maria, 1972- editor.
Title: Optimizing health literacy for improved clinical practices / Vassilios E. Papalois and Maria Theodosopoulou, editors.
Description: Hershey, PA : Medical Information Science Reference, [2018] | Includes bibliographical references.
Identifiers: LCCN 2017028081| ISBN 9781522540748 (hardcover) | ISBN 9781522540755 (ebook)
Subjects: | MESH: Health Literacy
Classification: LCC RA427.8 | NLM WA 590 | DDC 362.1--dc23 LC record available at https://lccn.loc.gov/2017028081

This book is published in the IGI Global book series Advances in Medical Technologies and Clinical Practice (AMTCP) (ISSN: 2327-9354; eISSN: 2327-9370)

British Cataloguing in Publication Data
A Cataloguing in Publication record for this book is available from the British Library.

For electronic access to this publication, please contact: eresources@igi-global.com.

Advances in Medical Technologies and Clinical Practice (AMTCP) Book Series

Srikanta Patnaik
SOA University, India
Priti Das
S.C.B. Medical College, India

ISSN:2327-9354
EISSN:2327-9370

Mission

Medical technological innovation continues to provide avenues of research for faster and safer diagnosis and treatments for patients. Practitioners must stay up to date with these latest advancements to provide the best care for nursing and clinical practices.

The **Advances in Medical Technologies and Clinical Practice (AMTCP) Book Series** brings together the most recent research on the latest technology used in areas of nursing informatics, clinical technology, biomedicine, diagnostic technologies, and more. Researchers, students, and practitioners in this field will benefit from this fundamental coverage on the use of technology in clinical practices.

Coverage

- Telemedicine
- Biomechanics
- Diagnostic Technologies
- Patient-Centered Care
- Medical informatics
- Biometrics
- E-Health
- Neural Engineering
- Clinical Nutrition
- Clinical Studies

IGI Global is currently accepting manuscripts for publication within this series. To submit a proposal for a volume in this series, please contact our Acquisition Editors at Acquisitions@igi-global.com or visit: http://www.igi-global.com/publish/.

The Advances in Medical Technologies and Clinical Practice (AMTCP) Book Series (ISSN 2327-9354) is published by IGI Global, 701 E. Chocolate Avenue, Hershey, PA 17033-1240, USA, www.igi-global.com. This series is composed of titles available for purchase individually; each title is edited to be contextually exclusive from any other title within the series. For pricing and ordering information please visit http://www.igi-global.com/book-series/advances-medical-technologies-clinical-practice/73682. Postmaster: Send all address changes to above address.

Titles in this Series

For a list of additional titles in this series, please visit: www.igi-global.com/book-series

Multifunctional Nanocarriers for Contemporary Healthcare Applications
Md. Abul Barkat (K.R. Mangalam University, India) Harshita A.B. (K.R. Mangalam University, India) Sarwar Beg (Jubilant Generics, India) and Farhan J. Ahmad (Jamia Hamdard, India)
Medical Information Science Reference • copyright 2018 • 602pp • H/C (ISBN: 9781522547815) • US $265.00 (our price)

Biomedical Signal and Image Processing in Patient Care
Maheshkumar H. Kolekar (Indian Institute of Technology Patna, India) and Vinod Kumar (Indian Institute of Technology Roorkee, India)
Medical Information Science Reference • copyright 2018 • 312pp • H/C (ISBN: 9781522528296) • US $265.00 (our price)

Next-Generation Mobile and Pervasive Healthcare Solutions
Jose Machado (University of Minho, Portugal) António Abelha (University of Minho, Portugal) Manuel Filipe Santos (University of Minho, Portugal) and Filipe Portela (University of Minho, Portugal)
Medical Information Science Reference • copyright 2018 • 286pp • H/C (ISBN: 9781522528517) • US $245.00 (our price)

Innovative Research in Thermal Imaging for Biology and Medicine
Ricardo Vardasca (University of Porto, Portugal) and Joaquim Gabriel Mendes (University of Porto, Portugal)
Medical Information Science Reference • copyright 2017 • 340pp • H/C (ISBN: 9781522520726) • US $210.00 (our price)

Internet of Things and Advanced Application in Healthcare
Catarina I. Reis (Polytechnic Institute of Leiria, Portugal) and Marisa da Silva Maximiano (Polytechnic Institute of Leiria, Portugal)
Medical Information Science Reference • copyright 2017 • 349pp • H/C (ISBN: 9781522518204) • US $210.00 (our price)

Integrating Biologically-Inspired Nanotechnology into Medical Practice
B.K. Nayak (K.M. Centre for Post Graduate Studies, India) Anima Nanda (Sathyabama University, India) and M. Amin Bhat (Sathyabama University, India)
Medical Information Science Reference • copyright 2017 • 394pp • H/C (ISBN: 9781522506102) • US $190.00 (our price)

Recent Advances in Drug Delivery Technology
Raj K. Keservani (Rajiv Gandhi Proudyogiki Vishwavidyalaya, India) Anil K. Sharma (Delhi Institute of Pharmaceutical Sciences and Research, India) and Rajesh Kumar Kesharwani (National Institute of Technology, Warangal, India)
Medical Information Science Reference • copyright 2017 • 510pp • H/C (ISBN: 9781522507543) • US $215.00 (our price)

IGI Global
DISSEMINATOR OF KNOWLEDGE

701 East Chocolate Avenue, Hershey, PA 17033, USA
Tel: 717-533-8845 x100 • Fax: 717-533-8661
E-Mail: cust@igi-global.com • www.igi-global.com

Table of Contents

Detailed Table of Contents

Urbanization is one of the leading global trends of the twenty-first century impacting health. By 2050, over 70% of the world's population will live in cities facing health opportunities as well as challenges. Health literacy is a key attribute for urban settings entailing the knowledge, motivation, and competencies of citizens to access, understand, appraise, and apply information to manage health and interact with services related to health and wellbeing. Health literate citizens are an asset for communities and the cities at large and the investment in health literacy helps saving time, saving money, and saving lives. The health literacy agenda of the healthy cities network is introduced and examples are provided on how various healthy cities have implemented actions. Finally, recommendations are provided on how to create health literate settings.

The trajectory of health literacy has been shifting in an attempt to include the context of where patients receive their healthcare and treatment. Healthcare professionals and organizations that prioritize health literacy will redesign the way that they practice and deliver care to better align with the skills and abilities of those accessing care and services. This chapter suggests using the health literacy tapestry conceptual model along with the ten attributes of health literate healthcare organizations in a multifaceted approach to assess, plan, and implement sustainable health literacy strategies throughout the fabric of the entire healthcare organization.

Health literacy has been found to be linked to healthcare understanding and decision making. Therefore, it makes sense why individuals who do not understand clinical trials will be less likely to want to enroll in one. In fact, three major barriers found in the literature that prevent potential participants from enrolling in clinical trials include a distrust or negative perception, lack of understanding, and lack of accessible and affordable healthcare. Hence, there is a need to increase potential participants' healthcare understanding so that they can make the best healthcare decisions for themselves. Strategies suggested to help increase potential participants' health literacy include revising informed consent forms, utilizing culturally targeted statements, using a variety of material, and training investigative site personnel. These proposed strategies may help increase health literacy, which in turn could improve clinical trial recruitment. Furthermore, these strategies focus on different elements of health literacy and coupled together may bring the most improvement.

Modern healthcare needs to identify parameters for high-quality care. Quality improvement is the key for advancing in healthcare, and the new assessment tool shifts from a disease-centered outcome to a patient-centered outcome. Clinical outcome such as morbidity and mortality are directly connected and interdependent from patient-reported outcomes: well-informed patients who decide with their healthcare provider what treatment is best for them have better outcomes and higher patient satisfaction rates. These subjective data collected by rigorous, meaningful, and scientific methods and presented in a utilizable format can be used to create care objectives towards which both the surgeon and their patient can travel. Time has come to carry patient-centered outcomes from research into decision making and daily care plans. This chapter outlines a focus beyond life-prolonging therapy, aiming to minimize the negative effects of treatment, optimize quality of life, and align medical decisions with patient expectations.

This chapter focuses on the contribution of communication competences, used by healthcare professionals in the clinical relationship with patients, to improve therapeutic adherence through a better understanding of health instructions and, hence, higher competences in health literacy. It is a main and specific goal to construct a model of communication competences that includes the interdependent use of assertiveness, clear language, and positivity by the healthcare professional, validated by a focus group of specialists. The participants of focus group validate the model and most punctuate, in assertiveness, active behavior, ability to listen, and ability to openly speak; in clarity, the simple language, utilization of verbs; and in positivity, orientation to a positive behavior of the patient. The results confirm that the assertiveness, clear language, and positivity are pivotal and strategic elements to the optimization of health literacy and clinical practices, recognized in the literature and by the participants in the focus group.

Organ shortage is a worldwide persisting problem, as patients on waiting lists increase while actual donors cannot meet the demand for organs. Cultural and religious concerns, gaps of information, lack of medical procedure awareness and of understanding transplant-related terminology are some reasons why people refuse to donate organs. The medical, ethical, social, cultural, religious aspects of deceased organ donation (DOD) bring out the need for a systematic agenda of lifelong learning public awareness raising and health literacy on this issue. This chapter presents findings of a comparative research project in three European countries about how people learn about DOD and their suggestions for systematically promoting health literacy. A total sample of 1309 medical students, renal patients, and hospital administrative staff participated in a survey regarding attitudes, knowledge, sources of information, and communication about DOD. In addition, 51 participants took part in focus groups elaborating on their experiences and suggestions regarding health literacy about DOD.

Preface

We can begin to understand what health literacy is when we feel surprised, confused, stuck, or emotionally unable to further process a personal health problem. Healthcare professionals, specialists, family, friends, the Internet, books, and magazines are some of those to whom we ask for help to overcome our feelings of confusion when we are not sure what the health information we receive actually means to us, to our case.

Health literacy emerged as a term a few decades ago, but since then, the field is rapidly evolving. Its definitions show that it is a multi-faceted concept, which on one hand needs to be well defined, so that it can be measurable, and on the other hand, needs to be inclusive and reflective of its many facets. Health literacy is closely related to literacy skills -reading, writing, calculating and interpreting numbers- which are needed to understand health material and instructions, such as filling in a medical form or calculating the calories of a portion of food. It also involves a cluster of social skills and more advanced cognitive skills (Nutbeam, 2008). Information related to health and related decisions are relevant in other aspects of living and interrelated to other literacies, as seen in the expanded model suggested by Zarcadoolas et al (2005). According to that model, health literacy is examined in the four domains of fundamental literacy (reading, writing, numbers), science, civic and cultural literacies.

The need to promote health literacy is compelling, as even in literate societies, high percentages of people find health information and navigation in health systems challenging. Health literacy skills are measured at levels describing the levels of knowledge and skills in accessing, understanding, and applying health information at different contexts (Nutbeam, 2009). The European Health Literacy Survey (HLS-EU, 2012) conducted in eight European countries showed that the differences of health literacy are considerable among the countries, but about half of the respondents had limited health literacy. Among the findings of the survey, it was also reported that the risk of having limited health literacy was over 60% for respondents who had low educational background, financial trouble, more than one chronic illnesses and were older than 75 years old.

The role of healthcare organizations in health literacy is more closely examined in the last decade. Patient-centered care is often impeded due to the miscommunication between patients and health professionals. The complexity of the systems and, consequently, the demands they place on patients and their families, may exceed the skills of their users. The discussion paper *Ten Attributes of Health Literate Health Care Organizations* (Brach et al, 2012) suggests how health professionals as well as organizations can put health literacy at the forefront regarding their mission, infrastructure, policies, practices, and strategies, so they can deliver quality services to diverse populations. Schillinger and Keller (2012) suggested a framework in which attributes can address health literacy at five levels: organizational commitment, accessible educational and technology infrastructure, augmented workforce, policies and practices, and bi-directional communication. Embedding health literacy in the health systems and their operations means that it is a continuous effort, which needs training of the healthcare professionals, monitoring of the progress of health literacy activities, and overcoming barriers, such as lack of time for screening health literacy of patients (Brach, 2017; Palumbo, 2016). Health literacy is at the heart of modern sophisticated healthcare. From WHO (World Health Organisation) and the UNESCO Institute for Lifelong Learning (UIL) at a global level, to regional health policy makers, academics, governments, health care systems and hospitals -health literacy issues receive deep consideration as they can potentially affect us all and our quality of life.

Health literacy is a skill; our ability to access, process, understand and communicate health relevant information in an accurate, efficient, clear and simple way. Health literacy is also a civic right; it is our responsibility to fight health inequality and take responsibility to take care of our personal health and well-being -starting from an early age throughout our school years, professional life and lifelong learning journey.

Whether we live in a rural or urban environment, protection of health and prevention of disease is a birth right and a privilege. Global communications, personalised healthcare technology innovation and market-oriented restructuring of traditional healthcare organisations impact our theoretical models and definitions of health literacy.

On a more practical daily basis, the concept of health literacy becomes key in public education campaigns for the prevention and treatment of lifestyle related diseases such as obesity, diabetes, high blood pressure, drug addiction, sexually transmitted diseases, stress, depression, eating disorders, cancer, heart disease.

New viruses, environmental diseases and the health toll of extreme weather phenomena and natural disasters in tune with a culture of conflict and terrorism place the concept of health literacy right at the centre of current philosophical ethical debates and media headlines regarding the respect, preservation and survival of life.

This book presents a collection of different perspectives and trends. It addresses health literacy holistically seeing its different aspects, perspectives and methodologies as well as relationships with other areas, such as technology. It attempts to build bridges among health literacy needs, research and case studies, and highlight links between research and practice.

ORGANIZATION OF THE BOOK

The book is organized in 15 chapters, which we briefly present.

Chapter 1, "Health Literacy: A Key Attribute to Urban Settings," explains how health literacy for all can be achieved through health literate cities. It analyzes factors, challenges and trends affecting urban health and sustainable development as well as how empowered individuals and empowered communities can collaborate in effective partnerships adopting health literacy goals. It presents the WHO 2030 Agenda for Sustainable Development along with cases-examples of health literacy initiatives in Stoke-on-Trent, England, and Belfast and Galway, Ireland.

Chapter 2, "Weaving Health Literacy Strategies Throughout the Fabric of Healthcare Organizations," explores health literacy as a pillar of person-centered care and patient empowerment, engagement, and activation. Building on the 'Ten Attributes of Health Literate Healthcare Organizations', it introduces a conceptual framework, the Health Literacy Tapestry Model. This holistic approach describes antecedents and domains that influence the individuals, health professionals and health care organizations. The chapter also describes strategies of how the three domains of the Tapestry Model -oral, written, and environmental communication- can address issues of equitable health care and miscommunication.

Chapter 3, "Health Literacy in Non-Communicable Diseases: Context and Cases," addresses health literacy as a context and content specific concept. It discusses two cases on the East Coast of the US: health literacy about obesity in the New York City Department of Health and Mental Hygiene, Public Health Detailing Program and workers' mental health literacy, a research about understanding of mental health insurance benefits and understanding and attitudes regarding mental health services. It also presents an overview of health literacy approaches in Greece, analysing interconnecting health literacy initiatives.

Chapter 4, "Back to the Basics: The Importance of Considering Health Literacy in the Development and Utilization of Consumer E-Health Interventions," discusses the challenges of implementing eHealth interventions and the importance of including the health literacy component in them. It also describes strategies of patient empowerment and next generation interventions.

Chapter 5, "Uberization of Healthcare," highlights the role of technological and creative ideas in reaching out to audiences of different cultures and levels of health literacy. It presents the benefits and impact of various technological platforms taking into consideration the factors of time, cost, and audience engagement.

Chapter 6, "Increasing Health Literacy to Improve Clinical Trial Recruitment," presents the problem of insufficient enrolment in clinical trials and factors contributing to it. It suggests changes in the clinical trial process regarding informed consent forms, recruitment of minority populations, decision-making aids, and communication approach of investigative site personnel in order to increase the public's health literacy on this issue.

Chapter 7, "Health Literacy and Patient-Reported Outcomes," illustrates the role of patients in the improvement of healthcare. It explains how patient reported outcomes can be a platform of shared language between patients and health professionals, as it focuses on healthcare from the patient's experience and it provides a vehicle of patient empowerment and more active engagement in decision-making.

Chapter 8, "Healthy Thanks to Communication: A Model of Communication Competences to Optimize Health Literacy – Assertiveness, Clarity, and Positivity," explores elements of effective communication between healthcare professionals and patients. It presents a model of communication based on three key competences: assertiveness, clarity of language and positivity. It presents how these competences can advance the therapeutic relationship, promote better understanding and cooperation between patients and healthcare professionals.

Chapter 9, "Reflection and Understanding of Quality Management in Healthcare," expands on healthcare systems. It reviews characteristics of healthcare organizations in the USA, their current state and advocates continuous quality improvement to improve communication and promote patient-centered care. A collaborative approach of many stakeholders is emphasized as a way through which organizational leadership could be more efficient in its goals.

Chapter 10, Health Literacy in School," presents the importance of an introduction to healthcare in the school curriculum. It refers to the characteristics of selected health-related interventions regarding physical health and mental health.

Chapter 11, An Overview of Global Health Initiatives and Practices," discusses the impact of low health literacy. It presents examples of health literacy initiatives and provides bibliography focusing on studies in disease management.

Chapter 12, "Health Literacy and Ethnic Minority Populations," discusses challenges which patients of ethnic minority origin face in relation to the health system. Health literacy is seen in the context of collaboration between individuals, communities and healthcare organizations. They present community engagement initiatives in which health literacy is distributed within the community.

Chapter 13, "Health Literacy in the Development of Kidney Transplantation Programs in Low- and Middle-Income Countries," focuses on transplantation health literacy. It describes the ten years' experience of the UK charity organization Transplant Links in Africa, Asia, and the Caribbean in supporting kidney transplantation from living donors through mentoring and partnerships. It highlights areas of limited health literacy in this issue and suggests ways of addressing cultural differences in communication and promoting patient empowerment.

Chapter 14, Living Organ Donation: Role of Ethics for Improved Clinical Practice," discusses the role of ethics on informed decisions about living donors. It presents the sides of ethical dilemmas, that the physicians face, as well as ethical issues for the donors, such as the role of financial incentives and minor donors.

Chapter 15, "Health Literacy: The Way Forward to Increase the Rates of Deceased Organ Donation," discusses the importance of seeing health literacy in the framework of health and disease, life and death. It presents findings from a cross-cultural research project in the UK, the Netherlands, and Spain with medical students, renal patients, and hospital administrative personnel regarding the sources of information they use to get information about deceased organ donation, as well as their suggestions about future health literacy efforts in this issue.

Paraphrasing the original Latin saying 'in eadem es navi', we all sail in the same boat, only in a different cabin. Let an interdisciplinary and cross-cultural health literacy evidence-based exchange of ideas begin!

Vassilios E. Papalois
Imperial College, UK

Maria Theodosopoulou
Imperial College, UK

REFERENCES

Brach, C. (2017). The journey to become a health literate organization: A snapshot of health system improvement. *Studies in Health Technology and Informatics, 240*, 203-237. Retrieved from http://www.ncbi.nlm.nih.gov/pmc/articles/PMC5666686/

Brach, C., Keller, D., Hernandez, L. M., Baur, C., Dreyer, B., & Schyve, P. (2012). *Ten attributes of health literate health care organizations*. Washington, DC: Institute of Medicine of the National Academies.

HLS-EU Consortium. (2012). *Comparative report of health literacy in eight EU member states. The European health literacy survey HLS-EU.* Retrieved from http://www.health-literacy.eu

Nutbeam, D. (2008). The evolving concept of health literacy. *Social Science & Medicine*, *67*(12), 2072–2078. doi:10.1016/j.socscimed.2008.09.050 PMID:18952344

Nutbeam, D. (2009). Defining and measuring health literacy: What can we learn from literacy studies? *International Journal of Public Health, 54*(5), 303–305. doi:10.100700038-009-0050-x PMID:19641847

Palumbo, R. (2016). Designing health-literate health care organization: A literature review. *Health Services Management Research, 29*(3), 79–87. doi:10.1177/0951484816639741

Schillinger, D., & Keller, D. (2013). The other side of the coin: Attributes of a health literate health care organization. In L. M. Hernandez (Ed.), *How can health care organizations become more health literate? workshop summary* (pp. 69–96). Washington, DC: National Academy Press.

Zarcadoolas, C., Pleasant, A., & Greer, D. S. (2005). Understanding health literacy: An expanded model. *Health Promotion International, 20*(2), 195–203. doi:10.1093/heapro/dah609 PMID:15788526

Acknowledgment

We are most grateful to the editorial advisory board members Dr. Vassiliki Bouki (University of Westminster, UK), Professor Daniel Casanova (University of Cantabria, Spain), and Mr. Frank J.F.M. Dor (Imperial College, UK), for supporting with their well-known and widely respected experience and expertise this project.

We also wish to express our grateful thanks to the authors for their truly excellent contributions that made this book possible.

We also want to offer special thanks to IGI for providing us with this platform, and especially Ms Jordan Tepper for all her hard work, comments, and support.

Chapter 1
Health Literacy:
A Key Attribute for Urban Settings

Kristine Sørensen
Global Health Literacy Academy, Denmark

ABSTRACT

Urbanization is one of the leading global trends of the twenty-first century impacting health. By 2050, over 70% of the world's population will live in cities facing health opportunities as well as challenges. Health literacy is a key attribute for urban settings entailing the knowledge, motivation, and competencies of citizens to access, understand, appraise, and apply information to manage health and interact with services related to health and wellbeing. Health literate citizens are an asset for communities and the cities at large and the investment in health literacy helps saving time, saving money, and saving lives. The health literacy agenda of the healthy cities network is introduced and examples are provided on how various healthy cities have implemented actions. Finally, recommendations are provided on how to create health literate settings.

Health literacy is about rights, access, and transparency. It is about a new form of health citizenship, in which citizens take personal responsibility for health and become involved as citizens in social and political processes that address the root causes of health inequalities as well as inequalities in access to care. – Ilona Kickbusch

INTRODUCTION

Urbanization is one of the leading global trends of the 21st century impacting health. By 2050, over 70% of the world's population will live in cities facing health opportunities as well as challenges (World Health Organization, 2016b). Health literacy is a key attribute for urban settings to ensure health for all city dwellers. Health literacy entails the knowledge, motivation, and competency to find, understand, appraise and apply information to make judgment and make decisions in everyday life concerning healthcare, disease prevention and health promotion in everyday life to maintain and promote quality of life during

DOI: 10.4018/978-1-5225-4074-8.ch001

the life course (Sorensen et al., 2012). It is developed and implemented in a wide range of settings, for instance, at home, in communities, in schools, at work, and through activities and institutions in the wider society at large (Kickbusch, Wait, & Maag, 2005). Health literate citizens are regarded an asset for individuals, for communities and cities at large and along these lines the Surgeon General in the U.S. argued that health literacy can save lives, save money, and improve the health of million considering health literacy the currency of success for decision makers (Nielsen-Bohlman, Panzer, & Kindig, 2004).

This chapter highlights the role of health literacy as an attribute for cities and urban settings to ensure health for all. Firstly, the major challenges and trends influencing urban health are addressed. Secondly, it is explored how to develop health literate cities in practice by studying the implementation of health literacy strategies and actions by cities in the WHO Healthy Cities Network. Lastly, general recommendations are presented on how health literacy can be integrated as a key attribute for future health in cities and urban settings.

BACKGROUND

The good health of all its citizens is one of the most effective indicators of any city's sustainable development. According to the World Health Organization, healthy cities are environmentally sustainable and resilient. Cities with clean air, energy-efficient infrastructure, and widely accessible green spaces can attract more investment and businesses, create more jobs, and offer more opportunity to people from all walks of life. Healthy cities are socially inclusive being places where planning and policy-making can incorporate the views, voices, and needs of all communities. Health is not only an indicator for monitoring progress but a fundamental driver of sustainable development (World Health Organization, 2016b). Where people live affects their health and chances of leading flourishing lives. Hence, communities and neighborhoods that ensure access to basic goods, that are socially cohesive, that are designed to promote good physical and psychological wellbeing, and that are protective of the natural environment are essential for health equity (Marmot, Friel, Bell, Houweling, & Taylor, 2008).

Urbanization

The process of urbanization refers to the population shift from rural to urban areas and the ways in which each society adapts to the change (U.S. National Library of Medicine, 2017). The phenomenon has been closely linked to modernization, industrialization and the sociological process of rationalization. Urbanization can be seen as a specific condition at a set time (e.g. the proportion of total population or area in cities or towns) or as an increase in that condition over time. So urbanization can be quantified either in terms of, say, the level of urban development relative to the overall population or as the rate at which the urban proportion of the population is increasing. Urbanization creates enormous social, economic and environmental changes, which provide an opportunity for sustainability with the "potential to use resources more efficiently, to create more sustainable land use and to protect the biodiversity of natural ecosystems. Urbanization is not merely a modern phenomenon, but a rapid and historic transformation of human social roots on a global scale, whereby predominantly rural culture is being rapidly replaced by predominantly urban culture (Revolvy, 2017).

More than half of the global population now lives in urban settings and urbanization therefore can and should be beneficial for health (World Health Organization, 2016b). In general, nations that have high life expectancies and low infant mortality rates are also those where city governments and policies address the key social determinants of health. Within developing countries, the best local governance can help produce 75 years or more of life expectancy; with poor urban governance, life expectancy can be as low as 35 years. Better housing and living conditions, access to safe water and good sanitation, efficient waste management systems, safer working environments and neighbourhoods, food security, and access to services like education, health, welfare, public transportation and childcare are examples of social determinants of health that can be addressed through good urban governance (Knowledge Network on Urban Settings, 2008).

Social Inequalities in Urban Areas

Broader social factors affect the conditions in which we live, grow, work, and socialize. Socioeconomically disadvantaged and marginalized populations, such as new immigrants and ethnic minorities, in urban settings, are especially at risk of poor health due to their social conditions, or what practitioners call the social determinants of health. These social determinants of health are known to cause population health disparities and inequities. But the social determinants of health are also interconnected, dynamic and interdependent (World Health Organization, 2016a). A focus on health can unlock progress to reduce inequalities in urban areas, and expand access to services and opportunities. However, ensuring the health of urban residents goes well beyond the provision of health services. While universal access to health services is essential for maintaining and restoring good health, there is ample evidence linking the quality of urban environments with lifestyle and dietary habits, which are drivers of today's epidemics of obesity and diabetes. Urban policies, for example, that lead to increased air pollution contribute to premature deaths from strokes, heart attacks and cancers. Poorly managed waste and stagnant water provide breeding grounds for the mosquitoes that carry Zika and dengue fever, and outdated transport strategies can lead to increased traffic deaths and injuries. In turn, urban planning that places health upfront – by improving access to green and open spaces, for example, and controlling the sources of pollution – offers significant opportunities for improving the health, wellbeing and economic productivity of urban populations. Sustainable, health-promoting urban policies also reduce social inequalities by ensuring better access to housing, jobs, services, and education through efficient urban transit and inclusive neighborhood design. Notably, health is a unifying theme that can bring together a wide range of stakeholders at the city level. Diverse communities with different perspectives can be drawn into discussion and debate about the merits of certain plans and programs, as well as conversations that clarify trade-offs and the wider implications of policy choices when considering the impact of the social determinants for urban settings (World Health Organization, 2016b).

Health Literacy

For informed decision-making and evidence-based informed policy-making, health literacy is essential for all parties involved. As such, health literacy is, therefore, an attribute for timely, appropriate and transparent interaction between citizens and the health and social system (Sørensen & Brand, 2011). Essentially, high literacy rates in population groups benefit societies. Health literate individuals participate more actively in economic prosperity, have higher earnings and employment, are more educated and informed and contribute more to community activities and enjoy better health and well-being (Kickbusch, Pelikan, Apfel, & Agis, 2013). However, citizens and patients are often faced with complex information and treatment decisions when they access healthcare services, need to analyze relative risks and benefits, calculate medical dosages, communicate with healthcare providers, evaluate information for credibility and quality, interpret test result and locate health information (National network of libraries of medicine, 2017).

Research has revealed that low literacy leads to higher risk of death and more emergency room visits and hospitalizations. Health literacy may not be related to years of education or general reading ability; and a person who functions adequately at home or work may have limited health literacy in a healthcare related environment (Nielsen-Bohlman et al., 2004). Limited health literacy is associated with less participation in health-promoting and disease detection activities, riskier health choices (such as higher smoking rates), more work accidents, diminished management of chronic diseases (such as diabetes, HIV infection, and asthma), poor adherence to medication, increased hospitalization and re-hospitalization, increased morbidity and premature death (Kickbusch et al., 2013).

Limited health literacy follows a social gradient and can further reinforce existing inequalities, however how limited general literacy affects people's health cannot always be clearly separated from how limited health literacy affects people's health (Kickbusch et al., 2013). Some population groups are more vulnerable to possess inadequate health literacy such as for example the elderly, people with low levels of education, immigrant populations, minority populations, and low-income populations (Sørensen et al., 2015). The relationship between literacy and health is complex. Literacy impacts knowledge, health status, and access to health services. Several socio-economic factors impact health status such as income level, occupation, housing, and access to medical care. Poor and illiterate people are more likely to work under hazardous conditions or be exposed to environmental risk factors (National network of libraries of medicine, 2017). Building personal health literacy skills and abilities is a lifelong process. No one is ever fully health literate. Everyone at some point needs help in understanding or acting on important health information or navigating a complex system. Even highly educated individuals may find health systems too complicated to understand, especially when a health condition makes them more vulnerable (Kickbusch et al., 2013).

Capacity and competence related to health literacy vary according to context, culture, and setting. They depend on individual and system factors. These factors include communication skills, knowledge of health topics, culture and the specific characteristics of the health care, public health and other relevant systems and settings where people obtain and use health information. When these services or systems, for example, require knowledge or a language level that is too high for the user, health suffers (Kickbusch et al., 2013).

In addition to the effects of low health literacy on the individual, there are economic consequences of low health literacy to the society. Limited health literacy is associated with high health system costs. It is estimated that low health literacy represents between 7-17% of all healthcare expenditures in the US. By investing in health literacy and improvement of communication healthcare costs can be reduced and the quality of care increased (Vernon, Trujillo, Rosenbaum, & DeBuono, 2007).

Whereas this chapter focuses on the role of health literacy in general, it should be highlighted that specific types of literacies are important too when discussing urban health. In this regard, environmental health literacy is an emerging and evolving concept that bridges shared theories from the fields of risk communication, environmental health science, behavioral science, evaluation, communications, public health, and social science. It is important when for example considering the risk of natural and manmade disasters such as hurricanes, tornados, oil spills, and nuclear threats. Another example of literacy concerns digital health literacy or eHealth literacy which is the ability to seek, find, understand, and appraise health information from electronic sources and apply the knowledge gained to addressing or solving a health problem (Norman & Skinner, 2006). This is relevant when more and more cities digitalize services to their inhabitants and rely on citizens ability to navigate the Internet.

Cities: A Double-Edged Sword in the Context of Health and Sustainable Development

Cities serve as a double-edged sword in the context of health and sustainable development. On one hand, they are important engines of economic growth. On the other hand, cities are vulnerable to a number of social and environmental perils, particularly climate change-related risks and other natural disasters. Despite the challenges, well managed urban development could give rise to cities more conducive to economic growth and social inclusion, environmentally sustainable and resilient to climate change, and ensure health for all (International Development Finance Club., 2014).

The objectives of the chapter address the challenges and opportunities for urban health and sustainable development when applying the health literacy lens. As an example, the Healthy Cities movement will be studied more in detail, in particular with regards to the implementation of health literacy as a priority area in the overall strategic action planning. Lastly, future avenues are discussed and recommendations are made for the investment in health literacy and urban health.

HEALTH LITERACY AND SUSTAINABILITY IN URBAN SETTINGS

Urbanization is one of the leading global trends of the 21st century impacting health. By 2050, over 70% of the world's population will live in cities. According to the World Health Organization, the factors influencing urban health include urban governance; population characteristics; the natural and built environment; social and economic development; services and health emergency management; and food security. While urban living provides opportunities, it also brings challenges for improving health due to the exposure to many types of diseases such as infectious diseases: HIV/AIDS, tuberculosis, pneumonia, diarrhoeal diseases; noncommunicable diseases: asthma, heart disease, cancer and diabetes; and violence and injuries, including road traffic injuries (World Health Organization, 2016b).

To match these challenges health literacy as an asset for individual and communities will need to play a strong role. Investment in strengthening health literacy is likely to yield a substantial return on health and well-being at both the individual and community levels. Notably, people acquire and use personal health literacy based on the social environments in which they live, and social action can improve these environments. Combined with appropriate social resources, health literacy can become an asset that will support people in becoming more resilient (have a sense of adaptation, recovery and bouncing back despite adversity or change) and active for health: for example, by adopting healthier lifestyles or demanding their rights as patients as well as taking action to improve health in the community and contribute to sustainable development (Kickbusch et al., 2013).

Furthermore, health literacy is an important form of social capital. Communities benefit from the health literacy of their members, and community members benefit from community support and resources – such as self-help groups and neighborhood support – in enhancing their health literacy. Such characteristics make health literacy a part of people's cultural capital. Cultural capital is linked to health outcomes and people's opportunities to be active in their health. Possessing and applying cultural capital

– in the form of knowledge, values, norms, and skills – increases peoples' potential to pursue healthy lifestyles and is positively associated with peoples' health (Abel, 2008).

Health literacy means empowerment. Health literacy is rooted in the health promotion movement, with the aim to empower people as citizens, members of the workforce, consumers and patients so that they can better make decisions. Furthermore, health literacy builds resilience among individuals and communities about their health and improve their skills in managing themselves. Empowerment is both a process through which people gain more control over their lives, their health and its determinants and an outcome that reflects the ability of people – individuals or communities – to influence the world. Through empowerment, health literacy programmes can contribute to democratizing the health care system and to achieving a stronger commitment to health and well-being in communities and in society at large (Kickbusch et al., 2013).

Health literacy is a relational concept (Sørensen et al., 2015) that considers both an individual's level of health literacy and the complexities of the contexts within which people act (Kickbusch et al., 2013). Importantly, health literacy is not just about developing individual skills but also about the interaction between people and their environments and about enhancing their power and voice individually and with others. Health literacy programmes, for example, contribute to co-producing health by improving communication and by addressing the power balance between service users and providers or laypeople and specialists.

Health literacy, furthermore, is context specific and it has, therefore, different meanings in various sociocultural contexts relevant to health. Essentially, the health-literate settings approach recognizes the importance of context and is relevant for cities, schools, hospitals, workplaces, universities, prisons and other organizational settings. Healthy settings make a clear commitment to health and well-being and set out transparent strategies to reach that goal. The key principles of healthy settings include community participation, partnership, empowerment, and equity. As such health literacy is a key concept in health promotion and is a key dimension of healthy settings. Health-literate settings infuse awareness of and action to strengthen health literacy throughout the policies, procedures, and practices of the settings. They embrace strengthening health literacy as part of their core business and address the dynamics in the various settings: the educational setting, the school, the workplace, the market environment, the healthcare setting, mass media and communication and social media. In improving health literacy, the attention and resources must be focused on identifying and removing the barriers that constrain effective action (Kickbusch, 2004; Kickbusch et al., 2013). Lastly, to achieve widespread impact an inter-sectoral approach is recommended in recognition of health literacy not only being a topic for the health sector but supports a whole-of-society approach (Kickbusch et al., 2013; Public Health Association of British Columbia, 2012).

Healthy Cities

The WHO Healthy Cities project is an example of a long-term development project that seeks to place health on the agenda of cities around the world and to build a constituency of support for public health at the local level (Nutbeam, 1998). The project can be characterized as a social movement that employs an extremely wide range of political, social and behavioral interventions for the development and sustenance of urban population health. At all of these levels, the movement is inspired by ideological, theoretical and evidence-based perspectives. The result of this stance is a dynamic, complex and diverse landscape of initiatives, plans, programmes and actions (De Leeuw, 2009). In its 25 year history, the WHO European healthy cities movement has played a key role in the field of health promotion in Europe and beyond to decision-makers, politicians, citizens, and professionals in many sectors. The Healthy Cities movement origins from the idea of supportive environments which are one of the five core action areas of the Ottawa Charter on Health Promotion (World Health Organization, 1986). A healthy city can be defined as a city that is continually creating and improving those physical and social environments and expanding those community resources that enable people to mutually support each other in performing all the functions of life and in developing to their maximum potential (Nutbeam, 1998). The pre-requisites for developing healthy cities include political leadership by municipalities, vision and strategy, inter-sectoral collaboration and network (Tsouros, 2009).

Notably, the strategic goals of the WHO European Healthy Cities Network include

- Promoting action to put health high on the social and political agenda of cities,
- Promoting policies and action for health and sustainable development at the local level emphasizing addressing the determinants of health, equity in health and the principles of the European policies Health for All and Health 2020,
- Promoting inter-sectoral and participatory governance for health, health, and equity in all local policies and integrated planning for health,
- Generating policy and practice expertise, good evidence, knowledge and methods that can be used to promote health in all cities in the European Region,
- Promoting solidarity, cooperation and working links between European cities and networks of local authorities and partnerships with agencies concerned with urban issues,
- Increasing the accessibility of the WHO European Network to all Member States in the European Region.

In 2012, WHO European Member States adopted Health 2020 – the European policy framework supporting action across government and society for health and well-being (WHO Regional Office for Europe, 2013). In this regard, the cities of the WHO European Healthy Cities Network and national networks are considered key vehicles for delivering Health 2020 with opportunities for increased collaborative leadership across levels of government to gain improved health equity and health and well-being outcomes at all levels.

Linked to empowerment, health literacy was highlighted as a priority area in the most recent phase of the Healthy Cities strategic planning for 2014-2018. It was stated that empowerment is a multidimensional social process through which individuals and populations gain better understanding of and control over their lives. People are seen increasingly as the co-producers of their own health. Increased health literacy and access to good health-related information are prerequisites. Inadequate or problematic health literacy competencies in populations across Europe result in less healthy choices, riskier behavior, poorer health, less self-management and more hospitalization. Strengthening health literacy requires a life-course approach, is sensitive to cultural and contextual factors and is concerned with both individuals and the health literacy–friendliness of the settings within which people obtain and use their health information. Notably, healthy cities are a key setting for addressing health literacy. Through innovative partnerships with civil society including with communities of key populations at higher risk, healthy cities can advocate for and support health literacy strengthening programmes and services (Regional Office for Europe. World Health Organization, 2014). In response to the call for action, a number of cities implemented health literacy initiatives as part of their urban planning approach. Examples are provided in the following to illuminate various ways of adopting health literacy on the urban policy agenda.

Belfast, Northern Ireland

Health Literacy is a core theme for Belfast as part of the WHO Healthy Cities Network phase 2014-2018. The concept is highlighted within government policy in the Northern Ireland Executive's Making Life Better - a whole system framework for public health (2013-2023) (Department of Health, 2017). Making Life Better is the strategic framework for public health. It is designed to provide direction for policies and actions to improve the health and wellbeing of people in Northern Ireland and to reduce health inequalities. Health literacy is defined in the policy framework as the cognitive and social skills which determine the motivation and ability of individuals to gain access to, understand and use information in ways that promote and maintain good health. (World Health Organization, 2009). It is emphasized that health literacy means more than being able to read pamphlets; it empowers people to make healthier choices, decide to change their lifestyle and take action. Health literacy is dynamic, being influenced by both the individual and the healthcare system. Furthermore, the policy framework enhances that everyone has a personal responsibility for making decisions which can impact on their own health and wellbeing, but some may need more support than others, for example, when there are conflicting messages. Health and social care professionals including the independent Family Practitioner Services can help and guide people to make appropriate choices - the role of all professionals is not just about treatment when people are ill. It also encompasses supporting people to stay well and live more healthily, including those already living with a condition. This may be through giving them information and support about healthy living and guiding them to any further help they may need. The potential of the front-line workforce needs to be maximised. In many cases, it may be that individuals could be supported by a different service either within or outside of the health and social care system, or perhaps by a wider public or community-based service. It will be important that health professionals look to build linkages to support services beyond their own specialty, and beyond the health system to be able to signpost access to appropriate help. Improving health literacy aims to influence not only individual lifestyle decisions, and decisions about treatment and self-care, but also raise awareness of the determinants of health, and encourage individual and collective actions – at all levels of society - which may lead to a modification of these determinants. Improving health literacy needs to go beyond a narrow concept of health education and individual behavior, and address the environmental, political and social factors that determine health (Department of Health, 2017).

In preparation for taking forward a programme of work on health literacy, a working group was established with key partners to identify priorities for health literacy in Belfast, supported by Belfast Healthy Cities. A background paper was produced outlining the WHO definition of health literacy, evidence on the impact of health literacy on health and existing tools for measuring health literacy. A workshop was held to explore and develop a common understanding of health literacy within the context of Belfast. The workshop presented models of practice locally and from across the UK and Ireland. Through small group discussion, participants proposed suggestions for a way forward with partners and stakeholders in Belfast (Belfast Healthy City, 2014). The outcomes of the work included the development of a web-based resource that provides and highlights examples of local and international health literacy practice to enhance understanding. A template for evaluating and recording case-studies on health literacy was developed to provide information which may support the development of health literacy in policy and practice. A number of case studies, submitted by the working group, have been collated for reference and can be used to shape future practice in health literacy (Belfast Healthy City, 2017).

Stoke-On-Trent, England

Stoke-On-Trent is committed to building capacity in communities. Health literacy is about enabling people to take responsibility for their own health, their families' health and the communities health and wellbeing. To promote health literacy Stoke-on Trent as a healthy city will increase access to services and build community competency to practice health-promoting, health protecting and disease preventing behaviors alongside self and family care. A network of information champions and community-based information hubs will be developed through the city, alongside the development of Personalised Information Prescriptions.

Stoke-On-Trent has one of the lowest literacy levels in England (Skills for Life, 2003). The association between low literacy and poor health is reflected in this area, with high levels of long-term limiting illness affecting the city. Projects were made to alleviate this issue by developing a set of interventions that could support individuals to develop their skills to enable them to better understand health information and to navigate the healthcare system more effectively. For example, one project focused on diabetes management, with an intention to transfer key learning to other long-term health conditions. In this instance, two specific groups were prioritized: 1) Young men under 30 years of age, and 2) South Asian men. The results revealed that while all young men under 30 in the study could read, understand and interpret most health texts, more than half of the South Asian participants had health literacy scores which suggested that they could not, particularly those from the older age group. Findings from the qualitative research also reflected that although young men under 30 had adequate functional health literacy, they may have insufficient knowledge about diabetes and lack the motivation to translate knowledge into action due to a sense of indestructibility. As a result, pilot interventions were designed and implemented as part of the programme which included a peer mentoring scheme for South Asian men and the development of 'Ask Me Anything Cards' to encourage young men to actively ask questions about their condition. Further recommendations were raised including providing transition services for young adults; whole-family approaches and community links for South Asian groups; staff training to deliver clear messages; simplification of diabetes management; and joining up of patient support services within Stoke-On-Trent (Vida Estacio et al., 2012).

The Stoke-On-Trent City Council launched three movies to inform about health literacy. They explained about health literacy in general and why it is important; and provided information for patients, clients, and customers and for health professionals (Stoke on Trent City Council, 2017). In addition, to increase capacity building training on health literacy awareness was conducted for health professionals and frontline workers (Mills, 2017).

Galway, Ireland

To facilitate Galway Healthy Cities stakeholders in making evidence-informed decisions on the selection, implementation and evaluation of activities that will promote health literacy for people in Galway, a review of activities was undertaken. In this case, health literacy, as the discrepancy between an individual's health literacy skills and the demands and expectations placed on them by increasingly complex environments of health and social service provision. Health literacy has been consistently linked with population health outcomes. Its importance for health is reflected by its identification regionally as an action area by Galway Healthy Cities, nationally in the Healthy Ireland framework (The Department of Health, 2013), and internationally in the WHO Shanghai Declaration on Promoting Health in the 2030 Agenda for Sustainable Development (World Health Organization, 2016). The Healthy Ireland framework highlights health literacy as part of capacity building including to support and link existing partnerships, strategies and initiatives that aim to improve the decision-making capacity of children and young people through strengthening self-esteem, resilience, responses to social and interpersonal pressure, health and media literacy (including social media literacy). Furthermore, it is stressed to empower people and communities by addressing and prioritizing health literacy in the development of future policy, educational and information interventions (The Department of Health, 2013).

The review was comprised of three stages: an initial rapid synthesis of existing evidence on health literacy in the context of Healthy Cities through a scoping literature review, an online search of WHO European Healthy Cities websites and consultation with expert informants. The scoping review identified eight relevant articles which were reviewed. Themes identified included; 'Educational health literacy interventions', 'Healthcare, community and educational interventions' and 'Health literacy frameworks'. While these articles were identified as being relevant to the topic of health literacy interventions, particularly in healthcare settings, none referred to interventions carried out specifically in the context of Healthy Cities. The online search for Healthy Cities websites identified health literacy activities from five out of 24 sites which included: health literacy policies, workshops, and programmes. Information was not available regarding the effectiveness of the activities identified. The consultation with expert informants provided some further information on activities already identified and highlighted others. Overall the findings revealed that there are limited activities undertaken for the promotion of health literacy in the context of Healthy Cities (Sixsmith & O'Shea, 2016).

Essentially, the Healthy Cities Network promotes health literacy as a way to advance urban health. However, only a few cities have yet documented their efforts. Although, the three cases from Belfast, Stoke-on-Trent and Galway are not fully evaluated, they provide guidance on how city councils can start up the process of integrating health literacy as part of their strategic planning and services in practice. The key challenge for urban settings is to develop health literacy responsiveness which describes the way in which services, environments, and products make health information and support available and accessible to people with different health literacy strengths and limitations(Dodson, Good, & Osborne, 2015). Progress can be measured with performance-based and self-reported health literacy measurement tools (Boston University, n.d.) and assessment and audits related to organizational and system change (Dodson et al., 2015; Health Service Executive & National Adult Literacy Agency, 2009). The future will show to which degree healthy cities and urban settings eventually adopt health literacy responsiveness as part of their strategic planning and practical implementation for individuals and in communities.

The WHO Shanghai Declaration on Promoting Health in the 2030 Agenda for Sustainable Development

Internationally, the WHO Shanghai Declaration on Promoting Health was adopted in 2016 (World Health Organization, 2016). The declaration focused on three key areas: healthy cities, health literacy and good governance. It recognized that cities and communities are critical settings for health and emphasized that health is created in the settings of everyday life - in the neighborhoods and communities where people live, love, work, shop, and play. Health is one of the most effective markers of any city's successful sustainable development and contributes to making cities inclusive, safe and resilient for the whole population. Together with city leaders, the toxic combination of rapid rural-to-urban migration, global population movements, economic stagnation, high unemployment, and poverty as well as environmental deterioration and pollution must be addressed. It is not acceptable that city residents in poor areas suffer ill-health disproportionately and have difficulty accessing health services. Commitments were provided by the high-level decision-makers to:

- Apply fully the mechanisms available to government to protect health and promote wellbeing through public policies;
- Strengthen legislation, regulation, and taxation of unhealthy commodities;
- Implement fiscal policies as a powerful tool to enable new investments in health and wellbeing - including strong public health systems;
- Prioritize policies that create co-benefits between health and wellbeing and other city policies, making full use of social innovation and interactive technologies;
- Support cities to promote equity and social inclusion, harnessing the knowledge, skills, and priorities of their diverse populations through strong community engagement;
- Re-orient health and social services to optimize fair access and put people and communities at the center (World Health Organization, 2016).

Notably, the Shanghai declaration stressed that health literacy empowers and drives equity as health literacy empowers individual citizens and enables their engagement in collective health promotion action. A high health literacy of decision-makers and investors supports their commitment to health impact, co-benefits and effective action on the determinants of health. Health literacy is founded on inclusive and equitable access to quality education and life-long learning. It must be an integral part of the skills, and competencies developed over a lifetime, first and foremost through the school curriculum. The commitments made included to:

- Recognize health literacy as a critical determinant of health and invest in its development;
- Develop, implement and monitor inter-sectoral national and local strategies for strengthening health literacy in all populations and in all educational settings;
- Increase citizens' control of their own health and its determinants, through harnessing the potential of digital technology;
- Ensure that consumer environments support healthy choices through pricing policies, transparent information, and clear labeling (World Health Organization, 2016).

With the Shanghai Declaration, the high-level participants, followed in the footsteps of previous initiatives such as the Alma Ata declaration (International Conference on Primary Health Care, 1978), the Ottawa charter (World Health Organization, 1986) and the "Health for All policy framework (WHO Regional Office for Europe, 1999); and pledged to accelerate the implementation of the sustainable development goals (SDGs) through increased political commitment and financial investment in health promotion.

SOLUTIONS AND RECOMMENDATIONS

Cities are recommended to carry forward asset-based active citizenship into creating resilient communities as outlined by Health 2020. Furthermore, evidence of local action to promote health literacy should be further synthesized to complement current WHO guidance (Kickbusch et al., 2013) with local factors ensuring successful implementation along with implementation of the value of broader inter-sectoral partnerships in primary prevention (Green, Jackisch, & Zamaro, n.d.).

According to WHO (Kickbusch et al., 2013) a health-literate city:

- Recognizes at the highest political level the importance of becoming and remaining health literate and gives this priority through policies and interventions;
- Strives systematically to improve the health literacy of its people, its communities, various social groups and its institutions and services;
- Has leaders who understand the high relevance of health for the well-being of the city overall and the need to continually invest in and enhance the social assets of the city, including health literacy, community resilience, community empowerment and participation and social networking;
- Is committed to inter-sectoral work across government because decision-makers in many sectors understand the high relevance of health and seek health co-benefits and synergy in their policies in cooperation with the health sector;
- Provides individuals and communities with skills and knowledge because healthy people and communities are one of the key assets of cities;
- Aids citizens in navigating through the health, education and social service systems, making the healthy choice the easier choice in settings under city jurisdiction;
- Uses a range of media to deliver consistent and understandable messages and applies plain-language principles;
- Regularly reviews programmes encourage innovation and adapts services to the health literacy requirements of the most vulnerable people;
- Works with the private sector and the many voluntary organizations in the city as well as adult learning institutions to improve the overall level of health literacy in the city;
- Regularly measures the levels of health literacy in the city; and
- Is committed to accountability and transparency.

FUTURE AVENUES OF HEALTH LITERACY AND URBAN LIVING

At its core, health literacy as a key attribute to advancing health in urban settings is about creating the opportunities for urban residents to lead healthier, safer and more fulfilling lives. The health literacy strategies should not merely aim to reduce the burden of health literacy in a certain urban setting. Rather, it should regard the investment in health literacy an asset to unlock the full potential of the urban environment to enable citizens to lead healthy lives while they live, learn, work, play and interact in their city. The city infrastructure, which concerns the physical, social and governance structures are tools which can enhance health literacy, public health, and wellbeing. However, the design needs to be timely and appropriate to serve urban living (World Health Organization, 2016b). Yet, recognizing health as a core city value and have a wide variety of relevant stakeholders acting adequately upon their responsibility is multifaceted and extensive process. First, it demands understanding and embracing a concept of health which goes beyond the absence of disease, hence encompassing physical, social, and mental well-being. Second, it requires a composite apprehension of the influence of the environmental, biological, social, and political determinants of health. Third, it is important to constantly argue the case that health is imperative to people, society, and socio-economic development (Tsouros, n.d.). Whereas health sector actors can provide the relevant evidence, know-how and guidance on good practices to inform and shape healthy urban planning for the 21st century, the role of decision-makers and engaged citizens are crucial to help cities around the world embrace a systems approach to their interlinked environmental, economic and health challenges, supporting coordination between sectors and across the governance, finance, planning and outreach processes (World Health Organization, 2016b).

CONCLUSION

Urbanization will play a significant role in future health. Recognizing that the impact of low health literacy is underestimated and that it instead can be fruitful for urban development to regard health literacy an asset will be crucial for health and sustainability of city dwellers. Additionally, health literacy is closely linked to empowerment and social capital and as such it can be the catalyst to strengthen cohesion and interaction in communities and cities. The examples from the WHO Healthy Cities Network reveal that so far it is mostly the English-speaking countries that have been active investors in health literacy at city level and some city councils find it easier to implement actions than others. By ensuring capacity building among citizens as well as professionals working at system levels it is possible to bridge the gap of limited health literacy. However, it requires buy-in from all stakeholders involved to ensure that health literacy is indeed implemented – in policy as well as practice. Maximizing the impact of health literacy will support a better living in urban settings and in turn drive change towards economic growth and sustainability.

REFERENCES

Abel, T. (2008). Cultural capital and social inequality in health. *Journal of Epidemiology and Community Health, 62*(7), e13–e13. doi:10.1136/jech.2007.066159 PMID:18572429

Belfast Healthy City. (2014). *Health Literacy workshop Report*. Belfast, Ireland: Author.

Belfast Healthy City. (2017). *Health Literacy Case Studies*. Retrieved June 15, 2017, from http://www.belfasthealthycities.com/health-literacy-case-studies

Boston University. (n.d.). *Health Literacy Tool Shed*. Retrieved February 12, 2017, from http://healthliteracy.bu.edu/

De Leeuw, E. (2009). Evidence for Healthy Cities: reflections on practice, method and theory. *Health Promotion International, 24*(suppl 1), i19–i36.

Department of Health. (2017). *Making Life Better - Strategic Framework for Public Health*. Retrieved June 15, 2017, from https://www.health-ni.gov.uk/articles/making-life-better-strategic-framework-public-health

Dodson, S., Good, S., & Osborne, R. (2015). *Health literacy toolkit for low and of middle-income countries: a series of information sheets to empower communities and strenghten health systems*. New Delhi.

Green, G., Jackisch, J., & Zamaro, G. (n.d.). *Healthy cities as catalysts for caring and supportive environments and 3 Friuli Venezia Giulia*. Regional Health Trust for Purchasing and Shared Services. 10.1093/heapro/dav037

Health Service Executive. (2009). *National Adult Literacy Agency*. Dublin: Literacy Audit for Healthcare Settings.

International Development Finance Club. (2014). *Investing in Sustainable Cities: Challenges and Opportunities*. Author.

Kickbusch, I. (2004). Health and citizenship: The characteristics of 21st century health. *World Hospitals and Health Services*, *40*(4), 12–14. PMID:15751547

Kickbusch, I., Pelikan, J., Apfel, F., & Agis, T. (2013). *Health literacy: the solid facts*. Copenhagen: World Health Organisation Regional Office for Europe.

Kickbusch, I., Wait, S., & Maag, D. (2005). *Navigating health. The role of health literacy*. Alliance for Health and the Future, International Longevity Centre-UK.

Knowledge Network on Urban Settings. (2008). *Our cities, our health, our future Acting on social determinants for health equity in urban settings*. Kobe, Japan: Author.

Marmot, M., Friel, S., Bell, R., Houweling, T. A., & Taylor, S. (2008). Closing the gap in a generation: Health equity through action on the social determinants of health. *Lancet*, *372*(9650), 1661–1669. doi:10.1016/S0140-6736(08)61690-6 PMID:18994664

Mills, H. (2017). *Health Literacy Training In Stoke-On-Trent An overview of 2 training courses on offer*. Retrieved June 15, 2017, from http://slideplayer.com/slide/8888367/

National network of libraries of medicine. (2017). *Health literacy*. Retrieved June 16, 2017, from https://nnlm.gov/professional-development/topics/health-literacy

Nielsen-Bohlman, L. T., Panzer, A. M., & Kindig, D. A. (2004). *Health Literacy: A Prescription to End Confusion. San Fransisco*: The National Academies Press.

Norman, C. D., & Skinner, H. A. (2006). eHealth Literacy: Essential Skills for Consumer Health in a Networked World. *Journal of Medical Internet Research*, *8*(2), e9. doi:10.2196/jmir.8.2.e9 PMID:16867972

Nutbeam, D. (1998). Health Promotion Glossary. *Health Promotion International*, *13*(4), 349–364. doi:10.1093/heapro/13.4.349

Public Health Association of British Columbia. (2012). An inter-sectoral approach for improving health literacy for Canadians. A discussion paper. Victoria: Author.

Regional Office for Europe, World Health Organization. (2014). WHO European Healthy Cities Network Phase VI 2018) of the WHO European Healthy Cities Network: Goals and requirements. Copenhagen: Author.

Revolvy. (2017). *Urbanization*. Retrieved June 17, 2017, from https://www.revolvy.com/main/index.php?s=Urbanization

Sixsmith, J., & O'Shea, G. (2016). Health Literacy for Healthy Cities (HL4HC). Galway, Ireland: Academic Press.

Skills for Life. (2003). *The Skills for Life survey: A national needs and impact survey of literacy, numeracy and ICT skills*. Author.

Sørensen, K., & Brand, H. (2011). Health literacy: The essential catalyst for the responsible and effective translation of genome-based information for the benefit of population health. *Public Health Genomics*, *14*(4–5), 195–200. doi:10.1159/000324241 PMID:21734433

Sørensen, K., Pelikan, J. M., Röthlin, F., Ganahl, K., Slonska, Z., Doyle, G., ... Schyve, P. (2015). Health literacy in Europe: Comparative results of the European health literacy survey (HLS-EU). *European Journal of Public Health*, *25*(6), 1053–1058. doi:10.1093/eurpub/ckv043 PMID:25843827

Sorensen, K., Van den Broucke, S., Fullam, J., Doyle, G., Pelikan, J., Slonska, Z., & Brand, H. (2012). Health literacy and public health: A systematic review and integration of definitions and models. *BMC Public Health*, *12*(1), 80. doi:10.1186/1471-2458-12-80 PMID:22276600

Stoke on Trent City Council. (2017). *Stoke on Trent City Council - Health Literacy on Vimeo*. Retrieved June 15, 2017, from https://vimeopro.com/inspiredfilm/stoke-on-trent-city-council-health-literacy

The Department of Health. (2013). Healthy Ireland. A framework for improved health and wellbeing 2013-2025. Dublin, Ireland: Author.

Tsouros, A. (2009). City leadership for health and sustainable development: The World Health Organization European Healthy Cities Network. *Health Promotion International*, *24*(Suppl 1), i4–i10. doi:10.1093/heapro/dap050 PMID:19914987

Tsouros, A. (n.d.). City Leadership for Health and Well-being: Back to the Future. *Journal of Urban Health: Bulletin of the New York Academy of Medicine, 90*. 10.1007/s11524-013-9825-8

U.S. National Library of Medicine. (2017). *Urbanization*. Retrieved June 17, 2017, from https://meshb.nlm.nih.gov/record/ui?ui=D014507

Vernon, J., Trujillo, A., Rosenbaum, S., & DeBuono, B. (2007). *Low health literacy: Implications for national policy*. Academic Press.

Vida Estacio, Saidy-Khan, Karic, McKinley, Sargeant, Murray, ... Wydell. (2012). Action on health literacy in Stoke-on-Trent: Engaging South Asian men and Young men with Diabetes. Stoke-on-Trent, UK: Academic Press.

WHO Regional Office for Europe. (1999). *Health 21. The health for all policy framework for the WHO European region*. Copenhagen: WHO Regional Office for Europe.

WHO Regional Office for Europe. (2013). *WHO European Ministerial Conference on the Prevention and Control of Noncommunicable Diseases in the Context of Health 2020 Ashgabat Declaration on the Prevention and Control of Noncommunicable Diseases in the Context of Health 2020*. Ashgabat: Author.

World Health Organization. (1986). *The Ottawa Charter for health promotion*. Geneva: WHO.

World Health Organization. (2009). *Nairobi Call To Action*. Geneva: WHO.

World Health Organization. (2016). Global report on urban health: equitable, healthier cities for sustainable development. Kobe, Japan: WHO.

World Health Organization. (2016). Health as the pulse of the new urban agenda: United Nations conference on housing and sustainable urban development, Quito, October 2016. Geneva: WHO.

World Health Organization. (2016). Shanghai Declaration on Health Promotion in the 2030 Agenda for Sustainable Development. Geneva: WHO.

KEY TERMS AND DEFINITIONS

Determinants of Health: The determinants of health include the social and economic environment, the physical environment, and the person's individual characteristics and behaviors.

Health Literacy: The knowledge and skills to manage health in everyday life.

Health Literate Organization: An organization sensitive to health literacy matters.

Health Literate Setting: A setting sensitive to health literacy matters.

Health Literate Society: A society sensitive to health literacy matters.

Healthy City: A healthy city is continually creating and improving the physical and social environments and expanding the community resources that enable people to develop their fullest potential.

Urban Health: The health of people living in urban areas.

Urbanization: The population shift from rural to urban areas and the ways in which each society adapts to the change.

Chapter 2
Weaving Health Literacy Strategies Throughout the Fabric of Healthcare Organizations

Terri Ann Parnell
Health Literacy Partners, LLC, USA & Stony Brook University, USA

ABSTRACT

The trajectory of health literacy has been shifting in an attempt to include the context of where patients receive their healthcare and treatment. Healthcare professionals and organizations that prioritize health literacy will redesign the way that they practice and deliver care to better align with the skills and abilities of those accessing care and services. This chapter suggests using the health literacy tapestry conceptual model along with the ten attributes of health literate healthcare organizations in a multifaceted approach to assess, plan, and implement sustainable health literacy strategies throughout the fabric of the entire healthcare organization.

INTRODUCTION

This chapter will describe how the integration of health literacy strategies is essential to the provision of safe and equitable care for all patients. Only 12% of American adults have achieved the health literacy skills needed to understand health information and adequately access or navigate the complex health care system (Kutner, Greenberg, Jin & Paulson, 2003). Limited health literacy is also a concern for the general population in European countries where approximately one third of the population exhibits similar limited health literacy skills (HLS-EU Consortium, 2012). Previously, limited health literacy had been mostly attributed to an individual users skill, however recently there has been an increasing appreciation of the contributory role that health care providers and organizations have in enhancing an individual's health literacy. Even when looking at the evolving health literacy landscape, many have focused primarily on the health care professional's role as an effective communicator to patients. The significant contributions

DOI: 10.4018/978-1-5225-4074-8.ch002

that health care organizations can have in enhancing a patients' ability to understand health information and improve their ability to navigate the complex health system have not been included (Annarumma & Palumbo, 2016). Weaving health literacy strategies throughout the fabric of all heath care organizations will enhance alignment of complex organizational demands with the skills and support needed for all individuals accessing health care. Ultimately, this will foster and promote the provision of equitable health care for all (Logan et al., 2015).

This chapter explores knowledge and skills that will enhance the reader's ability to:

1. Understand the significance of integrating health literacy into a health care organization's mission, operations and quality initiatives;
2. Understand the importance of health literacy relative to person-centered care, patient safety, engagement and activation;
3. Define organizational health literacy strategies that will lessen the burden for individuals accessing health care and lastly;
4. Discuss the need to include patients and community members in health literacy efforts that meet the needs of all populations being served.

BACKGROUND

While the concept of health literacy was introduced several decades ago, the definition has continued to evolve (Berkman, Davis, & McCormack, 2010). Early definitions focused primarily on ability of individuals to apply reading and mathematical skills in a health care context (AMA Ad Hoc Committee, 1999) such as the constellation of skills required to function in the health care environment. This includes for example, the ability to read and comprehend medication bottles or appointment slips. A second early definition that focused on an individual's skills, originally developed by Ratzan and Parker (2000) and later used by the Institute of Medicine, is the degree to which individuals have the capacity to obtain, process, and understand basic health information and services needed to make appropriate health decisions (IOM, 2004).

More recently, health literacy has been viewed as being multi-dimensional and dependant upon individual and system factors, including communication skills and knowledge of laypersons and professionals, along with the culture and demands of health care situations and systems (Pleasant et al., 2016).

The effectiveness of health literate health care organizations will increase, as health literacy becomes accepted as a multi-dimensional, fluid, interwoven concept. Awareness of the importance of health literacy has evolved to a focus on the relationship or product of individual skills and the health literacy related burden placed upon individuals by complex health care organizations (Altin & Stock, 2015). Even individuals that are educated and literate when in their familiar environment and area of expertise may find themselves experiencing low health literacy when asked to comprehend and make informed decisions when placed in an unfamiliar environment where medical terms are used (Protheroe, Nutbeam & Rowlands, 2009). A health literate health care organization aligns and creates a culture and environment that engages and empowers all individuals so that they can successfully access and benefit from the wide range of health care services available (Brach et al., June 2012).

As health care systems become more complex, patients must become further engaged in a variety of tasks and skills in order to successfully manage their health care (DeWalt & McNeill, 2013). Most health-related interactions, such as managing a chronic illness or a complex medication regimen, require proficient health literacy skills. The skills necessary for a patient to access and navigate throughout the complex health care environment, understand and follow through with health care instructions and then comprehend insurance coverage related to the encounter requires a proficient level of health literacy. Partnering with patients to achieve safe, person-centered, equitable care cannot occur unless systems change to enhance alignment of the health care demands with the skills and abilities of those accessing health care and services.

In 2012, the Board on Population Health and Public Health Practice of the Institute of Medicine's Roundtable on Health Literacy published a perspective paper that suggested attributes of health literate health care organizations and systems (Brach et al., June 2012). This perspective paper informs ten organizational attributes with suggestions on how to attain each attribute, but is not prescriptive in nature, as it is understood that not all suggestions would be applicable to every type of health care organization. Attainment of the suggested attributes requires more than increased health literacy awareness. It necessitates a foundational knowledge of health literacy with an emphasis on organizational integration for sustainable culture change.

Furthermore, organizational health literacy is an essential component for attaining increased patient empowerment and engagement (Annarumma, Palumbo & Cavallone, 2016). Engaging patients in their own health care foundationally relies on health literacy (Koh, Brach, Harris & Parchman, 2013). Others have shared that health literacy is a crucial strategy for empowerment which will enhance a person's control over their health and well-being and also increase an individual's ability to seek information and responsibly participate (Kirkbush, Wait & Magg, 2006). Protheroe et al. (2009) reported limited health literacy as a significant barrier to a patient's ability to participate in health care in England. A suggested multi-prong approach includes interventions designed to increase patient knowledge and empowerment in addition to enhancing awareness and sensitivity of health care providers to the challenges faced by those with low literacy (Paasche-Orlow & Wolf, 2007).

As the need for improved health literacy continues to grow as an international priority, it is imperative that health care organizations partner with patients so that person-centered care is provided for everyone. Health literate health care organizations are those that implement strategies that universally make it easier for all patients to navigate, understand, and use health information and services so that they can adequately manage their health (Brach et al., June 2012). Health literate organizations also understand that all individuals, even those who may ordinarily have adequate health literacy, may experience low health literacy when in an unfamiliar environment, when experiencing anxiety or pain or when under acute stress. Organizational and systemic initiatives that raise awareness, educate and incorporate health literacy throughout the fabric of all processes are unquestionably needed. It is imperative that health systems be redesigned so that they can accommodate to the unpredictability of low health literacy (Rudd, 2010).

THE HEALTH LITERACY TAPESTRY

The Health Literacy Tapestry illustrated in Figure 1, is a conceptual framework highlighting the rich, dynamic, and complex nature of health literacy (Parnell, 2015).

Figure 1. The health literacy tapestry
© 2014 Springer Publishing Company. Used with permission.

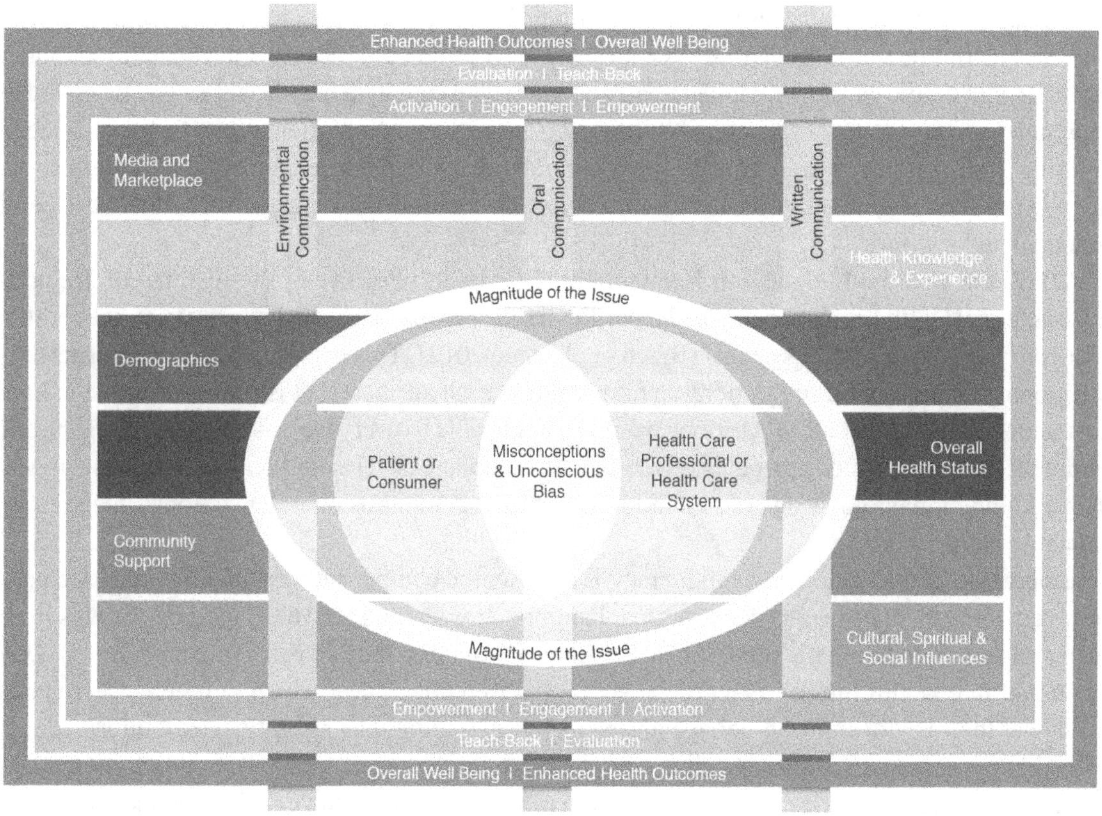

A tapestry can be defined as something that resembles a richly and complexly designed cloth; anything with variegated or complex details or an intricate combination of things or sequence of events (American Heritage Dictionary, 2012). Health literacy is a complex concern that is dynamic and changes for each individual depending upon each specific health context. The Health Literacy Tapestry illustrates a holistic approach with six interwoven "threads (antecedents) and three "fibers" (domains) that have an impact upon both the individual and the health professional or health care system (Parnell, 2015). The main fibers (domains) of health literacy include oral communication, written communication and environmental communication, which encompasses access and navigation. The "threads" (antecedents) represent the weaving of each individual's life experiences and can change over time

There are six interwoven threads. The first is the demographic thread, which includes race, ethnicity, age, gender and preferred language. The overall health status thread represents how individuals view their general health and their health beliefs and also includes their visual, hearing and cognitive abilities. The four remaining threads are self-explanatory and include the health experience and knowledge thread, the community support thread, the cultural, spiritual and social influences thread and lastly, the media and marketplace thread. Individual skills associated with each of the threads can be cultivated or enhanced over time with exposure to similar experiences and education or possibly diminish due to the specific health context or cognitive changes (Parnell, 2015).

The health care professional/system and the patient/ health consumer spheres come together at the center of the model, each with their own misconceptions and unconscious biases. For example, a patient may feel that the physician is someone not to be questioned because it would be disrespectful, or they may not accept free communication assistance services such as translators or qualified interpreters because of the misconception that there is a fee for the service. In regard to unconscious bias, health care professionals have often expressed that they can tell who has low health literacy by looking at the person or by reviewing their education level and occupation. While there is a disparate prevalence of low health literacy among adults over 65 years of age, minority groups, those with lower socioeconomic status, less education and limited English proficiency (USDHHS, 2010), education level or socioeconomic status alone do not define a person's level of health literacy.

The magnitude of the issue circumscribes all three domains, the patient/health consumer and the health care professional/health care system, as all components of health literacy are a cross cutting priority impacting individuals, health care professionals and health care organizations. Health literacy targeted strategies have been widely researched such as speaking and writing in plain language, revising consent and clinical forms, educating health care professionals, and using the teach-back method. However, implementing a organization or system wide approach to health literacy strategies may be the most effective way to address low health literacy (Murphy-Knoll, 2007; Wynia & Osborn, 2010).

The Health Literacy Tapestry model has recently been expanded to include the concepts of patient empowerment, engagement and activation as a necessary component essential to achieving enhanced health outcomes and overall well-being. Patients and their families need to be engaged as partners as well as advocates in their care in order to foster positive health outcomes. Health literacy is also an essential component for enhancing patient empowerment (Palumbo, Annarumma, Adinolfi, Musella, Piscopo, 2016). Empowering patients is an important priority for health care systems. Enhanced care will be delivered when patients take on more responsibility with self-management of chronic disease and even promoting their overall health and wellness. When patients feel confident in their ability to follow through with medical instructions and health care skills they are more likely to fully participate in managing their overall health (Smith, Curtis, Wardle, von Wagner & Wolf, 2013). Activation represents the patient's willingness and ability to manage their health. It has been demonstrated that individuals who are more activated are significantly more likely to participate in preventative measures such as annual checkups and immunizations and more healthy behaviors than those that are less activated (Hibbard & Greene, 2013). Smith et al. (2013) reported that health literacy and patient activation were often more positively associated with health outcomes than known correlates such as ethnicity and age (p.5).

Incorporating a measure of the professional's success in imparting health information to the patient by using the teach-back method is a way to respectfully assess patient comprehension. Asking the patient or family member to explain in their own words the information that was provided is a way to improve effective communication and enhance patient outcomes (Schillinger et al, 2003).

The Health Literacy Tapestry illustrates the complex, dynamic and multidimensional components of health literacy. Encouraging the provision of person-centered care by weaving health literacy strategies throughout the fabric of health care organizations will assist in enhancing patient engagement and activation, improve health outcomes and overall well being (Parnell, 2015).

ORGANIZATIONAL HEALTH LITERACY STRATEGIES

The trajectory of health literacy has been shifting towards including the context of where patients receive their health care and treatment. The U.S. National Action Plan to Improve Health Literacy (2010) reported that health literacy was a foundational component of successful interactions between patients and health care professionals and therefore highlighted suggested strategies for professionals and organizations to advance this goal. Since health literacy is context-related, the organizations, offices, and clinics where patients receive care can affect a patient's ability or inability to access, navigate, obtain and understand health information and services. Brach et al. (January 2012) described the concept of a health literate organization as an organization that makes it easier for everyone to navigate, understand and use information and services to take care of their health. Shortly thereafter, ten attributes of health literate heath care organizations were proposed with suggested guidelines and strategies to assist organizations in achieving their goals as listed below (Brach et al., June 2012).

Ten Attributes of Health Literate Health Care Organizations

1. Has leadership that makes health literacy integral to its mission, structure, and operations.
2. Integrates health literacy into planning, evaluation measures, patient safety, and quality improvement.
3. Prepares the workforce to be health literate and monitors progress.
4. Includes populations served in the design, implementation, and evaluation of health information and services.
5. Meets the needs of populations with a range of health literacy skills while avoiding stigmatization.
6. Uses health literacy strategies in interpersonal communications and confirms understanding at all points of contact.
7. Provides easy access to health information and services and navigation assistance.
8. Designs and distributes print, audiovisual, and social media content that is easy to understand and act on.
9. Addresses health literacy in high-risk situations, including care transitions and communications about medicines.
10. Communicates clearly what health plans cover and what individuals will have to pay for services.

Health care organizations that make health literacy a priority begin with an organizational assessment. It is a starting point that helps establish accountability and identifies best practices that can be shared with others and also assists in identifying opportunities for improvement. Involving and engaging health literacy stakeholders from all departments will assist with implementing your health literacy strategy, creating positive internal challenges and hard wiring the strategies for sustainability. Some helpful organization health literacy assessment tools include the Health Literacy Universal Precautions Toolkit (Brega et al., 2015), Building Health Literate Organizations: A Guidebook to Achieving Organizational Change (Abrams, Kurtz-Rossi, Riffenburgh & Savage, 2014) and the Health Literacy Environment of Hospitals and Health Centers (Rudd & Anderson, 2006). Using your assessment data will assist in reviewing and revising policies and with integrating health literacy across all quality and patient safety initiatives. Comparing and contrasting the health literacy assessment data with other patient experience data, language assistance data and the organizations community needs assessment will provide a thorough assessment as you begin your organizational health literacy journey.

The remainder of this chapter will discuss suggested health literacy organizational strategies based on the attributes of health literate health care organizations grouped across the three domains of the Health Literacy Tapestry; oral communication, written communication and environmental communication. Suggestions will be offered from the patient/health consumer perspective and the health care professional/organization perspective as well as from my personal experience integrating health literacy, culture and language assistance services across a large U.S. integrated health care system.

1. Oral Communication

Communication is the foundation of health care. In fact, every health care encounter depends on effective communication (Wynia & Osborn, 2010, p.103) and effective communication between health care providers and patients is a patient safety issue (Auerbach et al., 2016). In addition, effective communication is one way to build a trusting relationship with patients and families, have them be engaged and be active participants in their heath care (Parnell, 2015).

Health Care Professional / Health Care Organization

Health care professionals can implement several strategies to enhance effective oral communication. Effective communication begins with asking patients about their preferred language. Although a patient may be fluent in several languages, there may be a preference for one specific language when discussing health care. Requesting language assistance resources such as qualified interpreters when appropriate is essential for effective communication and patient safety (The Joint Commission, 2010). This is also the time to respectfully ask about other communication needs that may require auxiliary aids and services to assist with effective communication.

Plain language is communication your patients can more easily understand when it is heard or read, or communication designed to meet the needs of the intended audience, so that they can find what they need, understand and use the information (Plain Language Association International, 2011). Plain language is helpful for everyone, not only individuals with low health literacy. It is using common, every day words that most people will understand. In addition to using plain language, all health care professionals in a health literate health care organization should incorporate the teach-back method to ascertain if their teaching was understood. The teach-back method is not a quiz of the patient, but rather a way to evaluate how well the health care professional did teaching the patient. The health care professional should accept the burden by stating for example, "when you get home, what will you tell your family about your new medication schedule? I want to be sure I was clear with my instructions." Ending a teaching session by asking, "what questions do you have for me?" rather than "do you have any questions?" is more likely to encourage your patient to speak up and ask a question.

Health literate health care organizations implement and integrate health literacy strategies throughout the fabric of their organization. Health literacy becomes an organizational value that is part of the mission and vision. The organization creates a culture that makes clear, effective communication a priority across all areas and all communication channels (Brach et al., June 2012, p.6). It may do so by including education on health literacy, plain language and teach-back in new employee orientation, stressing that this is just as important as any other patient safety initiative.

It adapts a health literacy universal precautions approach by all staff assuming that all patients may have difficulty understanding health information and instructions. They identify physicians willing to be health literacy champions (Brach, Dreyer, Schillinger, 2013) and nurse leaders that can help bridge the health literacy gap between patients and providers (Parnell, 2014). To assist with sustainability, the organization develops metrics for effective communication that are monitored and regularly shared with all departments. They report success as best practices so that other departments can learn and possibly adapt a similar initiative. An organization that prioritizes health literacy will allocate financial and human resources (Brach et al., June 2012). Some examples may include full time roles and responsibilities for health literacy, a focus on hiring staff that reflect the populations they are providing care for or expanded language or communication assistance services to meet the needs of their diverse patient population.

Patient / Health Consumer

Addressing the delivery of equitable health care requires the collection of race, ethnicity and preferred language data from patients (IOM, 2009). A health literate health care organization educates its staff to respectfully collect this important data. In addition, patients religious and spiritual preferences should be collected and documented so that the health care team can provide culturally and linguistically appropriate care. When appropriate, patients should be offered free language and communication assistance services. An important aspect when offering these services to patients is to explain to them that they do not have to pay for this service. As our patient population becomes increasingly diverse, health care organizations must offer qualified professional interpreter services to patients and their families. Documenting data on a patient's race, ethnicity and preferred language is a fundamental step in identifying populations that are most at risk.

The Ask Me 3® initiative from the National Patient Safety Foundation® encourages patients to always ask three questions of their health care providers in an effort to help them obtain the information they need to be healthy (National Patient Safety Foundation, n.d.). The three questions are:

1. What is my main problem?
2. What do I need to do?
3. Why is it important for me to do this?

With practice, patients can be encouraged to self-initiate the teach-back method. This is helpful to patients who find that their clinician doesn't routinely incorporate teach-back in their discussions. For example the patient may say, "Beginning tomorrow, you want me to start taking my heart pill with my breakfast and walk for fifteen minutes each day. Is that correct?" It is best for all health care professionals to always incorporate teach-back with every patient, however if it is not done this is a suggested way for patients to speak up and check for understanding.

2. Written Communication

Written materials should never take the place of a respectful, effective conversation about medication management, discharge instructions or health information between the patient and his health care professional. They should however be used as understandable and clear references for the patient and family at a later time. Although written information is extensively used in health care, research findings have indicated that the majority of health related materials are written at levels that far exceed most average high school graduates skills and ability (Rudd, 2010). These complex written materials place a significant burden on the person reading the information. Health care organizations can implement policies, procedures and strategies to lessen that burden for all patients and families.

Health Care Professional / Health Care Organization

Although patient-centered communication is most often thought of between a patient and a health care professional, a health literate health care organization must also be responsible for how they communicate information in all written materials, patient forms and organizational signage (Epstein & Street, 2007). Organizations can begin by reviewing existing policies and procedures to ensure that they support the values and mission of a health literate organization. For example, reviewing policies such as general patient and family education, patient rights and responsibilities, translation and vital documents will set the standard and expectation of all staff in the organization. Once staff are educated about the policies there is accountability that will assist with culture change and sustainability. When designing written, audiovisual, social media or patient portal content the established policies will encourage all stakeholders to involve diverse audiences in the development process so that the information is clear, understandable and easy to act on (Brach et al., June 2012). Assigning oversight and responsibility for review of all patient education materials, and a process for development and ongoing monitoring will assist in delivering consistent person-centered health information. The Healthy People 2020 goal to improve the health of populations includes increasing the proportion of people who report that their health care providers always gave them easy to understand instructions about their illness or health conditions so that they knew what to do (Office of Disease Prevention and Health Promotion [ODPHP], 2016). In addition, having available staff to assist patients with filling out forms is another way to support a health literate organization. Acknowledging cultural and linguistic preferences for the organizations patient population will ensure that the written information is respectful and relevant for everyone. Allocating financial and human resources to assist with a quality translation process is necessary to develop written materials in all identified languages. When organizations start on their health literacy journey it can seem overwhelming at first. While all written communication materials should be developed with health literacy and plain language key principles, prioritizing high risk topics or departments such as informed consent or palliative care, can assist organizations with addressing written communication in complex areas that require precise communication.

Patient / Health Consumer

In an effort to bridge the communication gap that so often occurs between health care professionals and patients, health care organizations should provide written health information and patient education in a way that meets their patients cultural, linguistic and health literacy needs.

Despite mandates and federal acts requiring print materials to be written in a clear, concise, and understandable manner, research results documenting a mismatch between written materials on the Internet or in text, serve as a crucial limitation to access of information and more importantly the ability to act upon the information (Schwartzberg, VanGeest & Wang, 2005). Organizations can make resources on their websites and portals more accessible for patients by applying user-centered design principles and carrying out usability testing with a variety of end-users including persons with low literacy skills. In addition, the organization can also collect useful feedback from the people that use the services. They can even reach out to patients and offer training on how to use the portal. This should be offered respectfully without stigma and shame, and can assist in increasing the number of patients accessing the portal and hopefully increase those that are more engaged in their care and treatment.

All written health information that is provided to the community must meet their cultural, linguistic and health literacy needs. One size does not fit all, therefore an article about new services or screenings may need to be revised several times for publication in periodicals for different communities. All too often, attention is solely placed on the written content by having it translated into the common language of the community. However, the illustrations or photographs must also be representative of the community for which it is intended. The written information should be inviting to patients and community members and they should be able to easily identify with the information and illustrations.

3. Environmental Communication

Visiting a health care organization is most often a time of stress, fear and anticipation for the majority of people, which makes access and navigation more difficult under the best circumstances. Patients, caregivers, friends and family can experience undue stress and confusion in many of these settings (Lee & Bauer, 2013). Assessing your organization's environment is a foundational activity that will assist in understanding the barriers that may exist and help you plan strategies to enhance access to health information and services for everyone.

Health Care Professional / Health Care Organization

Health literate health care organizations consider a wide range of priorities that will enhance access to health information and assistance with navigation (Brach et al., June 2012). These organizations identify strengths as well as potential barriers to access and navigation. The approach can be as varied as each organization and can be implemented with key health literacy champions, diverse teams or even invited health literacy experts from outside your organization. Whichever assessment approach you select, you will want to be certain to include patients, volunteers or community members to capture their challenges and unique perspectives.

Creating a shame free environment and educating all health care professionals and staff to anticipate patient and family needs is essential in a health literate environment. A shame free environment is one where all staff anticipates patient needs and encourages individuals to ask questions when needed (Parnell, 2015). Health literate organizations place a priority on resources to assist patients such as trained multi-lingual volunteers and staff to assist visitors. Other resources that can help patients find and also navigate their way through an organization are external and internal signage, kiosks in lobby's and waiting areas, and printed maps. With hospitals continuing to serve an increasingly diverse population, it is essential that signage and all resources be understandable to everyone.

Developing an internal organizational committee of a broad range of stakeholders is helpful in assessing, planning, and implementing strategies that continue to enhance the health literacy environment. Health care professionals can and should contribute, as they are keenly aware of how their patients and families access, navigate and experience the overall facility. The health literacy environment and the wayfinding experience significantly impact patient-centered care, patient satisfaction and can also assist in improving the bottom line (Lee & Bauer, 2013).

Patient / Health Consumer

Just as we encourage health care organizations to prioritize signage, it is important that the wording used for the signs remain consistent throughout the organization (Rudd & Anderson, 2006). This will positively impact a patient's ability to navigate throughout your organization. Signage will be more easily understood when written in plain language and if labeling is consistent through out the organization (Parnell, 2015.) For example, the heart center should always be called "heart center" and not "cardiac center", "cardiology center" or "cardiothoracic center" elsewhere in the organization. Another example is to refer to the "lab" consistently and not refer to it in other locations as laboratory or phlebotomy. The overhead and wall signage should be clear and large enough for patients to easily read. They should also incorporate the languages of the patient population seeking care and treatment. The proper signage can make your patients and visitors feel welcomed and comfortable just as improper or poor signage can make the patient experience confusing and frustrating.

Wayfinding kiosks that are in the languages of the patient population are another patient resource that is especially helpful if they have the ability to print the information so the patient can take it with them for reference. Organizational staff such as navigators or volunteers should be available to assist patients and visitors to lessen the literacy demands in complex health organizations. A health literate health care organization prioritizes the training of all staff to be of assistance in creating a shame-free environment that encourages everyone to ask questions or directions when needed.

In addition to signage, other materials can be used to contribute to an organizations wayfinding program such as furniture, open spaces, statues, art, and other landmarks. These resources provide visual landmarks that can be useful to patients as wayfinding tools. Health literate health care organizations use a multifaceted approach to lessen the burden placed on individuals navigating though their organization by providing clear, easy to understand signage, architectural design and staff resources (Groene & Rudd, 2011).

CONCLUSION

Health care organizations and systems have become increasingly complex. While it is essential for patients to have the health literacy skills to obtain information, make informed decisions and navigate through their health care experience, it is equally essential that the health care organizations and the professionals that provide the care also be health literate. Health care professionals and organizations will need to adapt their way of practicing and delivering care to always be health literate. Although many health care professionals are informed and even dedicated to meeting patients where they are to address their health literacy needs, the impact of their efforts will go unrealized if their health care organization is not supportive of their practice (Palumbo & Annarumma, 2014). Without the proper policies and infrastructure to support professionals, organizations will not be able to provide health literate patient care (Brach, Dreyer, & Schillinger, 2013). A collaborative effort by professionals, patients and organizations that focuses on patient empowerment, engagement and activation will be necessary to transform the way health care is delivered and ultimately enhance health outcomes. By using the Health Literacy Tapestry (Parnell, 2015) along with the Ten Attributes of Health Literate Health Care Organizations (Brach et al., June 2012), organizations can begin to weave health literacy throughout the fabric of their entire health care organization.

REFERENCES

Abrams, M. A., Kurtz-Rossi, S., Riffenburgh, A., & Savage, B. A. (2014). *Building health literate organizations: A guidebook to achieving organizational change*. Retrieved May 11, 2017 from http://www.healthliterateorganization.org

Ad Hoc Committee on Health Literacy for the Council on Scientific Affairs, American Medical Association. (1999). Health literacy report of the council on scientific affairs. *Journal of the American Medical Association*, *281*(6), 552–557. doi:10.1001/jama.281.6.552 PMID:10022112

Altin, S., & Stock, S. (2015). Health literate healthcare organizations and their role in future healthcare. *The Journal of Nursing Care*, *4*(2). doi:10.4172/2167-1168.1000238

American Heritage Dictionary of the English Language. (2012). (4th ed.). Retrieved April 25, 2017 from http://www.wordnik.com/words/tapestry

Annarumma, C., & Palumbo, R. (2016). Contextualizing health literacy to health care organizations: Exploratory insights. *Journal of Health Management*, *18*(4), 611–624. doi:10.1177/0972063416666348

Annarumma, C., Palumbo, R., & Cavallone, M. (2016). Empowering patients by empowering health care organizations: a comparative study. In *Proceedings of 19th Toulon-Verona International Conference*. University of Huelva.

Auerbach, A. D., Kripalani, S., Vasilevskis, E. E., Sehgal, N., Lindenauer, P. K., Metlay, J. P., ... Fletcher, G. (2016). Preventability and causes of readmissions in a national cohort of general medicine patients. *JAMA Internal Medicine*, *176*(4), 484–493. doi:10.1001/jamainternmed.2015.7863 PMID:26954564

Berkman, N. D., Davis, T. C., & McCormack, L. (2010). Health literacy: What is it? *Journal of Health Communication*, *15*(S2), 9–19. doi:10.1080/10810730.2010.499985 PMID:20845189

Brach, C., Dreyer, B., & Schillinger, D. (2013). Physicians' role in creating health literate organizations: A call to action. *Journal of Internal Medicine*, *29*(2), 273–275.

Brach, C., Dreyer, B., Schyve, P., Hernandez, L. M., Lemerise, A. J., & Parker, R. (2012). *Attributes of a Health Literate Organization*. Washington, DC: National Academy of Sciences.

Brach, C., Keller, D., Hernandez, L. M., Baur, C., Parker, R., & Dreyer, B. … Schillinger, D. (2012). *Ten Attributes of Health Literate Health Care Organizations*. Washington, DC: National Academy of Sciences. Retrieved April 26, 2017 from http://iom.edu/~/media/Files/Perspectives-Files/2012/ Discussion-Papers/BPH_Ten_HLit_Attributes.pdf

Brega, A. G., Barnard, J., Mabachi, N. M., Weiss, B. D., DeWalt, D. A., Brach, C., . . . West, D. R. (2015). *AHRQ Health Literacy Universal Precautions Toolkit* (2nd ed.). AHRQ Publication No. 15-0023-EF. Rockville, MD. Agency for Healthcare Research and Quality.

DeWalt, D. A., & McNeill, J. (2013). *Integrating health literacy with health care performance measurement*. Washington, DC: Institute of Medicine.

Epstein, R. M., & Street, R. L., Jr. (2007). Patient-Centered Communication in Cancer Care: Promoting Healing and Reducing Suffering. National Cancer Institute, NIH Publication No. 07-6225.

Groene, O., & Rudd, R. E. (2011). Results of a feasibility study to assess the health literacy environment: Navigation, written and oral communication in ten hospitals in Catalonia, Spain. *Journal of Communication in Healthcare*, *4*(4), 227–237. doi:10.1179/1753807611Y.0000000005

Hibbard, J. H., & Greene, J. (2013). What the evidence shows about patient activation: Better health outcomes and care experiences; fewer data on costs. *Health Affairs*, *32*(2), 207–214. doi:10.1377/hlthaff.2012.1061 PMID:23381511

HLS-EU Consortium. (2012). *Comparative report of health literacy in eight European member states.* The European Health Literacy Survey-hls-eu. Retrieved April 26, 2017 from https://www.healthliteracyeurope.net/hls-eu

IOM (Institute of Medicine). (2004). *Health literacy: A prescription to end confusion.* Washington, DC: The National Academy Press. Retrieved from http:www.iom.edu/Reports/2004/Health-Literacy-A-Prescription-to-End-Confusion.aspx

IOM (Institute of Medicine). (2009). *Race, Ethnicity, and Language Data: Standardization for Health Care Quality Improvement.* Washington, DC: The National Academies Press.

Kickbusch, I., Wait, S., & Magg, D. (2006). *Navigating health. The role of health literacy.* London: International Longevity Centre-UK.

Koh, K. K., Brach, C., Harris, L. M., & Parchman, M. L. (2013). A proposed health literate care model would constitute a systems approach to improving patients' engagement in care. *Health Affairs*, *32*(2), 357–367. doi:10.1377/hlthaff.2012.1205 PMID:23381529

Kutner, M., Greenberg, E., Jin, Y., & Paulson, C. (2003). The health literacy of America's adults: results from the 2003 National Assessment of Adult Literacy. Washington, DC: National Center for Educational Statistics; NCES publication no.2006-483.

Lee, D., & Bauer, C. *(2013). Wayfinding elements in the environment of care.* Health Facilities Management. Retrieved May 14, 2017 from http://www.hfmmagazine.com/articles/284-signs-of-change

Logan, R. A., Wong, W. F., Villaire, M., Daus, G., Parnell, T. A., Willis, E., & Paasche-Orlow, M. (2015). *Health literacy: A necessary element for achieving health equity.* Discussion Paper. Institute of Medicine. Retrieved April 26, 2017 from http://www.nam.edu/perspectives/2015/Health-literacy-a-necessary-element-for-achieving-health-equity

Murphy-Knoll, L. (2007). Low health literacy puts patients at risk: The Joint Commission proposes solutions to national problem. *Journal of Nursing Care Quality*, *22*(3), 205–209. doi:10.1097/01.NCQ.0000277775.89652.30 PMID:17563587

National Patient Safety Foundation. (n.d.). *Ask Me 3: Good questions for good health.* Retrieved May 11, 2017 from http://www.npsf.org/?page=askme3

Office of Disease Prevention and Health Promotion. (2016). Heart disease and stroke. In *Healthy People 2020.* Retrieved May 14, 2017 from https://www.healthypeople.gov/2020/topics-objectives/topic/health-communication-and-health-information-technology/objectives

Paasche-Orlow, M. K., & Wolf, M. S. (2007). The causal pathways linking health literacy to health outcomes. *American Journal of Health Behavior, 31*(Suppl 1), S19–S26. doi:10.5993/AJHB.31.s1.4 PMID:17931132

Palumbo, R., & Annarumma, C. (2014, August). The importance of being health literate: An organizational health literacy approach. *17th Toulon-Verona International Conference Proceedings*.

Palumbo, R., Annarumma, C., Adinolfi, P., Musella, M., & Piscopo, G. (2016). The Italian health literacy project: Insights from the assessment of health literacy skills in Italy. *Health Policy (Amsterdam), 120*(9), 1087–1094. doi:10.1016/j.healthpol.2016.08.007 PMID:27593949

Parnell, T. A. (2014). Nurse leader strategies, health literacy, and patient outcomes. *Nurse Leader, 12*(6), 49–52. doi:10.1016/j.mnl.2014.09.005

Parnell, T. A. (2015). *Health Literacy in Nursing: Providing Person-Centered Care*. New York, NY: Springer Publishing Company.

Plain Language Association International (PLAIN). (2011). Retrieved May 10, 2017 from http://plainlanguagenetwork.org/plain-language/what-is-plain-language/

Pleasant, A., Rudd, R. E., O'Leary, C., Paasche-Orlow, M. K., Allen, M. P., Alvarado-Little, W., ... Rosen, S. (2016). *Considerations for a new definition of health literacy. Discussion Paper*. Washington, DC: National Academy of Medicine. Retrieved from http://nam.edu/wp-content/uploads/2016/04/Considerations-for-a-New-Definition-ofHealth-Literacy.pdf

Protheroe, J., Nutbeam, D., & Rowlands, G. (2009). Health literacy: A necessity for increasing participation in health care. *The British Journal of General Practice, 59*(567), 721–723. doi:10.3399/bjgp09X472584 PMID:19843420

Ratzan, S. C., & Parker, R. M. (2000). Introduction. In C. R. Selden, M. Zorn, S. C. Ratzan, & R. M. Parker (Eds.), *National Library of Medicine current bibliographies in medicine: Health literacy. NLM Pub. No. CBM 2000-1*. Bethesda, MD: National Institutes of Health, U.S. Department of Health and Human Services.

Rudd, R. (2010). Improving Americans' health literacy. *The New England Journal of Medicine, 363*(24), 2283–2285. doi:10.1056/NEJMp1008755 PMID:21142532

Rudd, R. E., & Anderson, J. E. (2006). *The health literacy environment of hospitals and health centers*. Harvard School of Public Health. Retrieved May 11, 2017 from https://cdn1.sph.harvard.edu/wp-content/uploads/sites/135/2012/09/healthliteracyenvironment.pdf

Schillinger, D., Piette, J., Grumbach, K., Wang, F., Wilson, C., Daher, C., ... Bindman, A. B. (2003). Closing the Loop: Physician Communication With Diabetic Patients Who Have Low Health Literacy. *Archives of Internal Medicine, 163*(1), 83–90. doi:10.1001/archinte.163.1.83 PMID:12523921

Schwartzberg, J. G., VanGeest, J., & Wang, C. (2005). *Understanding health literacy: Implications for medicine and public health*. American Medical Association.

Smith, S. G., Curtis, L. M., Wardle, J., von Wagner, C., & Wolf, M. S. (2013). Skill Set or Mind Set? Associations between Health Literacy, Patient Activation and Health. *PLoS One*, *8*(9), e74373. doi:10.1371/journal.pone.0074373 PMID:24023942

The Joint Commission. (2010). *Advancing Effective Communication, Cultural Competence, and Patient- and Family-Centered Care: A Roadmap for Hospitals*. Oakbrook Terrace, IL: The Joint Commission.

U.S. Department of Health and Human Services, Office of Disease Prevention and Health Promotion. (2010). *National Action Plan to Improve Health Literacy*. Washington, DC: Author.

Wynia, M. K., & Osborn, C. Y. (2010). Health Literacy and Communication Quality in Health Care Organizations. *Journal of Health Communication*, *15*(2), 102–115. doi:10.1080/10810730.2010.499981 PMID:20845197

Chapter 3
Health Literacy in Non-Communicable Diseases:
Contexts and Cases

Christina Zarcadoolas
Hunter College, USA

Barbara K. Kondilis
Hellenic American University, Greece

ABSTRACT

The chapter highlights some of the methods used to embed health literacy principles into patient outreach and education materials about non-communicable diseases: chronic conditions including mental health conditions. A person's or population's understanding and engagement with health represents its health literacy. Health literacy is a form social capital. The authors use an ecological, socially contextualized model of health literacy and demonstrate how it guides the structure and content of health education material in case examples from New York City, United States, and Greece in Europe. While the specific methods used in these cases vary, the essential principal is that it is critical to identify and build on information about an individual's health literacy contextualized in the individual's or group's socio-cultural and lived experiences. Only this way can an individual's or group's health literacy be advanced so that they can engage in behavior changes for both short- and long-term health outcomes.

INTRODUCTION

We are witnessing the making of a perfect storm. Social trends, local and global, are challenging the effectiveness of our health care system as well as patients' abilities to effectively manage their health information. The first trend is the growing number of individuals with one or more chronic conditions, particularly among underserved populations. Currently in the U.S. one-fifth (21%) of middle-aged adults have at least one chronic condition and the number of people managing chronic conditions is likely to increase given the growth in the older population, especially the "oldest old" (Freid, Bernstein, & Bush, 2012). The second trend is the growing diversity of the population and growing health inequality. The

DOI: 10.4018/978-1-5225-4074-8.ch003

prevalence of chronic conditions is higher among underserved and minority populations (US Surgeon General, 2001; Sullivan Commission, 2005; Kessler, 2009). The third trend is the exponential growth of sources and modalities of health information available to patients. For example, patient-accessible Electronic Medical Records (EMRs) and Personal Health Records (PHRs) are proliferating in both small and large clinical practices and health care delivery systems in the US (ONC, 2015). So too, the number of health websites and eHealth and mHealth applications is also exploding. There are more than 40,000 medical, health and fitness apps available for smartphones and growing (Miller, 2013). All these trends present opportunities and challenges to patients, especially those who are underserved, under-educated, low health literate and ethnic minorities.

As clinicians have less time to spend with patients, and as medicine becomes more complex, patients are called upon to be more engaged and knowledgeable about their care. Patients and health consumers routinely have difficulty understanding information and performing routinely healthcare related tasks. These tasks include: tracking medical appointments, understanding health insurance coverage and medication and medication-taking regimens, understanding complex health conditions well enough to make informed decisions about behaviors and treatment options. These highlight the need for healthcare professionals and educators to understand as much possible about a patient's health literacy and how this is impacting how the patient can "manage" their health.

It is not uncommon for a patient with hypertension to say, "I can tell when my pressure is high because I get a headache" or for the asthmatic to say, "I only have asthma when I have an asthma attack." These remarks reveal much about the patient's understanding of their health (their health literacy). Dr. Ethan Halm, who studied a population of adult, underserved, asthmatics, found that these patients had either a functional understanding of the chronic nature of their condition, or they had an "episodic" understanding of their asthma. Episodic understanding describes the phenomenon of a person with a chronic health conditions who believes they only have the condition when they have symptoms. Halm's patients were less likely to perceive the importance of information about the use of inhaled corticosteroids and other means to "manage" their condition, and they had poor management of their condition (Halm, Mora, & Leventhal, 2006).

Unfortunately, the need to have patients play an active role in managing their health information and health has not been matched by health information and health management tools that are understandable to patients and reflect the health literacy and life experience of patients, especially underserved populations with low literacy and/or low health literacy (Lustria, Smith, & Hinnant, 2011; Sarkar et al., 2011). It is essential that health information and health information management tools are usable, useful and address the unique needs of the widest possible range of patient and provider populations (Britto et al., 2009; Krist & Woolf, 2011; Lazar, 2007). In order to achieve optimal outcomes, patients need to be health literate about their conditions (Baur, 2010; Davis et al., 2002; Koh et al., 2012; Schillinger, et al., 2003).

The lack of understanding of basic health and science information coupled with poor understanding of how to manage and treat a condition are fundamental characteristics of low health literacy. Almost thirty years of compelling evidence shows that low health literacy is associated with poorer patient engagement and management of their health, and poorer health outcomes. Low health literacy has been referred to as "the silent killer" (Zarcadoolas, Pleasant and Greer, 2005). A recent report by the European Centre for Disease Prevention and Control (ECDC) (Sixsmith, Doyle, D'Eath, & Barry, 2014) highlighted the 'evolving' concepts of health literacy, that "health literacy must be embedded in all population-level health initiatives at both a national and European level" (p. 3), calling among other things to have capacity-building partnerships and citizen-centered health communication efforts. Though the focus of the ECDC report was mainly on communicable diseases, the report explicitly noted that these concepts of health communication easily transfer and apply to non-communicable diseases. A report on health literacy published for the World Health Organization, Regional Office for Europe (Kickbusch, Pelikan, Apfel, & Tsouros, Eds, 2013) indicates that more than 75% of all deaths are caused by one of four chronic diseases: cancer, heart disease, diabetes and respiratory disease, and that non-communicable diseases frequently result in chronic conditions. Health literacy plays a critical role in helping people better manage their chronic disease especially as they grow older. Fifty-two percent of people below the age of 65 have one or two chronic health conditions (Kickbusch et al., p. 12). That number rises to 62% for those aged 65–74 years, and roughly 80% of the population aged 85 and older (Kickbusch et al.).

The U.S. and Greece, while geographically distant, share some important health related problems. On one side of the world, the U.S. population, especially in the country's major urban areas, is increasingly diverse and unequal. Changes in health care systems have accentuated gross disparities in access as well as understanding and engagement in personal and population health. On the other side of the world, Greece is in the midst of an ongoing economic crisis. The first issue is the growing number of individuals with one or more chronic conditions. Chronic health conditions require a patient to understand their illness, engage in medication adherence, behavior modifications and other treatment guidelines and protocols in order to manage their condition. These all require an adequate degree of health literacy. The second issue is a growing diversity of the population, characterized by race and ethnicity data in the U.S., and in Greece, characterized by an influx of migrants and immigrants (by legal and illegal means) over the last years. The third issue is the exponential growth of sources and modalities of health information available to patients, both formal (Electronic Medical Records) and informal (social media).

In looking at the U.S. data on chronic conditions, nearly one-fifth (21%) of middle-aged adults have at least one chronic condition (Freid, Bernstein, & Bush, 2012), and the number of people managing chronic conditions is likely to increase given the growth in the older population, especially the "oldest old." In the U.S. and around the globe another trend is the growing diversity of the population as characterized by race and ethnicity data. In the U.S., the Hispanic population will more than double, from 53.3 million in 2012 to 128.8 million in 2060, and the Black population is expected to increase from 41.2 million to 61.8 million over the same period (U.S. Census Bureau, 2012). There persists a disparity between the health of Whites and non-minority groups and the health of Blacks, Hispanics and other ethnic and racial minorities. Rates of chronic conditions are higher among Hispanics and Blacks, and individuals in these groups are also more likely than Whites to experience health disparities (CDC, 2013). The changing landscape of European countries and the fact that many migrants score lower on literacy and health literacy measures is important to note when looking at health disparities. The WHO European Region estimates that there are 75 million migrants, making up 8% of the European population (Kickbusch et al., 2013).

This is no exception for smaller countries such as Greece that have seen their national ethnic composition change drastically within the last five to ten years, and whose micro and macro systems, particularly educational and medical systems, will need specialized training in handling migrant issues. The impact of economic and social problems, including continued unemployment, poverty, social exclusion, and homelessness due to severe austerity policies have affected both morbidity and mortality including the rise in trends related to mental health (depression and suicides), substance abuse, and infectious diseases in Greece (Kondilis, Giannakopoulos, Gavana, Ierodiakomou, Waitzkin, & Benos, 2013). Similar impacts of economic and social determinants have been identified by researchers concerning dental care (Kentikelenis, Karanikolos, Pananicolas, Basu, McKee, & Stuckler, 2011). Some medical authors compare those trends to similar data from 1980s and 1990s of down-trodden post-communist controlled countries now part of the European Union (Kondilis et al., 2013). Researchers cite problematic trends related to chronic diseases such as diabetes, due to lack of access to proper care and services both in the public and private sectors (Kondilis et al., 2013). Though in the short-term state expenditures are reduced, researchers imply dubious consequences to long-term public health and healthcare for those living in Greece (Simou & Koutsogeorgou, 2014), and one group appropriately sub-titled their paper "Omens of a Health Tragedy" (Kentikelenis, et al., 2011) citing problematic health trends in all areas of both chronic and communicable diseases.

The growth in prevalence of chronic conditions coupled with the generally low health literacy of millions highlights the importance of developing patient education and public health outreach materials that are relevant and effective for the target population. The goal of the chapter is to demonstrate how an ecological, more socially contextualized model of health literacy can be used to develop outreach and educational tools that inform patients and contribute to advancing their overall health literacy. We use case examples in health promotion that focus on non-communicable diseases - chronic conditions including mental health conditions. Cases are from New York City, U.S., and Greece in Europe.

BACKGROUND

Health Literacy

Health literacy refers to the wide range of skills and competencies that people develop to seek out, comprehend, evaluate and use health information and concepts to make informed choices, reduce health risks and increase quality of life (Zarcadoolas, Pleasant, & Greer, 2005; Zarcadoolas, Pleasant, & Greer, 2006). Societal contexts differ in terms of level of health literacy affected by scientific knowledge, culture and community practices relating to health and/or related policies and accessing necessary services (Kondilis et al., 2012; Lahana, Pappa, & Niakas, 2011). People's health literacy is largely impacted by home, school, community and psycho-social influencers including their age, lived experience, culture, educational background, and technology.

Health numeracy, a part of health literacy, is the degree to which individuals can access, process, interpret, communicate and act on numerical, quantitative, graphical, biostatistical and probabilistic health information needed to make effective health decisions (Golbeck, et al, 2005). Low health literacy is linked to poor health decisions, increased health risks and poorer health outcomes (Nielsen-Bohlman et al, 2004). Low health literate patients have poor patient management of chronic diseases, poorer adherence to medication and treatments, higher rates of hospitalization, and poor health outcomes (Kirsch, Jungeblut, Jenkins, & Kolstad,1993; Nielsen-Bohlman et al., 2004; Rudd, 2002; Schwartzberg, Van Geest, & Wang, 2005). The sobering statistic is that more than 50% of the adults in the U.S. are low health literate and at greater risk of poor health management and disease prevention (Kirsch, et al., 1993; Nielsen-Bohlman, Panzer, & Kindig, 2004).

Experts in reading and information processing, including the readability of portal information, have amply demonstrated that linguistically "simplified" texts are often not more understandable (Charrow & Charrow, 1979; Davison et al., 1980; Duffy & Kabance, 1982; McNamara, Kintsch, Butler-Songer, & Kintsch, 1996; Kintsch, 1994). A recent discussion paper for the World Health Organization Working Group on Non-Communicable Diseases indicates literacy is both task- and skills-based. It is not a fixed asset but rather content and context specific. Health literacy affects both clinical care and public/community health. Thus, health literacy is both a personal and population asset (Nutbeam, 2017). Both a person's fundamental literacy and health literacy play an important role in what information they seek out, understand and then use, as well as their health outcomes (Nielsen-Bohlman et al., 2004; Schwartzberg et al., 2005; Davis, Williams, Marin, Parker, & Glass, 2002; McCray, 2005; Schillinger et al., 2003). Other factors influencing the effectiveness of health information are a patient's access, attitudes and skill with using communication technology – the internet, e-health tools and social media (technological literacy) (ITEA, 2007). As communication technology plays more of a role in health and healthcare delivery we see the increase in challenges to the privacy and security of personal health information when using eHealth tools (Agarwal & Khuntia, 2009; Atienza et al., 2014; Westin, 2012). We will use both the ecological model of health literacy combined with user-centered design for both the New York City cases and Greece examples, to demonstrate how the readability of information found on the internet, can be re-engineered to be optimally accessible to users.

Hundreds of articles published over the last 25 years demonstrate that much of the global population has low health literacy and several studies look at patterns of health literacy in populations via the European Health Literacy Survey HLS-EU (Sorensen et al., 2015; Sorensen et al., 2013; Kickbusch et al., 2013). The European Health Literacy Survey (HLS-EU) findings indicate that nearly half of all adults in the eight participant European countries have inadequate or problematic health literacy skills that adversely affect their health literacy (Sørensen et al. 2015). The Greek term for health literacy (translated as "Εγγραματοσύνη Υγείας" in short) was coined by a Greek national advisory panel during the creation of the HLS-EU as this is a relatively new research area for Greece (Kondilis, Magoulas, Ioannidi, & Agrafiotis, 2012). The HLS-EU findings indicate a tendency for Greeks to fall in the middle range of being fairly "health literate" overall when compared to the rest of the European sample. Regarding the EU health literacy model dimensions of health care, disease prevention, and health promotion in the range of "inadequate" health literacy – 43%, 42%, 46% were respective of Greece; 49%, 59%, 70% for Bulgaria (Spain was the highest with 52% in the "problematic/inadequate" category in the health care dimension, while Bulgaria was the highest in the other two dimensions); lowest was 25%, 26%, 36% respectively for the Netherlands (Sørensen et al.). The HLS-EU for Greece indicates that the sampled population seems to be confident in the information they receive and understand from their doctor, pharmacist, the media, or other source of social support, and consider themselves able to access the necessary healthcare services. Researchers however point out that subjective perceptions including self-efficacy and belief in effective communication are factors unaccounted for in such statistics. This suggests that "the Greek population has a tendency to overvalue their abilities or to present an idealized self-image which does not necessarily correlate with their actual or objectively evaluated abilities" (p. 9) (Kondilis et al., 2012).

Environments can greatly contribute to efforts related to non-communicable diseases. The economic crisis hit the U.S. in 2008 and Greece in 2009. Many people lost access to consistent healthcare and preventive services. The negative health consequences and even suicide is well documented (Kentikelenis, et al., 2011; Kondilis et al., 2013; Simou & Koutsogeorgou, 2014; WHO, 2009; Commonwealth Fund, 2014; PBS, 2017; Newsweek, 2015).

Science and Technology Literacy

In addition to low health literacy, the overall science literacy of the U.S. public is very low (National Science Foundation, 2003). People with low science literacy have difficulty understanding basics of the scientific process, evidence and science technology. According to the 1995 Science and Engineering Indicators, 12% of the 2,000 American adults surveyed qualified as well-informed, 25% qualified as moderately well-informed, and 63% not informed about science. More recently, in 2001, half of Americans surveyed reported that humans lived at the same time as dinosaurs, and 2/3 of those surveyed could not explain what it means to study something scientifically (National Science Foundation, 2003). Approximately three out of four adults in Europe and the U.S. are unable to read and understand news of information that uses basic science constructs (Lewenstein, 1992; Shen, 1975).

Non-Communicable Health Conditions

The growth in prevalence of chronic conditions foregrounds the importance of effective and efficient health information management by patients, and better health outcomes. Persons with non-communicable and chronic conditions are faced with the task of integrating complex information from a wide variety of sources over the course of their illness. As the prevalence of chronic conditions increases, management complexity intensifies, heightening the potential for poor outcomes (U.S. Department of Health and Human Services, 2010). In order to achieve optimal outcomes, patients with chronic conditions must effectively manage their health information and be actively engaged in their health care self-management (Bodenheimer et al, 2002; Newman, Steed, & Mulligan, 2004). Access to relevant, understandable health information when a patient needs it, and in the modality/format desired, has the potential to have a positive influence on engaging patients in their care, and help them to make better decisions about their health. Patients are working to integrate and manage complex health information using varied modalities – print, web-based, mobile, apps, PHRs, SMS, among other tools, devices and artifacts. Those management tasks are fraught with challenges and potential pitfalls.

Public health officials, health providers, schools and the media have been communicating health information for generations. Yet the effectiveness of these efforts continues to be examined and questioned. In the 1980s increasing attention was placed on the gap information content and what patients and the public actually understood and could act on, as these were the early years of health literacy research (Davis et al, 1990; Gazmarian, 1999; Parker et al., 1995; Williams et al, 1995). Initially health literacy was equated with a patient's abilities to "read" and understand health information, but it has since been demonstrated that health literacy entails much more than functional literacy skills (Nutbeam 2017; Niels-Bohlman, 2005; Nutbeam, 2000; Zarcadoolas, 2006). The last decade has seen the growth in more *ecological* models of health literacy that encompass issues of lived experience, culture and modality (Freedman, Bess, Tuker, Boyd, Tuchman, & Wallston, 2009; Nielsen-Bohlman et al., 2004; Nutbeam, 2000; Pleasant & Kuruvilla, 2008; Zarcadoolas et al., 2006).

Living well in our contemporary and ever more global society requires that we have competency in a range of types of literacies: among them fundamental reading literacy, science literacy, computer-technological literacy, financial literacy. The field of "new literacy studies" (NLS) places literacy behaviors squarely in social contexts (Street, 1993). Literacy is understood primarily as a socio-cultural phenomenon rather than simply a cognitive process. Fundamental to NLS is the assumption that we can best understand literacy practices, including reading and writing, when we conceptualize and examine them in broader social and cultural, historical, political, and economic contexts.

The New York City case studies that are included in this chapter incorporate an ecological health literacy model developed by Zarcadoolas, Pleasant & Greer (2004; 2006). This model focuses on four core literacies involved in health literacy: 1. *Fundamental literacy* (reading, writing, and numeracy) refers to the abilities to comprehend and produce written language and working with numbers; 2. *Science literacy* refers to levels of knowledge of science and technology, including some awareness of the scientific process; knowledge of fundamental scientific concepts, ability to comprehend technical complexity, an understanding of technology, and an understanding of scientific uncertainty are central aspects; 3. *Civic literacy/community literacy* refers to abilities that enable citizens to become aware of public issues, to participate in critical dialogue about public issues, and to become involved in decision-making processes; and 4. *Cultural literacy* refers to the abilities to recognize and use collective beliefs, customs, world-view, and social identity in order to interpret and act on information.

User-Centered Design

The New York City cases demonstrate how an ecological model of health literacy is combined with standard methods of user-centered design (UX). UX involves an early and continual focus on users and an iterative approach to design, whereby feedback from users, through focus groups and pilot usability testing, is used to modify the design as appropriate. This approach is consistent with current implementation science that advocates that research in intervention diffusion (e.g., the diffusion of EMRs) should engage target users in the process as "local participation" improves the adoption and sustainability of interventions (Krish, Lawrence, & Aron, 2008). It is well established in the human computer interaction and information systems literature that involving stakeholders in the design and development of technology applications enhances the likelihood of developing more usable systems (Leonard, 2004; Winkelman et al., 2005).

Poor usability of health information in many formats, including print, multi-media, and electronic, has been identified as a central problem for patients and health consumers (Nijland, van Gemert-Pijnen, Kelders, Brandenburg, & Seydel, 2011; Ashcraft, 2005; Stephanidis, 2001). Included are issues related to cultural differences (Marcus & Gould, 2000); personality differences (Hymes, 1974; Sapir, 1949); potential cognitive, motor and emotional impairments (U.S. Amendment to Section 508 Rehabilitation Act, 2000). Developers must also consider the features available to a consumer and – with the rise in mobile phone use as a primary access point to the Internet – developers must design highly 'plastic' systems that convert across display sizes, web browsers, mobile displays, languages, and support devices for disabled users. The New York City case studies to be discussed employ the methods of user-centered design as well as the ecological approach to health literacy.

Psycho-Education and Health Education

The user-centered approach aims to increase usability and level of audience engagement, and is most often used in the Greek case as it has been applied in North America in the fields of health education and health communication. As health literacy is "an important form of social capital" and empowers communities (Kickbusch et al., p. 2), the way we approach educating our patients, providers, workplaces, and the larger community is critical. The approach taken by providers in educating their patients about their illness, deciding upon a common treatment action, promoting access to care, socio-cultural variants, use of ICTs, public and private partnerships are important considerations that affect the health literacy of all (United Nations ECOSOC, 2011; Watson, Gallois, Hewett, & Jones, 2014). Lynn Payer, a medical journalist, writes in her book *Medicine and Culture* (Payer, 1996, *Rev. ed.)* about the differences in how illness is viewed and treated in the U.S. and Europe. Though her generalizations to some seem to reflect more of the medical versus non-medical models, she highlights how different countries spend their money on healthcare, and her viewpoint as expressed in her book, not only reflects the late 1980s to mid-1990s, but gets at the larger historical issue of medical training and treatment for such chronic condition like heart disease and cancer.

MAIN FOCUS OF THE CHAPTER

How to Read the New York City Case Studies and Examples

One of the pressing challenges in health communication is to develop ways to present health information in easily understood formats (Ancker & Kaufman, 2007; Ancker, et al., 2006; Cosmides & Tooby, 1996). Health information of many kinds is often linguistically inaccessible to under-served populations (Doak & Doak, 2002; Root & Stableford, 1999) and not delivered in modalities and contexts conducive to uptake and use (Lipkus, Samsa, & Rimer, 2001; Nelson et al., 2009; Schwartz, et al., 1997).

The two New York City cases presented address: 1. adult obesity and 2. worker mental health literacy.

1. Addressing Obesity Through Health Literacy

This case study (2008) describes the methods that were used to develop the adult obesity education materials for both health providers and patients for the New York City Department of Health and Mental Hygiene (DOHMH) Public Health Detailing Program. DOHMH is one of the largest public health agencies in the world, serving more than 8 million New Yorkers of diverse ethnic, cultural and economic backgrounds. The Public Health Detailing Program is a primary care provider outreach initiative modeled on pharmaceutical detailing. The Public Health Detailing Program ran from 2003 until 2011 and then was resumed in 2016. More than 20 topics over 40 campaigns have been developed to promote clinical preventive services and chronic disease management.

In the case discussed in this chapter, researchers worked with DOHMH to gather provider and patient attitudes and perceptions regarding overweight and obesity, in order to develop the Kit materials. The individuals participating in this study were healthcare providers and their frontline staff practicing in low-income communities in New York City, and overweight men and women residing in low-income communities recruited through the local district public health offices in Manhattan, Brooklyn, and the Bronx.

2. Worker Mental Health Literacy

This case study describes research conducted to identify what workers from a large self-insured, self-administered entity on the East Coast of the U.S. understood about their mental health benefits and to explore their understanding and attitudes about seeking mental health services. The goal of the project was to use the information gathered to help develop outreach and worker education materials about mental health. The self-insured entities were the 1199 Service Employees International Union (SEIU) Benefit Funds, serving members of the SEIU, United Healthcare Workers East. 1199SEIU is the largest healthcare workers' union in the United States, and the Benefit Funds are among the largest labor-management funds in the U.S., providing a range of comprehensive benefits to 400,000 working and retired healthcare industry workers and family members. Members work in the hospital nursing home and home care industries, as well as in pharmacies, freestanding clinics and other healthcare settings. The Funds collaborated with the National Alliance on Mental Illness in NYC (NAMINYC) and Hunter College School of Public Health to conduct this project.

Highlights From the Greek "Case" of Health Literacy and Non-Communicable Diseases

As Greece looks to emerge from this dark period of economic and social crises (Kentikelenis et al., 2011), a central question in public health is how can the population (re) engage in practicing good preventive care and how individuals and communities can practice more preventive health, and invest in curtailing the growing threats of chronic conditions such as hypertension, diabetes, and poor mental health. Prevention and education programs for non-communicable diseases like mental health illnesses have been sparse or lacking altogether. An example from the mental health area is the Open-the-Doors global network anti-stigma program operating in over 20 countries including Greece just over a decade (Stuart, 2008; Oikonomou-Lalioti, n.d.). Another example is the qualitative research done with both mental health providers and users of the mental health system who describe difficulties in accessing and providing necessary care due to large case-loads or financial barriers to care in the prefecture of the island of Crete pursuant to the economic crisis (Triliva, Fragkiadaki, & Balamoutsou, 2013). This and other research helps build a stronger case for the individual-community importance in addressing any health literacy roadblocks.

Studies on aspects of health literacy, such as sources of health information, include one by Vardavas, Kondilis, Patelarou, Akrivos, & Falagas (2009) with adolescents in Athens and Crete. The study results revealed a gender difference in girls seeking more sources of health information when compared to boys, and the overall results indicate the youth (N=369) are insufficiently informed on major health issues. The authors recommend better health education programming be done for youth in schools to promote healthier lifestyles and to help prevent both chronic and infectious diseases. The majority of the sample indicated preference in consulting with their family and physician over other sources like the internet, for health information, as well as the majority of the girls in the sample indicating that they are significantly less comfortable talking with their doctor ($p<.001$) than their boy counterparts are. Elements of trust are implied in building relationships with healthcare professionals, since schools in Greece do not have continual healthcare access including on-site school nurses (Vardavas et al.). The use of ICTs could enhance both the training of healthcare professionals as well as provide more useful information for patients making healthcare decisions for Greeks as well as those traveling to Greece, particularly in hard-to-reach areas as implied by researchers (Lahana, et al., 2011; Mougiakakou, et al., 2011; Chronaki, et al., 2006).

Greece has one of the largest per-capita access to pharmacies in Europe as well as the highest per capita ratio of patients to dentists in Europe; specifically, 126 dentists for every 100,000 inhabitants in Greece (Eurostat Statistics Explained, 2017). Ironically, due to the cost of dental services, less Greeks and other Europeans use these services due to economic and financial issues (Eurostat). Furthermore, an article by a practicing pharmacist (Gkiourda, 2017) indicates the importance of pharmacists in Greece in helping patients deal with chronic illness, since local community pharmacists know the medical history of their patients (e-records tracking medicines are becoming more commonplace). Gkiourda (2017) indicates that pharmacists are well-trained and description given of paying individual attention to their "patient-human" (*ασθενή - άνθρωπο*). In turn, pharmacists describe being better-motivated to guide their patients towards improved self-care and patient-provider relations, as patients with their provider's input then make better decisions for their health and chronic disease outcomes.

Though there have not been many cases relating to health literacy formally written up, it is clear that those persons who are older, particularly middle-age to elderly, those who suffer from poor physical and mental health, access more services including emergency room, often have other co-morbid chronic illnesses, and higher costs for an already economically disadvantaged society (Lahana et al., 2011; Kondilis et al. 2012; Simou & Koutsogeorgou, 2014; Sorensen et al., 2015). Non-governmental organizations in Greece such as Praxis or Prolepsis often help both economically disadvantaged and other marginalized groups access care and work on chronic health issues, build networks for better collaboration, and highlight community strengths. Local colleges and universities such as Hellenic American University/ Hellenic American College in Athens, address issues of social and personal responsibility through required or on-going courses such as "Global Citizen Seminar" and "Developing the Global Citizen" which include health literacy concepts and general information on health issues where students and faculty focus group participants indicated the multi-disciplinary approach to be very useful to young people who are constantly interacting in person or on-line with interpersonal issues which in turn affect their personal and community 'health' ranging from environmental issues such as second-hand smoke to corporate social responsibility, to name a few (Kondilis, 2016). All the afore-mentioned efforts in combination strengthen social capital for a future goal by providers and educators to improve health literacy at the individual and group level.

Addressing Obesity Through Health Literacy

The New York City Department of Health and Mental Hygiene (DOHMH) is one of the largest public health agencies in the world, serving over 8 million New Yorkers of diverse ethnic, cultural and economic backgrounds. The DOHMH Public Health Detailing Program (PHD) is a primary care provider outreach initiative modeled on pharmaceutical detailing (Dresser, Short, Wedemeyer et al, 2012). PHD works with primary care providers, dentists, pharmacists and other clinical and community members to improve patient care relating to key public health challenges. Health Department representatives ("reps") promote clinical preventive services and chronic disease management through the delivery of brief, targeted messages to health care providers, community stakeholders and staff at their practice sites. During the visits, the reps distribute Detailing "Action Kits" that contain clinical tools, provider resources and patient education materials to promote evidence–based best practices.

The following case study describes the methods that were used to develop the Adult Obesity Action Kit in 2008. Researchers worked with the DOHMH to gather provider and patient attitudes and perceptions regarding overweight and obesity, in order to develop the Action Kit materials. The individuals participating in this study were healthcare providers and their frontline staff practicing in low-income communities in New York City, and overweight men and women recruited through the local district public health offices, now known as Neighborhood Health Action Centers, located in Manhattan, Brooklyn, and the Bronx.

Setting the Stage

Overweight and obesity are chronic conditions affecting approximately 68% of adults and 31.7% of children ages 2–19 in the United States (Ogden, Carroll, Curtin, 2010). Between 1999-2000 and 2013-3014 there was a significant increase in obesity in both adults and youth (30.5 percent to 37.7 percent adults and 13.9 percent to 17.2 percent children) (Ogden, Carroll, Fryar, et al., 2015). The case presented here is situated in New York City where the prevalence of overweight and obesity in neighborhoods, when stratified by socio-economic status and race, was, at the time of development, among the highest in the nation. In 2008, in the historically minority and at-risk populations in East Harlem, Central Harlem, and Central Brooklyn, 31% of adults were obese; in South Bronx, 33.8% of adults were obese; while only 21% of residents were obese in all other neighborhoods of New York City. (DOHMH, 2008; Karpati, Kerker, Singh et al., 2004)

Psycho-social, cultural and environmental issues are often closely related as contributing factors to overweight and obesity. A growing literature shows that an area's income and availability of food and physical activity resources are related with obesity. Recent research in New York City, for example, has illustrated obesity to be significantly associated with neighborhood-level factors, particularly the availability of supermarkets and food stores, fitness facilities, percent of commercial land use and area income (Black et al., 2010). A separate data analysis of neighborhood food environment and areas in New York City calculated the lowest scores of food availability and access within East and Central Harlem and North and Central Brooklyn, areas with the highest proportions of Black residents and the lowest median household incomes, meanwhile finding the most favorable "food desert" scores on the Upper East Side, a predominantly white, middle and upper-income area (Gordon, et al., 2011). On a more inter-personal level, there can be challenges of trust between healthcare providers and patients, and recent research in childhood obesity has identified opportunity for improvement in the area of primary care providers' knowledge of obesity and their discussion with patients of behaviors that contribute to obesity (Spivack, 2010). Relatedly, interests of a family in food gratification, a gratification that is relatively inexpensive, parental satisfaction, and notions of weight, constitute other psycho-social and cultural issues in contributing factors to overweight and obesity (Kaufman & Karpati, 2007).

Health education messages to patients and the public about preventing and treating overweight and obesity are ubiquitous in the United States, and yet the alarming increases in prevalence of these conditions seem to demonstrate that they have had minimal impact on people's knowledge and behaviors. Therefore we must ask - Is there simply not enough information available for patients and consumers, not enough access to good information, or is there something more?

As stated in the introduction to this chapter, there is ample evidence from the field of health literacy that much health information for patients and the public is not tailored to the fundamental literacy or specific health literacy needs of the majority of the U.S. population (Nielsen-Bohlman, Panzer, Kindig, 2004; Schwartzberg, Van Geest, Wang, 2005; Zarcadoolas, Pleasant, Greer 2006). Some examples of health information routinely presented to patients and the public about overweight and obesity is information about BMI and weight, calorie intake, food labeling, food intake logs, as well as exercise, and the proliferation of apps and websites. To greater or lesser degree this information assumes that the user can read and interpret the material, including numbers in charts and graphs, has some basic understanding of nutrition science – food converting to energy, calories used by the body, and the information assumes the user can modify behaviors to manage weight better.

The DOHMH was mindful of the mismatch between content in traditional patient materials and patients' literacy levels and set out to develop materials for providers and consumers informed by patient health literacy about overweight and obesity and provider needs to help patients address overweight and obesity (Zarcadoolas, et al., 2011).

Case Description

This case describes four related field research activities used to inform the development of the Adult Obesity Action Kit:

1. Interviews with health providers of the patient/consumer target population
2. Focus groups with patients/consumers
3. Health Literacy Load analysis of existing outreach and education materials
4. Pilot testing to gather early responses to draft materials

The Adult Obesity Action Kit's target audience was: 1. health providers, and 2. overweight individuals whose healthcare providers practice in underserved communities.

1. Provider and Frontline Staff Interviews

Twelve healthcare providers were interviewed by the researchers, along with a total of twelve interviews with each provider's frontline staff. We asked providers about what they thought were the cause(s) of patients' weight problems, counseling techniques they used and success rates in helping patients achieve and maintain weight loss, and their ability to follow-up on weight-related issues. Additionally, we asked providers to describe the materials they would like to have on hand when they work with their patients on weight management. Speaking with frontline staff, we asked about their role in disseminating health education materials on weight management or other topics to patients, their comfort level reinforcing health messages, the supply of information in waiting areas to give to patients, and patients' comfort level with frontline staff discussing their health issues. The interviews lasted an average of 45 minutes.

Providers shared a broad range of opinions, ranging from why they thought their patients were overweight, to their ease or lack of ease in discussing weight with their patients. Most providers said they brought up overweight and obesity in the context of talking to their patients about co-morbid conditions such as diabetes, hypertension, and hyperlipidemia. Providers viewed their patients' weight as a crucial contributor to and persistent problem in treating such chronic illnesses. Providers noted a range of contributors to weight problems in their patients - cultural influences, limited environmental supports, mental health challenges, and socioeconomic status.

Frontline staff explained that providers do not generally instruct them to hand out health-related literature to patients; however, the frontline staff said that they would welcome the opportunity to hand out such material. All frontline staff said that materials should be culturally sensitive, interesting, inviting, and written and designed for the literacy level of their patients.

2. Patient/Consumer Focus Groups

A total of six focus groups were conducted with a total of 62 overweight men and women, 32 English speakers and 30 Spanish speakers, who were residents of three low-income communities in Manhattan, Brooklyn, and the Bronx. The local district public health offices in Manhattan, Brooklyn and the Bronx recruited participants by posting bilingual flyers in key areas of the neighborhoods. The focus groups were convened in all three targeted neighborhoods. Each group lasted about an hour and participants received $40 for their time.

The discussion was designed to explore attitudes and opinions about weight and health of obese and overweight persons living in these communities where the prevalence of chronic conditions such as obesity, overweight, and diabetes are high. Experienced moderators guided discussion using direct questions. The moderators asked individuals questions related to health literacy on obesity, their perceptions of its causes, their provider's role in helping with weight maintenance, and strategies the individuals use to manage their weight. We used a grounded theory model to analyze the data, and independent coders then used an iterative process to attain inter-code reliability. Each focus group was recorded and taped.

While most providers told us that they thought patients are uninformed about the mechanics of overweight and obesity, we found the focus group participants were very knowledgeable about the 'basics'. Almost unanimously, individuals named many of the common health risks and treatment guidelines associated with overweight and obesity.

Several themes emerged from the focus groups. They were:

- **Provider Messages are Discounted:** Individuals who expressed skepticism about the role of providers in weight loss said they heard messages from their physician as a "mantra" or "broken record," and many individuals said that physicians only discussed weight after they had diagnosed a co-morbid condition.
- **Culture Drives Eating:** Individuals at every focus group explained that culture drives their eating behaviors and the types of food they eat. They named their own "staple food," and discussed how hard it is to leave these foods out of "typical" meals – pasta for Italians, rice for Haitians and Panamanians. A person who identified as African-American shared that food is central as a gesture of hospitality in the home and every Sunday at church, and that the aroma and social invitation to collard greens, macaroni and cheese, ham or turkey, tends to be difficult to decline.
- **Emotional Eating and Self-Blame:** Individuals explained that they find it hard to manage what they eat when they feel depressed or anxious.
- **Poor Food Availability:** Almost all individuals said they believed that neighborhoods in poor communities conspire against healthy eating for both themselves and their children, citing the ubiquity of fast-food restaurants and the scarcity of convenient healthy food store options as a primary barrier to better nutrition.

3. Health Literacy Load Analysis

We triangulated the qualitative findings from the provider interviews and patient/consumer focus groups with analyses of the content, readability and health literacy levels of existing consumer messaging about overweight and obesity used previously by the DOHMH as well as from a sampling of materials from national health promotion and education entities. We modified methods of health literacy load analysis from text analysis methods developed by Zarcadoolas et al (Zarcadoolas, Pleasant, and Greer 2006; Zarcadoolas, Pleasant, and Greer 2005). The health literacy load analysis codes, categorizes, and analyzes text in terms of health literacy assumptions and demands. We conducted a structural and functional analysis of material and messages to clarify the likely demands of the material on consumer/patient comprehension and use. The product of this analysis was a list of vocabulary, slogans, framing techniques and interactive tools that could be "usability" tested with patients/consumers in subsequent response sessions.

- **Development of Obesity Action Kit**

With the collected information from providers, patients/consumers and the analysis of existing materials, the research team worked closely with the DOHMH PHD team to develop Action Kit tools. What we heard clearly led us to see that we needed to contextualize overweight and obesity in novel and relevant ways and develop messages in clear language that used cultural and civic literacy frames pertaining to overweight and obesity. We identified the overarching message that "small steps can make a big difference."

The objectives or key functions for the Action Kit's provider/clinical tools were:

1. To convey concise epidemiological information concerning overweight and obesity in New York City;
2. To frame the discussion of overweight and obesity in new, more constructive ways to resonate with patients;
3. To provide verbal coaching scripts for providers to help them speak in new ways to their patients about overweight and obesity. These scripts could help providers discuss: the sociocultural context of overweight and obesity, commitment-building to manage weight, and goal-setting for a plan of action and a segue to follow-up.

4. Pilot Testing New Material

To inform the final development of messages and tools to include in the Adult Obesity Action Kit, we collected responses to draft materials by conducting follow-up interviews with providers and response focus groups with consumers. We investigated how useable and useful they would be to patients through direct questioning and hands-on activities.

- **Final Action Kit**

The Adult Obesity Action Kit ultimately contained twelve items, including clinical tools, provider resources, and patient education materials. Some materials were adaptations of existing materials and some materials were newly designed tools in response to the identified themes.

The Adult Obesity Action Kit and some of its innovations included:

1. **What Is Your BMI Wall Poster:** The poster offers step-wise directions for a patient to learn how to calculate BMI – rather than merely defining BMI to the patient.

2. **My Plate Planner:** The Planner uses an illustration of a plate to list many popular and culturally appropriate foods eaten at breakfast, lunch, and dinner, and it offers tips on different methods of preparing different food groups, rather than only showing a patient what and how much food should go on a plate.
3. **Test Your Knowledge on Portion Sizes Flipchart:** The flipchart, adapted from the National Heart Lung and Blood Institute "Portion Distortion" (National Heart, Lung, and Blood Institute 2010), engages patients in a guessing game, optimizing the element of surprise, and places portion sizes in a greater historical/cultural picture at the same time the chart presents examples of food portion distortion. The participants with whom we tested the flip chart unanimously remarked upon the drastic increase in serving sizes and volunteered that they too have increased their portion sizes since their youth.
4. **Sugar in Soda Bottle Demonstration Prop:** The demonstration prop showed itself to be figuratively popping – the 17 teaspoons of sugar in the otherwise-empty 20-ounce soda bottle elicited dramatic exclamations such as "I'll never bring soda into the house again!" or "I've been poisoning my kids!"
5. **How to Lose Weight Health Bulletin:** A less surprising but no less serious material is the How to Lose Weight health bulletin, an established publication through the DOHMH that provides examples for providers to explain to patients that when they are addressing overweight and obesity, taking even small steps can lead to a big difference. The small steps include brief and easy-to-read tips for people to achieve healthier weight.
6. **Tips for Healthy Weight Loss Palm Cards (Small, Highly Portable Note Cards With Messages Printed Front and Back):** Similarly, the palm cards feature simple tips and empowerment statements for taking control of weight, for patients to use as daily reminders of easy-to-accomplish ways to improve diet and increase physical activity – and unlike more conventional education materials, these tips feature the reasoning or the "science" behind why a person should consider engaging in these activities.
7. **My Self-Management Goal Sheet for a Healthy Weight Sheet:** This sheet for providers asks patients to determine, based on their goal, when they will do an action, how often they will take the action, and where they will take the action. The sheet recognizes that setting realistic goals is crucial to maintaining motivation and is informed by the focus group participants' expressed desire for concrete action.
8. **Obesity Pocket Guide for Clinicians, Including a Coaching Script for Providers:** The Obesity Pocket Guide for Clinicians features statements providers can say to develop a non-judgmental alliance with their patients in discussing weight management. The Guide also offers providers statements designed to go beyond fundamental literacy needs to address civic and cultural elements such as social forces working against eating a healthy diet, learned eating habits associated with cultural norms, and other powerful psycho-social issues that often influence patient weight-loss success. We developed those statements based on participants' expressed need for "connection," "support," and "positive talk" from their providers. As an example, one statement the Guide offers is 'Think about the types of food you find most in your neighborhood. It's probably hard to avoid the McDonald's or the Popeye's or the Dunkin' Donuts. You have to defend yourself against unhealthy choices.'

Figure 1. Sample page from portion distortion flip chart

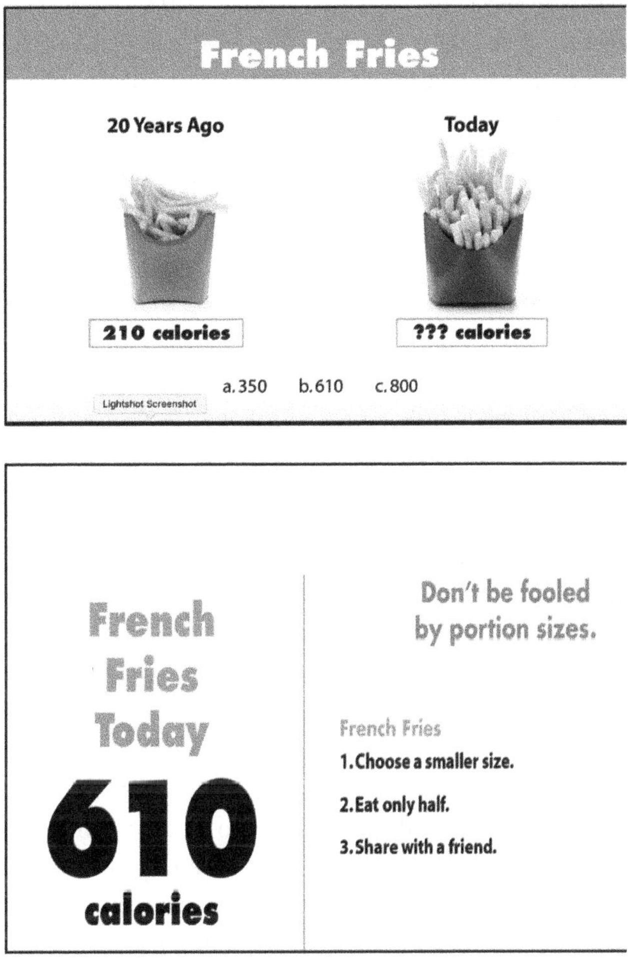
French Fries
20 Years Ago
Today
210 calories
??? calories
a. 350 b. 610 c. 800
Lightshot Screenshot
French Fries Today
610
calories
Don't be fooled by portion sizes.
French Fries
1. Choose a smaller size.
2. Eat only half.
3. Share with a friend.

SOLUTIONS AND RECOMMENDATIONS

This case study highlights both the importance of using an ecological model of health literacy and qualitative research activities to better understand your target audience. The providers and frontline staff interviews provided good insight into the barriers and opportunities to communicate with patients experienced by the providers. Likewise, the discussions with consumers sketched a picture of their basic health literacy about obesity and overweight, and demonstrated that consumers have a rich, nuanced understanding of some aspects of the interplay of society, culture, food and the needs of self.

Worker Mental Health Literacy

This case study describes a project that conducted research to identify what workers from a large self-insured entity on the East Coast of the U.S. understood about their mental health insurance benefits and to explore their understanding and attitudes about seeking mental health services. The goal of the project was to use the information gathered to help develop outreach and worker education materials about mental health. The self-insured entities were the 1199SEIU Benefit Funds.

1199SEIU is the largest local healthcare workers' union in the United States and the SEUI Benefit Funds are among the largest labor-management funds in the United States, providing a range of comprehensive benefits to 400,000 working and retired healthcare industry workers and family members. Members work in the hospital, nursing home and care industries, as well as in pharmacies, freestanding clinics and other healthcare settings. The Funds collaborated with the National Alliance on Mental Illness in NYC (NAMINYC) and Hunter College School of Public Health to conduct this project.

Setting the Stage

In the U.S., recent legislation[1] has paved the way for ending the long-standing insurance practices that discriminate against people with mental illness and drug and alcohol addictions from achieving parity for behavioral healthcare with medical-surgical healthcare coverage. Despite the removal of some of these structural barriers, mental health services in the U.S. are generally underused while there exists much untreated mental illness.

Untreated mental illness degrades the well-being of individuals and families, and also costs society as a whole (Michie, 2003; Peterson, Demerouti, and Bergström et al, 2008; Wieclaw, Agerbo, Mortensen et al., 2006). In the employment sector alone, lost productivity as a result of workers' poor mental health is estimated to cause losses of billions each year, depression alone costing employers over $44 billion annually (Stewart, Ricci, Chee et al, 2003). Occupational stress and workers' mental health problems can have the other serious consequences of increased absenteeism and high turnover (Jacobson, Aldana, and Goetzel, 1996).

Many factors may contribute to an individual's inability to recognize or respond to mental health needs including lack of effective public health outreach and education, and inadequate health literacy on the part of consumers (Wieclaw, Agerbo, Mortensen et al., 2006; Peterson, Demerouti, and Bergström et al, 2008). Research over the last two decades has demonstrated that poor comprehension and perception and attitudinal barriers play a central role in individuals not seeking mental health treatment (Michie, 2003; Department of Health and Human Services, National Institute for Occupational Safety and Health, 2008; Yassi, Pawson, and Leary et al, 2004). Researchers have concluded that apart from targeting structural barriers, increasing population mental health literacy is critical to the effort to enhance mental health care (Rosenbach, Lake, and Williams et al, 2009).

Worker mental health is a growing concern of corporate America (Wang, 2013; Holmes, 2016; Aetna, 2015) as well as among public health experts. The incidence of mental health problems is higher among healthcare workers than workers of any other occupational group (Wieclaw, Agerbo, Mortensen et al., 2006; Peterson, Demerouti, & Bergström et al,. 2008; Michie, 2003). Healthcare workers regularly experience high workloads, inadequate staffing, organizational changes, dealing with difficult and/or critically ill patients, and exposure to infectious and/or hazardous substances, which can increase their own risk of depression, anxiety, sleep problems and addiction, or exacerbate existing conditions (Department of Health and Human Services, National Institute for Occupational Safety and Health, 2008). Healthcare workers' low levels of well-being can pose a risk for patient safety and satisfaction; low-levels of well-being of healthcare workers has been associated with more errors, higher infection rates, and reduced patient satisfaction.

Case Description

As discussed in the introduction to this chapter, health literacy is defined as the ability to find, access, understand and use health information to make informed health choices (Jorm, 2000). Important components of health literacy are abilities to mediate science, civic and cultural information (Barrio, Palinkas, Yamada et al., 2008). Mental health literacy is the knowledge and beliefs about mental disorders that aid an individual to recognize, manage and prevent mental disorders (Jagdeo, Cox, Stein, et al., 2009). In this project we focused on 3 central aspects of mental health literacy:

- The ability to recognize a state of being as a potential mental health condition;
- The ability to know how to access professional services for a mental health condition;
- The ability to negotiate or mediate socio-cultural barriers to accessing healthcare.

The target audience was members of 1199SEIU Healthcare Workers East working in hospitals and nursing homes. All members have health coverage including general medical and behavioral/mental health benefits through the 1199SEIU Benefit Funds. Individuals were recruited to participate in one of four focus groups through their call center. Eligibility criteria were the following: being a member of 1199SEIU Healthcare Workers East; receiving health coverage including general medical and mental benefits through the 1199SEIU Benefit Funds; being between 18 and 70 years of age; and self-reporting English fluency. One of the four focus groups consisted largely of "delegates" - union members elected by peers in their department or floor to represent the interests of their colleagues. One of the six participants in the delegate group was not a delegate. Participation in all groups was fully voluntary, and participants received $40 per focus group plus one round-trip Metrocard. Researchers obtained IRB approval through Hunter College prior to commencing research activities.

Four focus groups with a total of 33 participants were conducted. Each focus group lasted approximately one hour and 15 minutes and was audiotaped with participant consent. Experienced moderators guided discussion using a combination of direct questions and reality-based scenarios that described three different individuals experiencing common mental/emotional problems – post-partum depression, emotional anxiety in a child, anxiety and work-related stress. Participants discussed what they thought might be the nature of the problem and what would be the best path of action. The researchers used a grounded theory model to analyze data from the focus groups. Independent coders used an iterative process to attain acceptable inter-coder reliability. Major and minor themes emerged, and we discussed them in collaboration with 1199SEIU Benefit Funds personnel.

Findings

The following section presents and discusses the major findings.

- **Sources of Information:** Workers reported using a range of ways to obtain benefit information – print, website, emails, outreach programs at job sites, and making phone calls to the Funds. Most wanted to be better informed about changes to coverage.
- **Health Coverage Literacy:** Without exception workers had no problem telling the moderators about what their health coverage was and how they could use it. Participants were quick to take out their Health Benefits ID cards to show how they can contact Member Services, and they knew the

process required for seeing a specialist. However most did not mention and did not know on direct questioning, what their mental health coverage was. The only exception was the delegate group, who did know the mental health services that were covered.

- **Embarrassment and Stigma:** All participants showed that they could identify the hypothetical character's general condition – depression, anxiety, stress. Some suggested that the hypothetical character might need professional help. However, participants were less likely to endorse seeking mental health services because the person could encounter disapproval from family, friends or co-workers and lead to stigma. Most participants, excluding those in the delegate group, said that mental health problems or conditions remain a taboo, a subject that is not discussed with others for fear of being labeled as crazy, judged by others, considered an unfit parent (for parents), and importantly, considered an unfit worker, as word of your "breakdown" always gets around in the workplace. Most struggled with how to deal with stigma personally and societally: "People see people seeing a psychologist or a psychiatrist as completely different; they just want to label you as crazy."

As the discussions of the scenarios proceeded, the workers had a difficult time linking possible root causes of the condition with circumstances. Workers commented on the scenario as if the symptoms themselves were the prevailing issue requiring treatment: "Welcome to the real world"; "Sounds like he needs a vacation"; "Bullying…having nightmares and staying away from school." There were also clear instances of a gender bias regarding who actually had a mental health condition. Women in two of the groups minimized the scenario of the male transit worker's symptoms of stress by focusing on the unfair situation in the workplace causing the stress, meanwhile two men defended the male transit worker and asserted he might need mental health services.

- **Privacy Concerns:** Workers reported both real and perceived concerns about privacy. While all participants knew that patient medical information should be kept confidential by law according to rules set by the Health Insurance Portability and Accountability Act, many said they believe that breaches of privacy among workers are common in the workplace. Participants described breaches of privacy as "everyone knowing" if a coworker has a health problem. Many participants expressed that they had experienced or seen a loss of privacy at the workplace—and some participants asserted that there is a need to reinforce that "HIPAA regulations are for workers, too!" Participants' privacy concerns emerged as a serious deterrent to seeking mental health services[2].
- **Accessing Services:** Another challenge that emerged during this study was the workers not knowing how to find a mental health care provider and the workers' mistrust in a mental health provider. While some workers said they could ask their primary care provider for a referral to a mental health provider, many participants expressed the belief that people would not seek mental health treatment because they do not know how to locate a provider.
- **Need for Education:** Participants in these focus groups unanimously felt that education, particularly on-site at places of employment, was critical to successful de-stigmatization of mental health issues, services and coverage. Many agreed that it was the responsibility of employers to make services and information regarding mental health more available, even when that meant personally approaching an employee to offer support or assistance. Perhaps most interesting, was the fact that many participants openly discussed their use of, or their desire to use mental health services and thus, their desire to learn more. However, they were stymied with coming up with specific

strategies or venues to achieve this goal of de-stigmatization. For example, if a worksite workshop or Wellness Member Assistance Program session was conducted, they questioned how a worker could attend without being stigmatized by simply attending. Likewise, workers questioned how they could avoid being noticed and stigmatized when picking up printed health information. Workers also expressed discomfort about speaking to a delegate to find out what services were offered.

Improving Outreach and Education to Workers

As we stated initially, the Funds wanted to better understand the mental health literacy of their workforce so that they could develop effective ways to communicate information about mental health benefits and services. Among the products that resulted from this research was the following:

"For Your Benefit: Health & Well-being of 1199SEIU Members." The Funds' member magazine is distributed quarterly to workers as a hard copy and posted on the Funds' website, and features health issues of importance from a member perspective. The full Fall 2012 issue of "For Your Benefit" featured findings from the study as well as information on mental health resources - how members can use their Funds' benefits to find the help that they themselves or someone they love, may need.

"Erasing the Stigma of Mental Health Issues," has the prominent position of the first article in the magazine and spans two full pages, 3-4. (See Figure 2) The article asserts that mental illness "is not the result of personal weakness, lack of character or poor upbringing"—but medical conditions that "are treatable and recovery is possible," and affirms that the Benefit Funds are "here to help." The article states that stigma surrounding mental illnesses and the worry of others' perception was one of the most common concerns raised by members of the focus groups when the 1199SEIU Benefits Funds recently partnered with Hunter College and NAMI-New York City Metro for a series of focus groups and surveys. The article encourages readers to seek services by stating that the Benefit Funds offer comprehensive coverage for treating mental health issues, depression and anxiety disorders, and highlights that the Wellness Member Assistance Program is staffed by social workers who can help assess a member's situation, "provide support and guidance for a variety of problems and work with you and your healthcare provider to develop a plan to meet your needs." Drawing from the focus group findings, the article discusses worker concerns about privacy and makes explicit that all conversations with the program's social workers are strictly confidential.

The issue also includes an article about the importance of recognizing depression both in new mothers and in teens, which the Funds' Executive Director calls "an increasingly common problem" in her introductory message.

This case demonstrates how field research with workers was central in identifying key issues that were barriers to accessing and using their mental health services. The Funds' commitment to address this issue is seen in their almost immediate (within one month) translation of the research findings into outreach tools and the commitment to establish longer-term goals of developing new corporate policies and programs.

In addition to focusing the member magazine issue on the study results, the Funds sought to address the fear of stigma and normalize mental health care by promoting a "whole member" approach to health in all communications that puts mental well-being on par with physical well-being. Communications, education and outreach initiatives have so far included:

Figure 2. Sample of Newsletter addressing mental health - SEIU1199

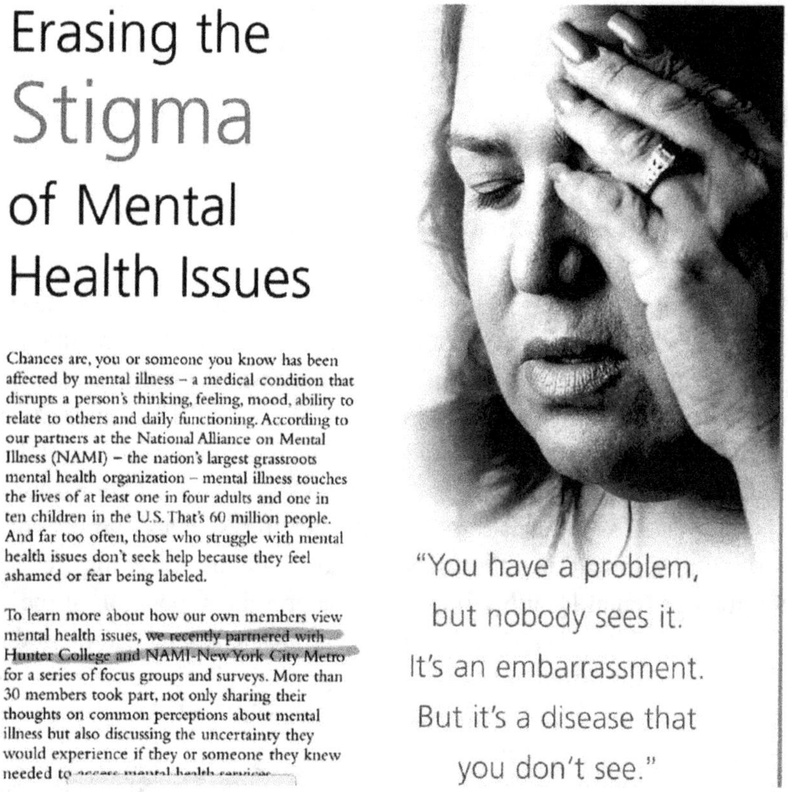

Erasing the Stigma of Mental Health Issues

Chances are, you or someone you know has been affected by mental illness – a medical condition that disrupts a person's thinking, feeling, mood, ability to relate to others and daily functioning. According to our partners at the National Alliance on Mental Illness (NAMI) – the nation's largest grassroots mental health organization – mental illness touches the lives of at least one in four adults and one in ten children in the U.S. That's 60 million people. And far too often, those who struggle with mental health issues don't seek help because they feel ashamed or fear being labeled.

To learn more about how our own members view mental health issues, we recently partnered with Hunter College and NAMI-New York City Metro for a series of focus groups and surveys. More than 30 members took part, not only sharing their thoughts on common perceptions about mental illness but also discussing the uncertainty they would experience if they or someone they knew needed to

"You have a problem, but nobody sees it. It's an embarrassment. But it's a disease that you don't see."

- Publishing an ongoing, regular feature in the member magazine, which addresses specific topics like stress relief or recognizing signs of anxiety in children, along with information about accessing the Funds' Wellness Member Assistance Program and mental health benefits.
- Providing Outreach Coordinators with information and materials on Wellness Member Assistance Program services and mental health benefits to help connect members with these services in the field.
- Introducing and promoting regular "Healthy Mind, Healthy Body" workshops to help members manage stress and anxiety at home and on the job.
- Updating member benefit materials to reflect a "whole member" philosophy, encompassing both mental and physical health.
- Emphasizing the confidentiality of Wellness Member Assistance Program and mental health services in all communications and outreach.

Health Literacy Approaches in Greece: Spinning a Stronger Network 'Web' for the Future

The United Nations Economic and Social Council (ECOSOC, 2011) has called for all countries to have common millennium development goals in increasing health literacy and empowerment in order to reduce disease burdens due to non-communicable diseases and promote access and partnerships at the local and macro levels -- Greece is no exception. Relative to countries such as the United States, Australia and England, the realization that adequate health literacy is essential for healthy individuals and a healthy country is more recently emerging both in Greece and the European Union during the last ten years or so (Kondilis et al., 2012; Sørensen et al., 2015). The efforts to acknowledge and address health literacy have been, in part, impeded by a very serious financial collapse in Greece starting in years 2009-2010 continuing to the present day. Unemployment has reached over 30% (youth at over 50%), depleted social security pensions, and austerity measures have led to what one reporter describes the Greek Prime Minister Tsipras choosing "slow pain rather than utter disaster" (Melvin, 2015). Recently collected national data is beginning to shed light on population health literacy in Greece and is likely to support existing programs and lead to new research, programs and policy to advance the public's health literacy.

The European Health Literacy Project (HLS-EU) started with a collaborative of European researchers, evolving into an eight-country study including Greece, and the project lasted between years 2009-2012 funded by the European Union (Sørensen et al., 2015). The thematic areas addressed by HLS-EU were cure and care, disease prevention, and health promotion (Sørensen et al., 2013). Part of the Comparative Health research program at CAPHRI, Maastricht University, HLS-EU was awarded the European Health Award Gastein in 2012 (Maastricht University CAPHRI, 2012). The HLS-EU findings for the Greek sample showed the population falling in the middle of having 'adequate' health literacy (Sørensen et al., 2015). Additional research in Greece documents the effects of the economic crisis on health including individual descriptions of insecurity for the future, depleted mental health, lack of access to proper healthcare, continued chronic health issues burdening particularly older citizens and those with special medical needs (Kentikelenis et al., 2011; Kondilis et al., 2013; Simou & Koutsogeorgou, 2014). The need for health promotion interventions in Greece including health literacy as one of the basic pillars of the public health policy agenda for the entire lifespan is necessary (Vozikis, Drivas, & Milioris, 2014; Kondilis et al., 2012; Vardavas et al., 2009). As research efforts in health literacy are relatively new, research funding is short-term, and any efforts to address patient and public health literacy, particularly for the poorest and underserved, falls at the discretion of community agencies and non-governmental groups, and healthcare providers. Meanwhile the health gap seems to be growing. Collaboration both among researchers of health literacy continues to be made both formally and informally in building a stronger "web" for the topic in Greece, Europe, and the US as evidenced from this chapter.

The term "health literacy" as defined by the Greek researchers on the European Health Literacy Project years, 2009-2012, (HLS-EU) use the Greek terms «εγγραματοσύνη υγείας» [eggramatosyni ygeias] (Kondilis et al., 2012) or a variation of it that translates to literacy on topics of health «εγγραματοσύνη σε θέματα υγείας». According to Greek mythology, Arachne, a mortal, contested the goddess Athena in a weaving contest, whereby Arachne's prowess landed her the blessing/curse to weave into eternity (Arachne: GreekMythology.com, 2017). By analogy, the emerging web of researchers and practitioners within and outside of Greece contribute important pieces to the collective web *network* defined as "an interconnected or interrelated chain, group, or system" (Merriam-Webster online Dictionary, 2017) appropriate to the individual and community efforts in Greece in gathering evidence, building collaborations, and taking action towards the future of health literacy. Weaving health literacy is the metaphor to highlight the Greek cases to be discussed in this section, emphasizing some of the work done by non-profits and educational institutions in Greece – the web creating the scaffolding on which more programs can emerge and innovate.

Available Data/Studies on Health Literacy for Greece

The HLS-EU included Greece as part of an eight-country European study, via an 86-question survey, including a functional health literacy test using the New Vital Signs (NVS) data was collected by Kantar TNS ICAP for Greece, part of the global research data collecting and consulting company Kantar TNS, who contract with the EU for the Eurobarometer data (Kantar TNS, n.d.). One thousand interviews were collected in each country for a total sample of 8,000 persons in all countries. Greece is a country of 10.82 million people where 35.4% of the population (3.8 million) lives in Athens, Attica, according to the Hellenic Statistical Authority (ELSTAT) (2017); the data collected by TNS in Metropolitan Athens composition was considered representative of the entire country's population (Kondilis et al., 2012). The HLS-EU results indicated that 55% of the Greek sample (N=1,000) fall in the "excellent' and 'sufficient' health literacy range and he segment of the population with the poorest scores of 'inadequate' health literacy for the countries, including Greece, fell among the under-educated, those reporting low incomes, those who considered their health status as "bad" and had long-term illnesses, including those over the age of 55 years. Existing data of older population groups, particularly those who suffer from co-morbid chronic illnesses (non-communicable disease), have poor physical and mental health, indicate that they access more services, including use of emergency services, at a cost higher to the Greek society which is already economically disadvantaged (Lahana et al., 2011; Kondilis et al. 2012; Simou & Koutsogeorgou, 2014; Sørensen et al., 2015).

Vozikis, Drivas, & Milioris (2014) conducted a health literacy study of over 1,500 university students (ages 18-24 years) in Greece, looking at determinants and association with self-perceived health, health behaviors and health risks, with a main focus on functional health literacy. They found a 'fair' to 'high'" total functional health literacy score for that population (Vozikis et al.). The World Health Organization report for Europe indicates that low literacy levels are common, and that children, adolescents, adults have limited literacy skills even in countries who are economically advanced with strong education systems (Kickbusch, et al., 2013). Roughly 92% of the Greek population is considered 'literate' according to past studies conducted by the country's national statistical center (ELSTAT), but evidence from studies of youth, including adolescents' self-report shows that they have many gaps in their knowledge of basic health matters including the need for more information in both communicable and non-communicable diseases (Vardvas et al., 2009). Adults sampled (N=100) report that they are more likely to trust selected healthcare providers, their family, and their friends as sources of health information in making necessary decisions for their health care, while more than half express not having adequate knowledge in navigating the public health system in Greece (Kondilis, Akrivos, Salloum, & Falagas, 2008). The research mentioned previously indicates a growing number of researchers in the area of health literacy, though much more work is needed both locally and nationally on the topic health literacy across the lifespan.

Access to Health Information

Printed health information has been a staple of public health communication around the world. So too in Greece. However, access to print health information, such as pamphlets, may be problematic in Greece. Studies have questioned if patients actually have access to print materials because pamphlets are often hidden from public view and the readability levels of these pamphlets may be too high for a substantial number of readers to understand (Kondilis, Akrivos, Soteriades, & Falagas, 2010). An over-reliance on printed information pamphlets, in the absence of explanation and guidance by health professionals, leaves people with low health literacy at considerable disadvantage (Manning & Dickens, 2006). Private clinics and hospitals, private practices, may keep their own electronic medical records, but this is not widespread, and only Greek pharmacies currently track publicly funded prescriptions including renewing these electronically. Access to electronically based health information or e-Health /mHealth in Greece and in other European countries seems to be more popular among younger people (Kummergold & Wynn, 2012; Chronaki et al., 2006). These services and tools such as the INTERMED platform are particularly useful for travelers (tourists) or citizens living in isolated areas (e.g. rural areas) in the Southeast Mediterranean countries of Greece, Italy, and Cyprus (Mougiakakou et al., 2011), although research has shown that Southern European countries including Portugal and Greece had significantly lower usage of the internet for obtaining health information (Andreassen et al., 2007).

The United Nations Economic and Social Council (ECOSOC, 2011) mentioned above, has also called for promoting better access to information communication technologies (ICTs). Studies have identified the use of ICTs to be useful for patients who use such tools to make health decisions (Greeks or those traveling to Greece, particularly in hard-to-reach areas) but also to enhance training of healthcare professionals (Lahana, et al., 2011; Mougiakakou, et al., 2011; Chronaki, et al., 2006). It is also notable that effective treatment for patients with chronic illness and their families often comes from local settings such as the community pharmacy (Gkiourda, 2017). Non-governmental organizations in Greece, such as Praksis (Praksis, n.d.) or Prolepsis (Partners in Prolepsis, n.d.) are often contracted and funded by national or international organizations, help both economically disadvantaged and other marginalized groups access care and work on several chronic health issues.

The Hellenic Forum on the Digital Future Conference, "Digital Policies for Human Capital & Development" (Ελληνικό Φόρουμ για το Ψηφιακό Μέλλον ημερίδα, "Ψηφιακές Πολιτικές για το Ανθρώπινο Κεφάλαιο και την Ανάπτυξη", March 2017), held a special session on digital health featuring speakers from higher education, field experts, and several political parties, who work on health research, policies, and related modes of delivery. The speakers highlighted the need for healthcare providers and educators to build their own e-skills for future e-health jobs, the need for the population majority in Greece to build information literacy skills to distinguish between "bad" and "good" health information, showcasing several on-line patient systems (e.g. "BioAssist SA) for elderly and chronically ill, oriented to help patients reduce emergency room visits and decrease mortality rates. Communication, including delivery and interpretation of a message, continues to be an important area on its own accord (Watson, Gallois, Hewett, & Jones, 2014). Health literacy efforts should start with youth in schools, universities, and communities (Vozikis et al., 2014; Marks, 2012; Marks, 2009), continue through adulthood (Kondilis et al. 2010; Kondilis et al., 2008), and account for training of healthcare professionals. One nationwide study of health psychologists in Greece (N=97) for example, indicated a need for training in order for these professionals to better provide psychotherapeutic interventions. Also problematic is the fact that many health psychologists don't have access to hospital-based libraries, since only a small number of hospitals in Greece have libraries, and some professionals are not familiar or proficient in using a personal computer (Kostagiolas, Samioti, Alexias, Kofiatis, & Niakas, 2012).

We cannot underestimate the role that non-governmental organizations (NGOs) or non-profits, colleges and universities are playing in substantially contributing to building the web of interconnected health literacy efforts in Greece. Efforts from NGOs like Prolepsis, public or private colleges and universities including the University Mental Health Research Institute (UMHRI) in Greek "Ερευνητικό Πανεπιστημιακό Ινστιτούτο Ψυχικής Υγιεινής" (Ε.Π.Ι.Ψ.Υ.) which is linked to the University of Athens Medical School, the Hellenic National School of Public Health Ε.Σ.Δ.Υ.), National and Kapodistrian

University of Athens, Harokopio University of Athens, and Hellenic American University/Hellenic American College in Athens (HAUniv/HAEC) are highlighted here[3].

Setting the Stage

The case examples discussed on the following section describe three areas including: 1. work done by Prolepsis in several areas relating to health literacy, 2. social and personal responsibility highlighting aspects of health literacy in undergraduate courses under the theme of "global citizen" by HAUniv/HAEC, and 3. efforts by UMHRI and a prefecture in Greece on mental illness. Health literacy, as highlighted in previous chapters in this volume, plays a key role in the development of material and looking at general outcomes of these institutions' community efforts.

1. Health Literacy and "Prolepsis"

The word "prolepsis" means *prevention* in Greek. The Institute of Preventive Medicine Environmental and Occupational Health Prolepsis, referred to as Prolepsis, has developed several projects that directly and indirectly relate to building health literacy targeting a variety of groups. Their most recent project in 2017 called MigHealthCare aims to produce a community-based care model to emphasize health promotion and prevention, integration, and a focus on reducing health inequalities for migrants, partnering with 14 universities, national authorities, and NGOs in ten European countries (Partners in Prolepsis, n.d.).

Major projects have included the Program on Food Aid and Nutrition Education called *Diatrofi,* for remote and rural areas in Greece. Initially, Iceland, Lichtenstein and Norway funded the program though the We are all Citizens Program, which is part of the EEA Grants mechanism for Greece (Partners in Prolepsis, n.d.) and ongoing funding via a Greek grant donor Stavros Niarchos Foundation between 2012-2016 (Partners in Prolepsis, 2013; Partners in Prolepsis, n.d.). This project started in December 2014, with 13 elementary schools in the areas of Xanthi, Imathia, Pierias, Thessaloniki, and Rodopi – all rural/remote areas in Greece – where the participating 1,115 students were provided with one free, healthy meal daily, educated on matters of health, nutrition and proper dietary habits with information materials targeted to them and their families. To date 18,000 students from over 100 schools across Greece have been reached through this program.

Prolepsis's aging and health literacy project, completed through the European Seventh Framework Programme (FP7) titled "Intervention Research on Health Literacy among Ageing Population" (IROHLA program), was launched 2012, lasting three years with 20 additional European partners (Partners in Prolepsis, n.d.). This project included the inauguration of Health Literacy Centre Europe, which aimed to function as a central portal of information and exchange of information beyond the IROHLA project. Their findings included the need to improve self-efficacy and the fact that the over age 75 group with low health literacy generally were a vulnerable group for low self-management abilities (European Union, 2017). Outcome goals were increasing health literacy through ICTs, creating government briefs on health literacy and how to include health literacy development in their programs, emphasis on self-management, medication adherence, the importance of good nutrition and physical activity for older persons, among others.

2. Health Literacy and the Global Citizen

The following case demonstrates how health literacy can be embedded into a much broader educational curriculum – teaching global citizenship. In a report by the Association of American Colleges and Universities (AAC&U) the idea of supporting liberal education and *global citizenship* includes analyzing the issue from multiple perspectives, focusing on experiential learning, being knowledgeable of values and real-world issues including inter-cultural issues, and taking action for positive individual and community change (Musil, 2006).

Hellenic American College is approved as a private institution by the Ministry of Education in Greece, and has signed a cooperation agreement with Hellenic American University enabling the College to offer the University's undergraduate and graduate degree programs at its facilities in Athens (Hellenic American College, n.d.). HAEC/HAUniv addresses global citizenship by designing a required undergraduate course under the category "interdisciplinary and intercultural studies" of General Education, in the form of weekly seminars over a one to one-and-a-half-year period between the years 2012-2015 "Global Citizen Seminars" evolving into a regular undergraduate general education course (non-required) titled "Developing the Global Citizen" starting Fall 2016. The aspect of social and personal responsibility was intertwined in the course, taught by interdisciplinary faculty, where all participating students (approximately 150 in all) over the years had to complete a pre-test on aspects of global citizenship (109 students completed), and worked on individual and group assignments including self-awareness exercises (journals, reflection sheets). Students reflected on the university's mission to "educate its students to be global citizens" (Hellenic American University, n.d.).

Issues related to *global citizenship* included civic engagement, the cyber-citizen (participation in and use of computer systems), health issues related to second-hand smoking, environmental issues (waste, recycling), preventing STDs/STIs/HIV, and other adhoc themes such as preventing bullying, dealing with vandalistic type graffiti (tagging etc.), preventing obesity and increasing physical activity were highlighted at an individual, community, and country level. The group assignment completed towards the end of the seminar or course on corporate social responsibility involved a local, regional, national and international issue such as Ebola with students assuming roles and short presentations. A general description of health literacy was shared with students as well as discussed with faculty teaching these sessions. Student and faculty perceptions were collected qualitatively and quantitatively as described briefly below, and analysis of the focus group discourse was formally presented at a European conference on discourse, identity, and borders (Kondilis, 2016).

Methods Used in "Global Citizenship" Course

Mixed methods utilizing focus group feedback and pre-surveys as part of an empirical study explored undergraduate student (N=9) and teaching faculty (N=15) perceptions of the concept of global citizenship, through participation (or lack thereof) in the Global Citizen Seminars (GCS). Feedback was collected in spring 2015 for the seminars, and one focus group (N=5) for the course was conducted in the fall of 2016. Each focus group was recorded and taped. The average age of students was 25 years and 67% have lived in another country outside their birthplace. Faculty focus group participants were GCS faculty and a total of three faculty focus groups were conducted composed of the total 15 participants, with an average age of 43 years, all of whom had lived outside their birthplace country, with higher education attained in European institutions mainly in Greece, but also in the United Kingdom and the U.S.

Semi-structured interviews included open-ended questions of what being a "global citizen" means, self-rankings for selected value rubrics of the AAC&U, falling under general categories of "personal and social responsibility," "intellectual and practical skills," and "integrative and practical skills." Within this context, many students indicated that their concept and awareness of responsibility in terms of the environment (recycling, corporate social responsibility, pollution including passive smoking) was increased, 3% indicated in self-reflections that they would consider 'quitting' smoking, nearly 100% in post-survey data indicated they were more aware of passive smoking issues, preventing STDs/STIs/HIV, and understanding corporate social responsibility. All students agreed that being an active and pro-active global citizen and being aware of related policies is one that all college students should be aware of. One student commented on global citizenship:

Going on that as far as being able to transcend your own cultural background and identities and be able to...learn and discover and know your place in the world and where you stand and how your actions, how your everyday actions affect other people around the world whether you are aware of it or not.

3. Addressing the Stigma of Mental Illness

The New York City case on mental health literacy demonstrated the role stigma plays in an individual's perception of mental health problems and seeking mental health services. Specific mental health prevention and education campaigns thus far have been sparse in Greece, particularly those that address the stigma of mental illness. Though groups like UMHRI or "Ε.Π.Ι.Ψ.Υ." (UMHRI - Ε.Π.Ι.Ψ.Υ., n.d.) began this work in the late 1990's, the crux of their work started over 12 years ago. Specifically, the Open-the-Doors global network anti-stigma program has been operating in over 20 countries including Greece since 1996 (Stuart, 2008) beginning with the Global Programme Against Stigma and Discrimination because of Schizophrenia, coordinated by UMHRI. From 2004 onwards, guided by the EU collaboration, UMHRI has been working on the issue of 'anti-stigma' of mental illness by primarily working with healthcare providers, patient and parental groups, and schools and universities. Factoring in what they know about people's perceptions of mental health, the group has been working towards building mental health literacy through general awareness trainings as well as educating healthcare providers on clinical assessment.

Given the severity and duration of the Greek economic crisis, recent studies are beginning to address mental health using a socio-cultural framework. Triliva, Fragkiadaki, & Balamoutsou, (2013) in one prefecture on the island of Crete, conducted a post-onset of the Greek economic crisis, addressing the key issues affecting access to necessary health care as related to mental illness. Triliva et al. conducted a qualitative study in Crete during the beginnings of the Greek crisis with the aim of creating more effective community partnerships. A focus group and one personal interview were conducted, focusing on services and needs of the mental health professions, using one psychiatric hospital (established in 2009) and one mental health center (established in 2007) including a participant group of three psychiatrists, three psychologists, three social workers, and one psychiatric nurse. The focus group discussions and interview lasted between one-and-a-half to two hours, results were audiotaped, transcribed and translated into English from Greek, and analyzed. The analysis of the data yielded three themes which researchers expressed "converge at many levels and appear to be going counter to the circumstances" (p. 6, Triliva et al.) geared to 1) forging partnerships for mental health, 2) extending the reach of mental health professionals, and 3) transforming professional identity through 'praxis' (actions). The group participants highlighted that support for the chronic service users was expanded from pharmacotherapy and psychotherapy to advocating for their rights and stigma reduction. Cost of services was cited as a problematic area for individuals and families in not accessing mental health services. Though this study began with addressing general community needs, from the perspective of the mental health professionals, the groups highlighted the community outreach interventions: The Family Support Group, a radio program discussing issues related to mental health, a community theatre performance and publication of their newsletter "Hearing Voices" playing an integral role in stigma reduction. Ultimately though not explicitly stated, these efforts worked toward increasing awareness of mental health and how to better access mental health services, thus, increasing the community's mental health literacy.

SOLUTIONS AND RECOMMENDATIONS FROM GREECE CASES

The above cases represent work done in Greece that has embedded health literacy principles and goals in its programming. To date, though Greek public entities in principle follow Healthy People 2020 and WHO goals for health literacy, there is no set national agenda that funds and promotes research or program development to address health literacy. Health literacy research that is done, is presented in national or international conferences; however, information is not always shared as NGOs and other institutions compete for research funding. Efforts have been made by this chapter's co-author to track the research that has been done, developing an initial task group on health literacy that first met in years 2015-2016. Collaborative efforts are underway among several educational institutions in Greece and Cyprus. Particular emphasis has been placed on coming up with mutually acceptable terms for the official translation of the term *health literacy* in the Greek language for Greece and Cyprus, with the ultimate goal of publishing a paper and finalizing this issue in 2018-2019. The project highlights discussed in previous sections involved multiple European partners, and some formal findings have already been shared either through publications or conference presentations. It is clear that cost and knowledge of interventions may determine how outreach is determined in the future. General recommendations for the evolving 'web' of health literacy in Greece include:

- Additional research and continued study of projects already started.
- Official translation of the term *health literacy* in the Greek language.
- Rigorous evaluation of existing programs to identify what works (e.g. baseline and post-intervention data) and publishing outcomes.
- Seeking available funding both at a national and European level to enhance program dissemination and overall community outreach.
- Broadening connections to include organizations and programs to better coordinate and relate issues to health literacy. This broadening could include youth leadership organizations, roundtables on public health literacy (including expanding the informal 'task group' on health literacy).

FUTURE RESEARCH DIRECTIONS

Collaboration and synthesis of information, in addition to sharing of 'good practices' however a culture defines those practices, is useful for the building blocks of health literacy. Researchers around the globe continue to share information as the authors have done here highlighting work already done in New

York City, and Greece, as communities continue to struggle with economic and social crises. Beyond the traditional healthcare workers and practitioners, it is clear that whom and what people trust for building on their health information is important and should continue to be explored in other studies.

CONCLUSION

A major challenge in individual and public health is for healthcare providers, public health officials, and companies/employers to effectively communicate complex health and science information to a diverse public (Nielsen-Bohlman, et al., 2004; U.S. Department of Health and Human Services, 2010; Nutbeam & Kickbusch, 2000). The manner in which health information is presented to patients/consumers is directly related to patient understanding and engagement (Epstein, Alper, & Quill, 2004; Nelson, Hesse, & Croyle, 2009; Trevena, et al, 2006). Given the increasing complexity of medicine, health systems, society and technology, it is essential that health information is usable, useful and addresses the unique needs of the widest possible range of patient populations (Britto et al., 2009; Krist & Woolf, 2011; Lazar, 2007; Wilson & Peterson, 2010). ECOSOC calls for all countries to have common millennium development goals in increasing health literacy and empowerment, including promote better access to information communication technologies, reduce disease burdens due to non-communicable diseases, and promote access and partnerships at the local and macro levels (ECOSOC, 2011).

There must be a clear imperative to place a patient/consumer's health literacy at the center when designing outreach and education. We must also be mindful of how people access and use information in their daily lives. Various cultures access information in various ways – via a range of healthcare providers such as pharmacists, community health workers, family, friends, and the ever-growing reach of advancing technology.

Literacy is not a fixed asset, but is both content and context specific (Nutbeam, 2017). This is particularly evident of countries experiencing austerity policies, affected by influxes and population trends. National and international policies and approaches to non-communicable diseases should seek to reduce health expenditures and maintain healthy societies. We hope the highlighted cases explicated some of these useful strategies. The authors highlighted two very different contexts in which researchers, employers, organizations, and institutions collaborated to advance people's health literacy. The issues raised affect all citizens around the globe, hence we, too, become 'global citizens' in sharing and combining the common threads of health literacy.

ACKNOWLEDGMENT

This research received no grant from any funding agency in the public, commercial, or not-for-profit sectors. The authors wish to acknowledge the assistance of the Psychology Department, Hellenic American University/Hellenic American College, The New York City Department of Health and Mental Hygiene, Public Health Detailing Program, Mount Sinai School of Medicine, and Hunter College School of Public Health, CUNY. We also thank Bridget Scallen for assistance in preparing this manuscript.

REFERENCES

Adoption of Electronic Health Record Systems among U.S. Non Federal Acute Care Hospitals: 2008-2014. (n.d.). Retrieved from https://www.healthit.gov/sites/default/files/databrief/2014HospitalAdoptionDataBrief.pdf

Aetna. (2015). *Mental Health, wellness, and corporate America.* Retrieved from https://news.aetna.com/2015/03/mental-health-wellness-corporate-america/

Agarwal, R., & Khuntia, J. (2010). *Personal Health Information and the Design of Consumer Health Information Technology: Background Report.* Prepared by Insight Policy Research under Contract No. HHSA290200710072T for the Agency for Healthcare Research and Quality U.S. Department of Health and Human Services. Retrieved from https://healthit.ahrq.gov/sites/default/files/docs/citation/AHRQ_Personal_Health_InfoFinalReport_FINAL508compliant.pdf

Ancker, J. S., & Kaufman, D. (2007). Rethinking health numeracy: A multidisciplinary literature review. *Journal of the American Medical Informatics Association, 14*(6), 713–721. doi:10.1197/jamia.M2464 PMID:17712082

Ancker, J.S., Senathirajah, Y, Kukafka, R., Starren, B. (2006). Design Features of Graphs in Health Risk Communication: A Systematic Review. *Journal of the American Medical Informatics Association, 13(*6).

Andreassen, H. K., Bujnowska-Fedak, M. M., Chronaki, C. E., Dumitru, R. C., Pudule, I., Santana, S., ... Wynn, R. (2007). European citizens' use of E-health services: A study of seven countries. *BMC Public Health, 7*(1), 53. doi:10.1186/1471-2458-7-53 PMID:17425798

Arachne: GreekMythology.com. (2017, July 11). Retrieved from https://www.greekmythology.com/Myths/Mortals/Arachne/arachne.html

Atienza, A. A., Zarcadoolas, C., Vaughon, W., Hughes, P., Patel, V., Chou, W. Y. S., & Pritts, J. (2015). Consumer attitudes and perceptions on mHealth Privacy and Security: Findings from a Mixed-Methods Study. *Journal of Health Communication*, 1-7.

Barrio, C., Palinkas, L., Yamada, A. M., Fuentes, D., Criado, V., Garcia, P., & Jeste, D. (2008). Unmet needs for mental health services for Latino older adults: Perspectives from consumers, family members, advocates, and service providers. *Community Mental Health Journal, 44*(1), 57–74. doi:10.100710597-007-9112-9 PMID:18026876

Baur, C. (2010). *National Action Plan to Improve Health Literacy.* U.S. Department of Health and Human Services, Office of Disease Prevention and Health Promotion.

Black, J. L., Macinko, J., Dixon, L. B., & Fryer, G. E. Jr. (2010). Neighborhoods and obesity in New York City. *Health & Place, 16*(3), 489–499. doi:10.1016/j.healthplace.2009.12.007 PMID:20106710

Bodenheimer, T., Lorig, K., Holman, H., Grumbach, K. (2002). Patient self-management of chronic disease in primary care. *Journal of the American Medical Association, 288*(19), 2469-2475.

Britto, M. T., Jimison, H. B., Munafo, J. K., Wissman, J., Rogers, M. L., & Hersh, W. (2009). Usability testing finds problems for novice users of pediatric portals. *Journal of the American Medical Informatics Association, 16*(5), 660–669. doi:10.1197/jamia.M3154 PMID:19567793

Centers for Disease Control and Prevention. (2013, November 22). Health Disparities & Inequalities Report. United States. Morbidity & Mortality Weekly Report (MMWR). *Supplement, 62*(Supplement No. 3), 1–187.

Centers for Disease Control and Prevention. (2016). *Heart Disease Fact Sheet.* Retrieved from: https://www.cdc.gov/dhdsp/data_statistics/fact_sheets/docs/fs_heart_disease.pdf

Centers for Disease Control and Prevention, Department of Health and Human Safety, National Institute for Occupational Safety and Health. (2008, July). *Exposure to stress: Occupational hazards in hospitals, 2008-136.* Retrieved from www.cdc.gov/niosh/docs/2008-136/pdfs/2008-136.pdf

Charrow, R. P., & Charrow, V. R. (1979). Making legal language understandable: A psycholinguistic study of jury instructions. *Columbia Law Review, 79*(7), 1306–1374. doi:10.2307/1121842

Chronaki, C.E., Kouroubali, A., Esterle, L., Orphanoudaki, E., Roumeliotaki, T., Stathopoulou, A., & Tsiknakis, M. (2006). eHealth consumer trends survey in Greece: Results of the 1st phase. *FORTH-ICS TR-365.*

Collins, S. R., Rasmussen, P. W., Doty, M. M., & Beutel, S. (2014). *Too High a Price: Out-of-Pocket Health Care Costs in the United States. Commonwealth Fund.* Retrieved from http://www.commonwealthfund.org/publications/issue-briefs/2014/nov/out-of-pocket-health-care-costs

Cosmides, L., & Tooby, J. (1996). Are humans good intuitive statisticians after all? Rethinking some conclusions from the literature on judgment under uncertainty. *Cognition, 58*(1), 1–73. doi:10.1016/0010-0277(95)00664-8

Davis, T., Crouch, M., Wills, G., Miller, S., & Abdehou, D. (1990). Gap between patient reading comprehension and the readability of patient education materials. *The Journal of Family Practice, 31*(5), 533–538. PMID:2230677

Davis, T., Williams, M., Marin, E., Parker, R., & Glass, J. (2002). Health literacy And cancer communication. *CA: a Cancer Journal for Clinicians, 52*(3), 134–149. doi:10.3322/canjclin.52.3.134 PMID:12018928

Davison, A., Kantor, R. N., Hannah, J., Herman, G., Lutz, R., & Salzillo, R. (1980). *Limitations of Readability Formulas in Guiding Adaptations of Texts. Technical Report (No. 162).* Champaign, IL: Center for the Study of Reading.

Doak, L., & Doak, C. (2002). *Pfizer Health Literacy Principles.* New York, NY: Pfizer, Inc.

Dresser, M., Short, L., Wedemeyer, L., Bredow, V. L., Sacks, R., Larson, K., & Silver, L. D. (2012). Public Health Detailing of Primary Care Providers: New York City's Experience, 2003–2010. *American Journal of Public Health, 102*(S3), S342–S352. doi:10.2105/AJPH.2011.300622 PMID:22690970

Duffy, T. M., & Kabance, P. (1982). Testing a readable writing approach to text revision. *Journal of Educational Psychology, 74*(5), 533–548. doi:10.1037/0022-0663.74.5.733

Epstein, R. M., Alper, B. S., & Quill, T. E. (2004). Communicating evidence for participatory decision making. *Journal of the American Medical Association, 291*(19), 2359–2366. doi:10.1001/jama.291.19.2359 PMID:15150208

European Union. (2007). *Final Report Summary - IROHLA (Intervention Research on Health Literacy among Ageing population).* Retrieved from http://cordis.europa.eu/result/rcn/184975_en.html

Freedman, D. A., Bess, K., Tucker, H., Boyd, D., Tuchman, A., & Wallston, K. (2009). Public Health Literacy Defined. *American Journal of Preventive Medicine, 36*(5), 446–451. doi:10.1016/j.amepre.2009.02.001 PMID:19362698

Freid, V.M., Bernstein, A.B., & Bush, M.A. (2012 July). Multiple chronic conditions among adults aged 45 and over: trends over the past 10 years. *National Center for Health Statistics Data Brief, Number 100*, 1-8.

Gazmararian, J. A. (1999). Health literacy among Medicare enrollees in a managed care organization. *Journal of the American Medical Association, 281*(6), 545–551. doi:10.1001/jama.281.6.545 PMID:10022111

Gkiourda, C. (2017). Αντιμετωπίζοντας τις χρόνιες παθήσεις στο φαρμακείο [Facing chronic diseases in the pharmacy]. Retrieved from http://www.y-o.gr/επικαιρότητα/634-αντιμετωπίζοντας-τις-χρόνιες-παθήσεις-στο-φαρμακείο

Golbeck, A., Ahlers-Schmidt, C., Paschal, A., & Dismuke, S. (2005). A definition and operational framework for health numeracy. *American Journal of Preventative Medicine, 29*(4), 375-376. doi: .10.1016/j.amepre.2005.06.012

Gordon, C., Purciel-Hill, M., Ghai, N. R., Kaufman, L., Graham, R., & Van Wey, G. (2011). Measuring food deserts in New York City's low-income neighborhoods. *Health & Place, 17*(2), 696–700. doi:10.1016/j.healthplace.2010.12.012 PMID:21256070

Halm, E. A., Mora, P., & Leventhal, H. (2006). No symptoms, no asthma: The acute episodic disease belief is associated with poor self-management among inner-city adults with persistent asthma. *Chest, 129*(3), 573–580. doi:10.1378/chest.129.3.573 PMID:16537854

Hellenic American College. (n.d.). *About Hellenic American College.* Retrieved from http://haec.gr/en/aboutus/about-haec-college

Hellenic American University. (n.d.). *Vision and mission.* Retrieved from http://hauniv.edu/about/charter-mission

Hellenic Statistical Authority (ELSTAT). (2017). *Greece in Figures.* Retrieved from http://www.statistics.gr/documents/20181/1515741/GreeceInFigures_2017Q2_EN.pdf/adec1d58-1d39-43ca-b07c-72a8a3741cb2

Holmes, L. (2016, May 16). What Happens When Major Companies Take Mental Health Seriously. *Huffington Post.* Retrieved from http://www.huffingtonpost.com/entry/mental-health-workplace_us_572b5a92e4b016f37894d142

International Technology Education Association. (2007). *Standards for Technological Literacy: Content for the Study of Technology* (3rd ed.) Retrieved from https://www.iteea.org/39197.aspx

Jacobson, B., Aldana, S., Goetzel, R., Vardell, K., Adams, T., & Pietras, R. (1996). The relationship between perceived stress and self-reported illness-related absenteeism. *American Journal of Health Promotion, 11*(1), 54–61. doi:10.4278/0890-1171-11.1.54 PMID:10163451

Jagdeo, A., Cox, B., Stein, M., & Sareen, J. (2009, November). Negative attitudes toward help seeking for mental illness in 2 population-based surveys from the United States and Canada. *Canadian Journal of Psychiatry, 54*(11), 757–766. doi:10.1177/070674370905401106 PMID:19961664

Jorm, A. F. (2000). Mental Health Literacy: Public Knowledge and beliefs about mental disorders. *The British Journal of Psychiatry, 177*(05), 396–401. doi:10.1192/bjp.177.5.396 PMID:11059991

Kantar, T. N. S. (n.d.). *Who we are*. Retrieved from http://www.tnsglobal.com/who-we-are

Karpati, A., Kerker, B., Mostashari, F., Singh, T., Hajat, A., Thorpe, L., ... Frieden, T. (2004). *Health Disparities in New York City*. New York: New York City Department of Health and Mental Hygiene. Retrieved from http://www.commonwealthfund.org/~/media/files/publications/other/2004/jul/health-disparities-in-new-york-city/karpati_disparities-pdf.pdf

Kaufman, L., & Karpati, A. (2007). Understanding the sociocultural roots of childhood obesity: Food practices among Latino families of Bushwick, Brooklyn. *Social Science & Medicine, 64*(11), 2177–2188. doi:10.1016/j.socscimed.2007.02.019 PMID:17383060

Kentikelenis, A., Karanikolos, M., Papanicolas, I., Basu, S., McKee, M., & Stuckler, D. (2011). Health effects of financial crisis: Omens of a Greek tragedy. *Lancet, 378*(9801), 1457–1458. doi:10.1016/S0140-6736(11)61556-0 PMID:21988763

Kerka, S. (2003). *Health Literacy Beyond Basic Skills*. ERIC Digest. ERIC Clearinghouse on Adult Career and Vocational Education Columbus.

Kessler, R., Aguilar-Gaxiola, S., Alonso, J., Chatterji, S., Lee, S., Ormel, J., ... Wang, P. (2009). The global burden of mental disorders: An update from the WHO World Mental Health (WMH) Surveys. *Epidemiologia e Psichiatria Sociale, 18*(1), 23–33. doi:10.1017/S1121189X00001421 PMID:19378696

Kickbusch, I. (2001). Health literacy: Addressing the health and education divide. *Health Promotion International, 16*(3), 289–297. doi:10.1093/heapro/16.3.289 PMID:11509466

Kickbusch, I., Pelikan, J. M., Apfel, F., & Tsouros, A. D. (Eds.). (2013). *Health literacy: The solid facts*. Copenhagen, Denmark: World Health Organization, Regional Office for Europe.

Kintsch, W. (1994). Text comprehension, memory, and learning. *The American Psychologist, 49*(4), 294–303. doi:10.1037/0003-066X.49.4.294 PMID:8203801

Kirsch, J. S., Junegeblut, A., Jenkins, L., & Kolstad, L. A. (1993). *Adult literacy in America: a first look at the results of the National Adult Literacy Survey (NALS)*. Washington, DC: Department of Education.

Koh, H. K., Berwick, D. M., Clancy, C. M., Baur, C., Brach, C., Harris, L. M., & Zerhusen, E. G. (2012). New federal policy initiatives to boost health literacy can help the nation move beyond the cycle of costly 'crisis care'. *Health Affairs (Project Hope), 31*(2), 434–443. doi:10.1377/hlthaff.2011.1169 PMID:22262723

Kondilis, B. (2016, September). *Student Discourses of Civic Engagement and Global Citizenship in a Time of Crisis in Greece.* Paper presented at the "Europe in Discourse: Identity, Diversity, Borders" 1st International Conference, Hellenic American College, Athens, Greece. Retrieved from http://europein-discourse.eu/2016-conference/conference-proceedings

Kondilis, B., Akrivos, P., Salloum, S., & Falagas, M. (2008, June). *Health literacy in Athens, Greece: Exploring sources of health information in adults.* EHMA Annual Conference, Athens, Greece. Retrieved from www.ehma.org/files/16.40%20B%20Kondilis.ppt

Kondilis, B., Akrivos, P., Soteriades, E., & Falagas, M. (2010). Readability Levels of Health Pamphlets distributed in Athens Hospitals & Health Centers. *Public Health, 124*(10), 547–552. doi:10.1016/j.puhe.2010.05.010 PMID:20832835

Kondilis, B., Magoulas, C., Ioannidi, E., & Agrafiotis, D. (2012, March). *The European Health Literacy Survey Greece.* Hellenic National School of Public Health. Retrieved from http://www.nsph.gr/files/006_Koinoniologias/HLSEU%20country%20report_Greece_2012_ENG.pdf

Kondilis, E., Giannakopoulos, S., Gavana, M., Ierodiakonou, I., Waitzkin, H., & Benos, A. (2013, April 18). Economic crisis, restrictive policies, and the population's health and healthcare: The Greek Case. *American Journal of Public Health,* e1–e8. doi:10.2105/AJPH.2012.301126 PMID:23597358

Kostagiolas, P. A., Samioti, F., Alexias, G., Korfiatis, N., & Niakas, D. (2012). Examining patterns of information behavior among healthcare professionals: A case study on health psychologists. *New Review of Information Networking, 17*(2), 108–119. doi:10.1080/13614576.2012.724300

Krish, S.R., Lawrence, R.H., & Aron, D.C. (2008). Tailoring an intervention to the context and system redesign related to the intervention: A case study of implementing shared medical appointments for diabetes. *Implementation Science,* 3-34. doi:10.1186/1748-5908-3-34

Krist, A. H., & Woolf, S. H. (2011). A vision for patient-centered health information systems. *Journal of the American Medical Association, 305*(3), 300–301. doi:10.1001/jama.2010.2011 PMID:21245186

Kummervold, P.E., & Wynn, R. (2012). Health information accessed on the internet: The development in 5 European countries. *International Journal of Telemedicine and Applications,* 1-3. doi:10.1155/2012/297416

Lahana, E., Pappa, E., & Niakas, D. (2011). Do place of residence and ethnicity affect health services utilization? Evidence from Greece. *International Journal for Equity in Health, 10*(16), 1–9. PMID:21521512

Lazar, J. (Ed.). (2007). *Universal usability: Designing computer interfaces for diverse user populations.* John Wiley & Sons.

Leonard, K. (2004). The role of patients in designing health information systems: The case of applying simulation techniques to design an electronic patient record (EPR) interface. *Health Care Management Science, 7*(4), 275–284. doi:10.100710729-004-7536-0 PMID:15717812

Lewenstein, B. V. (1992). The Meaning of 'Public Understanding of Science' in the United States after World War II. *Public Understanding of Science (Bristol, England), 1*(1), 45–68. doi:10.1088/0963-6625/1/1/009

Lipkus, I., Samsa, G., & Rimer, B. (2001). General performance on a numeracy scale among highly educated samples. *Medical Decision Making, 21*(1), 37–44. doi:10.1177/0272989X0102100105 PMID:11206945

Lustria, M. L., Smith, S. A., & Hinnant, C. C. (2011). Exploring digital divides: An examination of eHealth technology use in health information seeking, communication and personal health information management in the USA. *Health Informatics Journal, 17*(3), 224–243. doi:10.1177/1460458211414843 PMID:21937464

Maastricht University CAPHRI. (2012). *European health award for the HLS-EU project.* Retrieved from https://www.caphri.nl/european-health-award-hls-eu-project

Manning, D. I., & Dickens, C. (2006). Health literacy: More choice, but do cancer patients have the skills to decide? *European Journal of Cancer Care, 15*(5), 448–452. doi:10.1111/j.1365-2354.2006.00687.x PMID:17177901

Marks, R. (2009). Schools and health education: What works, what is needed, and why? *Health Education, 109*(1), 4–8. doi:10.1108/09654280910923345

Marks, R. (2012). *Health literacy and School-based education.* New York: Emerald.

McCray, A. T. (2005). Promoting health literacy. *Journal of the American Medical Informatics Association, 1*(2), 152–163. doi:10.1197/jamia.M1687 PMID:15561782

McNamara, D. S., Kintsch, E., Butler-Songer, N., & Kintsch, W. (1996). Are good texts always better? Interactions of text coherence, background knowledge, and levels of understanding in learning from text. *Cognition and Instruction, 14*(1), 1–43. doi:10.12071532690xci1401_1

Melvin, D. (2015, July 13). Between rock, hard place, Greece picks austerity. How did it get into this mess? *CNN.* Retrieved from http://www.cnn.com/2015/07/13/europe/how-greece-reached-this-point/

Merai, R., Siegel, C., Rakotz, M., Basch, P., Wright, J., Wong, B., & Thorpe, P. (2016). CDC Grand Rounds: A Public Health Approach to Detect and Control Hypertension. *MMWR. Morbidity and Mortality Weekly Report, 65*(45), 1261–1264. doi:10.15585/mmwr.mm6545a3 PMID:27855138

Michie, S., & Williams, S. (2003). Reducing Work Related Psychological Ill Health and Sickness Absence: A Systematic Literature Review. *Occupational and Environmental Medicine, 60*(1), 3–9. doi:10.1136/oem.60.1.3 PMID:12499449

Miller, J. D. (1983). Scientific literacy: A conceptual and empirical review. *Daedalus*, 29–48.

Miller, N. (2013). Apps for your smart phone. *Clinical Psychiatry News.* Retrieved from http://www.clinicalpsychiatrynews.com/views/blognosis/blog/apps-for-your-smartphone/ff1923da2e4f57803957d-bbb7fca029f.html

Mougiakakou, S. G., Kyriacou, E., Perakis, K., Papadopoulos, H., Androulidakis, A., Konnis, G., ... Koutsouris, D. (2011). A feasibility study for the provision of electronic healthcare tools and services in areas of Greece, Cyprus and Italy. *Biomedical Engineering Online, 10*(1), 49. doi:10.1186/1475-925X-10-49 PMID:21649924

Musil, C. M. (2006). *Assessing global leaning: Matching good intentions with good practice.* Washington, DC: Association of American Colleges and Universities.

National Heart, Lung, and Blood Institute (NHLBI). (2007). *Portion Distortion Interactive Quizzes Slides Sets.* Retrieved from https://www.nhlbi.nih.gov/health/educational/wecan/eat-right/portion-distortion.htm

National Science Foundation (NSF). (2003). *Science and engineering indicators.* National Science Board. Retrieved from www.nsf.gov/sbe/srs/seind93/chap7/doc/7d1a93.htm

Nelson, D., Hesse, B., & Croyle, R. (2009). *Making data talk: Communicating public health data to the public, policy makers and the press.* New York, NY: Oxford University Press. doi:10.1093/acprof:oso/9780195381535.001.0001

Network. (n.d.). Retrieved July 13, 2017 from https://www.merriam-webster.com/dictionary/network

New York City Department of Health and Mental. (2012). *Reversing the Epidemic: The New York City Obesity Task Force Plan to Prevent and Control Obesity.* Retrieved from http://www.nyc.gov/html/om/pdf/2012/otf_report.pdf

New York City Department of Health and Mental Hygiene, Bureau of Communications in cooperation with Bureau of Chronic Disease Prevention and Control. (2009). *Health Bulletin #51: How to Lose Weight.* Retrieved from http://www.nyc.gov/html/ doh/downloads/pdf/public/dohmhnews6-05.pdf

Newman, S., Steed, L., & Mulligan, K. (2004). Self-management interventions for chronic illness. *Lancet, 364*(9444), 1523–1537. doi:10.1016/S0140-6736(04)17277-2 PMID:15500899

Newsweek. (2015). *Many Insured Americans Can't Afford Health Care.* Retrieved from http://www.newsweek.com/many-americans-insured-cant-afford-health-care-334624

Nielsen-Bohlman, L., Panzer, A. M., & Kindig, D. A. (Eds.). (2004). *Health literacy: a prescription to end confusion.* Washington, DC: Institute of Medicine, National Academies Press.

Nutbeam, D. (2008). The evolving concept of health literacy. *Social Science & Medicine, 67*(12), 2072–2078. doi:10.1016/j.socscimed.2008.09.050 PMID:18952344

Nutbeam, D. (2017). *Discussion paper on promoting, measuring and implementing health literacy: Implications for policy and practice in non-communicable disease prevention and control (WHO GCM/NCD Working Group 3.3 2017).* University of Sydney.

Nutbeam, D., & Kickbusch, I. (2000). Advancing health literacy: A global challenge for the 21st century. *Health Promotion International, 15*(3), 183–184. doi:10.1093/heapro/15.3.183

Ogden, C., Carroll, M., Curtin, L., Lamb, M., & Flegal, K. (2010). Prevalence of high body mass index in US children and adolescents, 2007–2008. *Journal of the American Medical Association, 303*(3), 242–249. doi:10.1001/jama.2009.2012 PMID:20071470

Ogden, C., Carroll, M., Fryar, C., & Flegal, K. (2015, November). *Prevalence of obesity among Adults and Youth: 2014-2015.* NCHS Data Brief, No. 219. Retrieved from https://www.cdc.gov/nchs/data/databriefs/db219.pdf

ONC Office of the National Coordinator. (2015, April). *ONC Data Brief No. 23 April 2015.* Author.

Parker, R. M., Baker, D. W., Williams, M. V., & Nurss, J. R. (1995). The test of functional health literacy in adults: A new instrument for measuring patients' literacy skills. *Journal of General Internal Medicine*, *10*(10), 537–541. doi:10.1007/BF02640361 PMID:8576769

Partners in Prolepsis: Institute of Preventive Medicine Environmental and Occupational Health. (2013). *Diatrofi*. Retrieved from http://diatrofi.prolepsis.gr/en/

Partners in Prolepsis: Institute of Preventive Medicine Environmental and Occupational Health. (n.d.). *IROHLA – Intervention Research on Health Literacy among Ageing Population*. Retrieved from http://www.prolepsis.gr/new/en/Projects/39/IROHLA---Intervention-Research-on-Health-Literacy-among-Ageing.html

Partners in Prolepsis: Institute of Preventive Medicine Environmental and Occupational Health. (n.d.a). *Mig-HealthCare*. Retrieved from http://www.prolepsis.gr/new/en/Projects/50/Mig-HealthCare:-Strengthen-Community-Based-Care-to-minimize-health-inequalities.html

Partners in Prolepsis: Institute of Preventive Medicine Environmental and Occupational Health. (n.d.b). *Program on Food Aid and Nutrition Education – DIATROFI: Implemented in Remote and Rural Areas*. Retrieved from http://www.prolepsis.gr/new/en/Projects/44/Program-on-Food-Aid-and-Nutrition-Education---DIATROFI.html

Partners in Prolepsis: Institute of Preventive Medicine Environmental and Occupational Health. (n.d.c). *Who we are*. Retrieved from http://www.prolepsis.gr/new/en/Content/2/8/Who-we-are.html

Payer, L. (1996). *Medicine and Culture: Varieties of Treatment in the United States, England, West Germany, and France* (Rev. ed.). New York, NY: First Owl Books Edition.

Peterson, U., Demerouti, E., Bergström, G., Samuelsson, M., Åsberg, M., & Nygren, Å. (2008). Burnout and physical and mental health among Swedish healthcare workers. *Journal of Advanced Nursing*, *62*(1), 84–95. doi:10.1111/j.1365-2648.2007.04580.x PMID:18352967

Pleasant, A., & Kuruvilla, S. (2008). A tale of two health literacies: Public health and clinical approaches to health literacy. *Health Promotion International*, *23*(2), 152–159. doi:10.1093/heapro/dan001 PMID:18223203

Praksis. (n.d.). *About Praksis*. Retrieved from https://www.praksis.gr/en/about-praksis

Public Broadcasting System (PBS). (2017). *Health crisis: the uninsured*. Retrieved from http://www.pbs.org/healthcarecrisis/uninsured.html

Ratzan, S. C. (2001). Health literacy: Communication for the public good. *Health Promotion International*, *16*(2), 207–214. doi:10.1093/heapro/16.2.207 PMID:11356759

Root, J., & Stablefod, S. (1998). Easy-to-read consumer communications: A missing link in Medicaid managed care. *Journal of Health Politics, Policy and Law*, *24*(1), 1–26. doi:10.1215/03616878-24-1-1 PMID:10342253

Rosenbach, M., Lake, T., Williams, S. R., & Buck, J. (2009). Implementation of mental health parity: Lessons from California. *Psychiatric Services (Washington, D.C.)*, *60*(12), 1589–1594. doi:10.1176/ps.2009.60.12.1589 PMID:19952147

Royal College of Physicians. (2015 March). *Work and wellbeing in the NHS: why staff health matters to patient care.* Retrieved from https://www.rcplondon.ac.uk/guidelines-policy/work-and-wellbeing-nhs-why-staff-health-matters-patient-care

Rudd, R. E. (2002). A maturing partnership. *Focus on Basics*, *5*(c), 1–8.

Sarkar, U., Karter, A. J., Liu, J. Y., Adler, N. E., Nguyen, R., López, A., & Schillinger, D. (2011). Social disparities in internet patient portal use in diabetes: evidence that the digital divide extends beyond access. *Journal of the American Medical Informatics Association, 18*(3), 318-321. doi:.10.1136/jamia.2010.006015

Schillinger, D., Bindman, A., Wang, F., Stewart, A., & Piette, J. (2004). Functional health literacy and the quality of physician-patient communication among diabetes patients. *Patient Education and Counseling*, *52*(3), 315–323. doi:10.1016/S0738-3991(03)00107-1 PMID:14998602

Schillinger, D., Piette, J., Grumbach, K., Wang, F., Wilson, C., Daher, C., ... Bindman, A. (2003). Closing the loop: Physician communication with diabetic patients who have low health literacy. *Archives of Internal Medicine*, *163*(1), 83–90. doi:10.1001/archinte.163.1.83 PMID:12523921

Schwartz, L. M., Woloshin, S., Black, W. C., & Welch, H. G. (1997). The role of numeracy in understanding the benefit of screening mammography. *Annals of Internal Medicine*, *127*(11), 966–972. doi:10.7326/0003-4819-127-11-199712010-00003 PMID:9412301

Schwartzberg, J., VanGeest, J., & Wang, C. (Eds.). (2005). *Understanding health literacy: Implications for medicine and public health.* Chicago, IL: American Medical Association Press.

Shen, B.S.P. (1975). Science Literacy and the Public Understanding of Science. *Communication of Scientific Information*. 45-52. 10.1159/000398072

Simou, E., & Koutsogeorgou, E. (2014). Effects of the economic crisis on health and healthcare in Greece in the literature from 2009 to 2013: A systematic review. *Health Policy (Amsterdam)*, *115*(2-3), 111–119. doi:10.1016/j.healthpol.2014.02.002 PMID:24589039

Sixsmith, J., Doyle, P., D'Eath, M., & Barry, M.M. (2014). *Health communication and its role in the prevention and control of communicable diseases in Europe: Current evidence, practices and future developments.* European Centre for Disease Prevention and Control (ECDC Technical Report).

Sørensen, K., Pelikan, J. M., Röthlin, F., Ganahl, K., Slonska, Z., Doyle, G., ... Brand, H. (2015). Health Literacy in Europe: Comparative Results of the European Health Literacy Survey (HLS-EU). *European Journal of Public Health, 2015.* doi:10.1093/eurpub/ckv043 PMID:25843827

Sørensen, K., Van den Broucke, S., Fullam, J., Doyle, G., Pelikan, J., Slonska, Z., & Brand, H. (2012). Health literacy and public health: A systematic review and integration of definitions and models. *BMC Public Health*, *12*(1), 80. doi:10.1186/1471-2458-12-80 PMID:22276600

Sørensen, K., Van den Broucke, S., Pelikan, J. M., Fullam, J., Doyle, G., Slonska, Z., ... Brand, H. (2013). Measuring health literacy in populations: Illuminating the design and the development process of the European Health Literacy Survey Questionnaire (HLS-EU-Q). *BMC Public Health*, *13*(1), 1–22. doi:10.1186/1471-2458-13-948 PMID:24112855

Spivack, J. G., Swietlik, M., Alessandrini, E., & Faith, M. S. (2010). Primary care providers' knowledge, practices, and perceived barriers to the treatment and prevention of childhood obesity. *Obesity (Silver Spring, Md.)*, *18*(7), 1341–1347. doi:10.1038/oby.2009.410 PMID:19910934

Stewart, W., Ricci, J., Chee, E., Hahn, S., & Morganstein, D. (2003). Cost of Lost Worker Productive Work Time Among US Workers with Depression. *Journal of the American Medical Association*, *289*(23), 3135–3144. doi:10.1001/jama.289.23.3135 PMID:12813119

Street, B. V. (Ed.). (1993). *Cross-cultural approaches to literacy*. Cambridge, UK: Cambridge University Press.

The Sullivan Commission on Diversity in the Healthcare Workforce. (2004). *Missing persons: Minorities in the health professions*. Retrieved from http://www.aacn.nche.edu/Media/pdf/SullivanReport.pdf

Trevena, L. J., Davey, H. M., Barratt, A., Butow, P., & Caldwell, P. (2006). A systematic review on communicating with patients about evidence. *Journal of Evaluation in Clinical Practice*, *12*(1), 13–23. doi:10.1111/j.1365-2753.2005.00596.x PMID:16422776

U. S. Department of Health and Human Services. (2010). *National Action Plan to Improve Health Literacy*. U.S. Department of Health and Human Services, Office of Disease Prevention and Promotion. Retrieved from http://www.health.gov/communication/HLActionPlan/

United Nations Economic and Social Council (ECOSOC). (2011). Health literacy and the Millennium Development Goals: United Nations Economic and Social Council (ECOSOC) regional meeting background paper (Abstracted). *Journal of Health Communication*, *15*(Suppl. 2), 211–223. doi:10.1080/10810730.2010.499996 PMID:20845205

University Mental Health Research Institute (UMHRI) Ε.Π.Ι.Ψ.Υ. (n.d.). *About us*. Retrieved from http://www.epipsi.gr/index%20eng.htm

U.S. Census Bureau. (2012). *U.S. Census Bureau Projections Show a Slower Growing, Older, More Diverse Nation a Half Century from Now*. Retrieved from https://www.census.gov/newsroom/releases/archives/population/cb12-243.html

U.S. Department of Health and Human Services. (2001). *Mental health: Culture, race, and ethnicity—A supplement to mental health: A report of the Surgeon General*. Author.

Van Wert, R. (2017, June 8). Dichotomous endings: A physician's personal reflection [Blog Post]. Retrieved from http://healthaffairs.org/blog/2017/06/08/dichotomous-endings-a-physicians-personal-reflection/

Vardavas, C., Kondilis, B., Patelarou, E., Akrivos, P., & Falagas, M. (2009). Health literacy and sources of health education among adolescents in Greece. *International Journal of Adolescent Medicine and Health*, *21*(2), 179–186. doi:10.1515/IJAMH.2009.21.2.179 PMID:19702197

Vozikis, A., Drivas, K., & Milioris, K. (2014). Health literacy among university students in Greece: Determinants and association with self-perceived health, health behaviours and health risks. *Archives of Public Health*, *72*(1), 15. doi:10.1186/2049-3258-72-15 PMID:24987522

Wang, N. (2015, March 13). Mental Health: A New Priority in Corporate America. *US News & World Report.* Retrieved from https://www.usnews.com/news/articles/2015/03/13/mental-health-a-new-priority-in-corporate-america

Watson, B., Gallois, C., Hewett, D., & Jones, L. (2014). Culture and healthcare: intergroup communication and its consequences. Academic Press.

Westin, A. (2012). *National Partnership for Women & Families. Making IT Meaningful: How Consumers Value and Trust Health IT.* Retrieved from http://go.nationalpartnership.org/site/DocServer/HIT_Making_IT_Meaningful_National_Partnership_February_2.pdf

Wieclaw, J., Agerbo, E., Mortensen, P., & Bonde, J. (2006). Risk of affective and stress related disorders among employees in human service professions. *Occupational and Environmental Medicine, 6*(5), 314–319. doi:10.1136/oem.2004.019398 PMID:16621851

Williams, M., Parker, R., Baker, D., Parikh, K., Coates, W., & Nurss, J. (1995). Inadequate functional health literacy among patients at two public health hospitals. *Journal of the American Medical Association, 2714*, 1677–1682.

Wilson, C., & Peterson, A. (2010). *Managing Personal Health Information: An Action Agenda.* AHRQ Publication No. 10-0048-EF. Rockville, MD: Agency for Healthcare Research and Quality, U.S. Department of Health and Human Services.

Winkelman, W., Leonard, K., & Rossos, P. (2005). Patient-perceived usefulness of online electronic medical records: employing grounded theory in the development of information and communication technologies for use by patients living with chronic illness. *Journal of the American Medical Informatics Association, 12*(3), 306-314. doi:.10.1197/jamia.M1712

World Health Organization (WHO). (2009). *The Financial Crisis and Global Health.* Retrieved from http://www.who.int/topics/financial_crisis/financialcrisis_report_200902.pdf

Yassi, A., Pawson, D., Leary, T., Sikorski, J., Parent, D., & Gilbert, M. (2004). *Trends in workplace injuries, illness, and policies in healthcare across Canada: workers' compensation patterns and policy changes in healthcare organizations. Report for Health Canada Ottawa.* Ontario: Health Canada.

Zarcadoolas, C. (2010). The simplicity complex: Exploring simplified health messages in a complex world. *Health Promotion International.* doi:10.1093/heapro/daq075 PMID:21149317

Zarcadoolas, C., & Pleasant, A. (2008). Increasing Health Literacy. In J. C. Parker & E. Thorson (Eds.), *Healthcare Communication in the New Media Landscape.* New York, NY: Springer.

Zarcadoolas, C., Pleasant, A., & Greer, D. (2005). Understanding health literacy: An expanded model. *Health Promotion International, 20*(2), 195–203. doi:10.1093/heapro/dah609 PMID:15788526

Zarcadoolas, C., Pleasant, A., & Greer, D. S. (2006). *Advancing Health Literacy: a framework for understanding and action.* San Francisco, CA: Jossey-Bass.

Zarcadoolas, C., Sealy, Y., Levy, J., Dresser, M., Ponieman, D., Young, S. M., ... Silver, L. (2011). Health literacy at work to address overweight and obesity in adults: The development of the obesity action kit. *Journal of Communication in Healthcare, 4*(2), 88–101. doi:10.1179/175380611X13082296179316

ENDNOTES

1 See parity laws 1996 Mental Health Parity Act and the 2008 Paul Wellstone and Pete Domenici Mental Health Parity and Addiction Equity Act. At the time this chapter is being composed, much federal healthcare policy is in a precarious position due to certain politicians' attack.

2 The Health Insurance Portability and Accountability Act of 1996, or HIPAA, is federal legislation that provides data privacy and security provisions for safeguarding medical information. The HIPAA Privacy Rule set national standards to protect individuals' medical records and other personal health information.

3 ΕΠΙΨΥ has worked on several programs related to anti-stigma of mental illness starting in 2004; ESDY (ΕΣΔΥ) the Hellenic National School of Public Health was the main collaborator for the HLS-EU study between 2009-2012 along with a consultant from HAUniv/HAEC; Harokopio has been working on an ongoing nutrition and health literacy study the last years; Prolepsis has worked on IROHLA project on Aging and Health Literacy, and nutritional health literacy in its breakfast program "Diatrofi" discussed in this chapter.

Chapter 4
Back to the Basics:
The Importance of Considering Health Literacy in the Development and Utilization of Consumer E-Health Interventions

Reshma Prashad
York University, Canada

Mei Chen
Seenso Institute for Public Health, Canada

ABSTRACT

Health literacy is a critical foundation that needs to be considered prior to the development and deployment of consumer e-health technologies. The authors indicate the problems associated with the lack of effective health literacy strategies in current consumer e-health interventions and then present a patient-centered, disease-specific, task-relevant, and contextualized health literacy approach. The goal of such an approach is to help patients better understand their illnesses make sense of their health data, make informed decisions, and more effectively manage their health conditions. The authors make five recommendations concerning health literacy in order to make e-health interventions effective. They also describe next-generation health literacy interventions that take advantage of emerging technologies such as speech recognition, natural language processing, artificial intelligence, automatic translation, and augmented reality. Finally, the authors point out a research and development direction towards an intelligent, integrated, and connected consumer e-health solution.

DOI: 10.4018/978-1-5225-4074-8.ch004

INTRODUCTION

There has been a proliferation of technology utilization in healthcare over the last decade, particularly consumer health. One of the main reasons for this focus is the staggering increase in chronic illnesses and comorbidities, which leads to unsustainable healthcare costs (Curtis, Cheng, Rose & Tsai, 2011). Therefore, healthcare providers are utilizing eHealth interventions to collaborate with patients to help them manage their conditions to prevent exacerbations that are costly to the healthcare system. However, adoption and use of these consumer eHealth interventions by patients have been low. The main factors contributing to the low rate of adoption and utilization is health illiteracy, coupled with low digital literacy, language and cultural barriers of the intended users (Nutbeam, 2000).

Health literacy is of great importance to patients because they need to comprehend the health information presented to them in order to follow their doctor's instructions and actively participate in decision making about their health and wellbeing (Norman & Skinner, 2006b). Health literacy aids patients in proactively managing their conditions to prevent further exacerbations. Health literacy can also help patients in discerning the quality and credibility of health information available online to determine its applicability to their conditions (McCray, 2005). The lack of health literacy, on the other hand, negatively affects patients, their families, their caregivers and the overall healthcare system both in terms of clinical and financial outcomes.

This chapter discusses the significance of health literacy in facilitating optimal chronic disease management and in adopting consumer health technology. It first presents a background of the topic, followed by a discussion of the benefits of health literate patients. The challenges associated with the lack of considerations and effective health literacy strategies in current consumer eHealth interventions are addressed. Furthermore, the challenges concerning access limitations for people with disabilities and the lack of considerations about linguistic and cultural competency are discussed. Finally, practical strategies of how healthcare organizations can begin their journey of promoting health and digital literacy are recommended, and examples of effective health literacy interventions are provided.

BACKGROUND

The World Health Organization (WHO) defines chronic illnesses as conditions/diseases that persist for more than three months and cannot be cured with medications or vaccines (World Health Organization, 2017). Given that chronic illnesses do not disappear, healthcare organizations have to treat chronically ill patients on an ongoing basis for the rest of their lives. The cost of caring for chronically ill patients is economically unsustainable, and patients experience poor health outcomes as a result of receiving episodic care, this has a significant impact on the patient's quality of life (Wodchis, Dixon & Anderson, 2015).

Chronic diseases, such as heart disease, stroke, cancer, chronic respiratory diseases, and diabetes are the leading cause of mortality in the world, representing 60% of all deaths (World Health Organization, 2017). This invisible epidemic is an under-appreciated cause of poverty and hinders the economic development of many countries. In Canada, 68 billion dollars is spent annually on care for chronically ill patients, and that amount rises to 190 billion dollars when the indirect costs (sick days and loss of productivity) are added (Wodchis, Dixon & Anderson, 2015).

Current approaches to chronic disease management are ineffective and result in a low clinical value (Wodchis, Dixon & Anderson, 2015). In addition to suboptimal clinical effectiveness, chronic illnesses have a significant negative financial impact on both patients and the healthcare system. Effective and efficient chronic disease management is the first critical and essential step in transforming the healthcare system. A major shortcoming of current approaches is the collection of episodic data that is not beneficial to the proactive management of chronic conditions. Healthcare organizations have come to realize this and are therefore seeking ways to proactively engage patients via Consumer eHealth interventions in their homes and communities (Curtis, Cheng, Rose & Tsai, 2011).

Given healthcare organizations interest in engaging patients via consumer eHealth interventions (portals, mobile technologies) coupled with patients' interests in utilizing these technologies, health and digital literacy have become even more critical. However, many healthcare organizations have taken the wrong approach to engaging chronically ill patients as they have assumed that patients have both the health and digital literacy skills to accurately interpret and comprehend the complex health/medical information presented to them (Norman & Skinner, 2006b). Many research studies suggests that optimal benefits cannot be realized if patients are not provided with accurate and timely information from credible sources to inform their active participation and decision making in managing their chronic illnesses (Mancuso, 2009; Snowdown et al., 2015; Gruman, 2014). Discussed below are some of the benefits that can be achieved if healthcare organizations undertake the right approach to engaging, educating and empowering patients to utilize consumer eHealth interventions to manage their chronic conditions.

BENEFITS OF HEALTH LITERATE PATIENTS

Health literacy requires a complex combination of knowledge of ones' health and general health information (McCray, 2005). Patients need to not only understand their health status but also need to combine that with general health information to interpret its applicability accurately. Many studies show that patients with a lower socioeconomic status and low literacy levels choose to avoid utilizing consumer eHealth interventions due to a lack of health literacy and are further marginalized by a lack of support from their care providers in interpreting the information (Eng et al., 1998).

The effective and efficient management of chronic illnesses requires engaged and informed patients. This encompasses providing health information to patients to facilitate their understanding of the factors contributing to their health, knowledge about their conditions, informed decision making about available treatments (Snowdown et al., 2015). There are many benefits to patients being health and digitally literate, this includes increased interest, increased engagement, and increased compliance with treatment plans and ultimately increased the level of adoption and utilization of consumer eHealth interventions (Veenhof, Clermont & Sciadis, G, 2005). Discussed below are the benefits of promoting health and digital literacy to optimize the value of consumer eHealth interventions.

Patient Engagement

Healthcare organizations have recognized the need to engage patients in their care. Many studies have shown that engaged patients are more motivated and likely to conduct self-care (Wagner, 1998; Skinner, 2002). However, a critical factor in creating "engaged patients" is the ability to educate them about their illnesses, provide them with credible sources of health information in a timely manner and provide ongoing support throughout their journey (Wagner, 1998). Pairing the above strategies with providing access to their health records via portals or mobile devices have proven to be more effective than only providing them with access to their record via portals or mobile technologies (Snowdown et al., 2105). Ensuring that patients are health literate is foundational to the success of any eHealth initiatives in which patients are the end users (Norman & Skinner, 2006a).

Patient Education

Appropriate patient education is critical to the success of any consumer eHealth interventions. Many eHealth initiatives have produced less than optimal results because of the failure to acknowledge the importance of patient education (Parker, Baker, Williams & Nurss, 1995). Some of the critical factors that are often ignored or missed by healthcare organizations are the lack of consideration of the patient's health literacy level, lack of consideration for the patient's language, lack of consideration of the patient's age and lack of consideration for patients with disabilities.

When healthcare organizations do not consider the patient's health literacy level, they are not providing the patient with the full opportunity to benefit from the eHealth intervention. Raw medical data is mostly complex for the average patient population; therefore, when healthcare organizations do not break down the information to a reasonable literacy level, patient does not benefit from having access to the information (Norman & Skinner, 2006b). As a result, patients turn to the internet to help them interpret the data and are very likely to come across non-credible sources of health information that could be detrimental to them (Institute of Medicine, 2004). Unsuspecting patients can be led into buying non-prescribed harmful medications or could be given unprofessional medical advice that can cause harm. It is therefore vital that healthcare organizations take the responsibility of providing their patients with credible sources of disease-specific health information to help them improve their health literacy levels and ensure that benefits can be realized from having access to their health information. Healthcare organizations can help patients enhance their health literacy levels by ensuring that the health information provided is at a reasonable reading level and help patients to make connections with the data and their health (Veenhof, Clermont & Sciadis, G, 2005).

Patient Empowerment/Activation

One of the main goals of patient engagement via consumer eHealth interventions is to empower/activate patients to become active participants and decision-makers in their care. Patients that are engaged and empowered through education are more likely to have better health outcomes as a result of proactive management of their conditions. (Wagner, 1998). Additionally, they tend to comply better with treatment plans and have a better sense of control over the impact of the conditions on their lives.

Health literacy is the vehicle through which patients can be engaged, educated and empowered to take actions to change their behaviors and improve their health outcomes. It is, therefore, the responsibility of the healthcare organizations to ensure that patients are supported with disease-specific credible health information to inform their decision-making capabilities (Zelmer & Hagens, 2016). Informed decision-making is critical in the management of chronic conditions, as patients are constantly provided information upon which they have to make a decision. Therefore, clarification and support are essential for long-term behavioral changes and compliance to treatment plans. A lack of compliance is one of the critical factors influencing poor behavioral changes and subsequently health outcomes (Schulz & Nakamoto, 2013).

CURRENT CHALLENGES

Despite the promising benefits of utilizing consumer eHealth interventions for chronic disease management, the lack of health and digital literacy has significantly impeded the full propensity of the benefits that can be realized (Nielsen-Bohlman, Panzer & Kindig, 2004). The negative impacts of the lack of or low levels of health and digital literacy will be discussed in this section. Additionally, challenges with the lack of linguistic and cultural competency in eHealth will also be addressed. This subsection will focus on an in-depth discussion of these issues and the impacts on the management of chronic conditions. To put this discussion in context, the strategies currently used to promote health literacy in consumer eHealth interventions will be reviewed along with their benefits and limitations.

In general, health literacy education is lacking in all types of eHealth interventions. The majority of health-related technology developers do not consider health literacy when they develop their digital patient record systems, mobile health apps or self-monitoring devices, since their primary goal is to collect, store, and display personal health-related data (Gruman, 2014). As a result, when healthcare organizations deploy such technologies to empower consumers, they often provide access to patient record systems or other eHealth technologies without any health literacy component. Although consumers appreciate the timely access to their health data from patient record systems or their mobile devices, the most significant challenge they face is to make sense of the data and use it to manage their conditions (Zelmer & Hagens, 2016).

Some patients feel that health IT solutions fall short of providing them with the information they need. In particular they do not always help them to understand their situation (e.g., why is my new prescription medication making me itch), make informed choices, or guide changes in behavior or changes in their treatment (Eng et al, 1998). Many patients desire the right information at the right time, particularly information about what action they need to take to follow through on medical advice and information that allows them to make informed choices, improve their care and treatment outcomes (Gruman, 2014).

It has become clear to many healthcare organizations that have deployed eHealth technologies that a health literacy component is essential in helping patients to understand and use their health data to guide their self-care (Snowdown et al., 2105). These organizations either add some patient education materials copied from the Internet or add information from a licensed health information library for patients to browse. In such cases, the information provided is general and simplistic; it is an "add-on" rather than an integral part of the eHealth solution. This type of information can be browsed independently and often do not address a wide range of issues with which patients are concerned. In most cases, the health literacy component is inadequate and isolated from the tasks of making sense of the patient data, thus using such data does not always improve disease management, instead it results in the following problems.

Low Rates of Adoption

Low rates of adoption of eHealth interventions are profoundly influenced by a patient's level of health literacy (Rootman, 2003). Patients with low levels of health literacy who are not provided education or support through their healthcare providers are more likely to ignore the benefits of eHealth tools and therefore contribute to the low rates of adoption. For both the healthcare organizations and patients to benefit from the implementation of eHealth tools, health literacy levels need to be considered early in the development stage. Also, patients should be given the opportunity to provide feedback on both the education materials, as well as the usability of the eHealth tool (portals, mobile applications, etc.) (Zelmer & Hagens, 2016).

Low Rates of Sustained Utilization

Another challenge often faced by healthcare organizations that have implemented eHealth tools are low rates of sustained utilization (Curtis, Cheng, Rose & Tsai, 2011).

Some organizations have up to a 50% reduction in utilization rates within a three-month period (Kim et al., 2016). Many factors that contribute to these dismal results, two of the most critical factors being the patients' ability to comprehend the health/medical information presented to them and the second being the user-friendliness of the eHealth tool utilized (Kim et al., 2016).

Despite the fact that consumer digital health tools are being heavily implemented for over a decade now, healthcare providers are still not fully acknowledging the importance of the two factors mentioned above. Within the Canadian context, surveyed patients consistently rate these two factors as the most important when deciding to continue or stop utilizing an eHealth tool (Zelmer and Hagens, 2016).

Healthcare providers and organizations need to pay attention to these results if they intend to engage patients to become active participants in their care. Most importantly, patients should not be expected to comprehend and take action on complex health/medical information. Healthcare providers and organizations need to play an active role in ensuring that these two criteria are met to optimize patient adoption.

Lack of Linguistic and Cultural Competency Considerations

In the few cases where consumer eHealth interventions were targeted at marginalized patient populations, the lack of linguistic considerations further exacerbated the inequities and inequalities faced by this patient population (Sarkar et al., 2011). For example, despite the fact that a high percentage of marginalized patient populations includes immigrants whose first language is not English, minimal effort is placed on ensuring that literacy standards are met to accommodate these patient populations (Tieu et al., 2017).

The actions described above further exacerbate the discrimination faced by the patients who most need these interventions to aid the management of their conditions (Sarkar et al., 2011). Instructions and guidance materials are not translated to accommodate the populations whose first language is not English; as a result, minority/immigrant populations are excluded due to their cultural and language differences.

Similarly, some eHealth interventions promote disparities due to variances in education levels related to literacy (Cammaerts, 2003). Not only are marginalized and immigrant patients not able to understand the language utilized in some eHealth interventions due to language barriers, but they are also not able to comprehend the content of the message due to its complexity. The language in some eHealth interventions are too complex for marginalized patients with lower levels of education; they are not able to comprehend the instructions or medical results in the applications (Yamin et al., 2011). For example, one consumer eHealth intervention utilized in Canada provides only numerical cancer staging data to patients without providing a "legend" table explaining what the various stages are. Patients find this information confusing and turn to the Internet to help them with the classification. However the information the encounter is even more confusing to them. This results in less interest and participation from marginalized patient groups including immigrant populations.

Another area that is often ignored in eHealth interventions is cultural competency. This refers to one's ability to understand, acknowledge, and display sensitivity to another person's culture, traditions, or language. In a healthcare context, cultural competence is the providers and organizations ability to deliver health care services efficiently that meet the social, cultural and linguistic needs of patients (Yamin et al., 2011). A culturally competent healthcare system can help to improve clinical outcomes and quality of care. Cultural competency is a crucial indicator of whether patients from minority groups will uptake a specific technology or intervention (Cammaerts, 2003). Many eHealth interventions ignore cultural competency, for example, cultural impacts are not considered when solutions are designed to promote wellbeing.

Limitations for Seniors and People With Disabilities

Another form of discrimination faced by marginalized patients is ageism. Many eHealth interventions do not consider usability factors such as ease of use or size of text in the design of these applications; these factors cause challenges for patients (Tieu et al., 2017). As a result, patients with low vision or disabilities are automatically excluded from participating in the utilization of these interventions. In many cases, diabetes applications are failing to reach patients who may become blind as a result of diabetes (Sarkar, 2011). This defeats the purpose of the mobile diabetes applications which is to promote utilization of the tool to reduce further deterioration.

Consumer eHealth interventions can create limitations for people with disabilities, for example, if a patient is not able to see instructions on a mobile diabetes application, they should be provided with voice support when utilizing this type of technology (Sarkar, 2011). It is therefore vital that healthcare providers and healthcare organizations ensure that consumer eHealth interventions are accessible to patients with disabilities; this would provide an opportunity for equitable utilization of healthcare resources and eliminate the potential for exclusion as a result of physical and mental disabilities (Yamin et al., 2011). For example, if a patient has a tremor in his/her hand he/she may not be able to utilize a mouse pointer, therefore other options for selecting or pointing needs to be available for this patient to fully utilize the technology. The omission of these considerations provides further opportunities for discrimination and exclusion.

Seniors are another group of patients that consumer eHealth interventions can create challenges for. Seniors have multiple conditions and illnesses such as hand tremors, arthritis, cataracts and other physical challenges. As a result, consumer eHealth interventions can potentially cause exclusion to accessing healthcare services (Yamin et al., 2011). This further exacerbates current challenges for seniors and results in discouraging them from trying eHealth interventions that can be potentially beneficial to them. Also, consideration has to be made around costs to senior patients. Senior patients are unlikely to purchase expensive software or hardware. For example, in one study, senior patients preferred to use non-digital trackers to monitor their glucose because of the associated costs (Kim et al., 2016). Therefore, care providers and healthcare organizations need to reflect on this when considering various technologies and services for remote monitoring.

Limited Success With Consumer eHealth Interventions

Consumer eHealth interventions have been widely implemented and utilized for well over a decade now; however, many healthcare providers and organizations are reporting suboptimal results based on their expectations around adoption and sustained utilization (Zhao, Freeman & Li, 2016). For example, one of the oldest patient portals implemented in Canada is now ten years old and is still experiencing low sustained utilization due to the poor presentation of patients' medical records. Patients are not provided disease-specific credible sources of health information within the portal. Patients have to find information about the meaning of their health record on the web or clarify results with their healthcare providers.

Additionally, most of the health/medical information provided to patients via portals are still technically complicated in terms of language (Tieu et al., 2017). Patients would require a mid-level to a high level of medical knowledge to comprehend the information provided to them. Health/medical information is not provided to patients at an accessible reading level that is beneficial to patients of all cultural or educational backgrounds (Yamin et al., 2011). As discussed throughout this chapter, several factors contribute to poor results with eHealth interventions; these include a lack of considerations of patients/consumers health literacy levels, digital literacy levels, cultural backgrounds, education levels, disabilities, and age.

SOLUTIONS AND RECOMMENDATIONS

Consumer eHealth interventions are changing the nature of patient-physician interactions (Zelmer & Hagens, 2016). By leveraging these tools, healthcare organizations have the opportunity to provide patient-centered care, while achieving operational efficiencies. However, to achieve this goal, they have to consider health and digital literacy education and ensure it is an integral part of consumer eHealth interventions, before investing significant amounts of resources and effort in implementing and promoting eHealth tools. They can make use of a broad range of communication strategies to ensure that patients are trained to understand health information and its applicability to their health and wellbeing (Nutbeam, 2000). This will promote active engagement among patients and ultimately promote patient empowerment to become active participants in their care (Snowdown et al., 2015). Only through health and digital training can eHealth tools be utilized efficiently for patient benefit. This section will conclude by providing practical strategies of how healthcare organizations can begin their journey of educating and empowering patients through health and digital literacy to become active participants in their care and efficiently utilize consumer eHealth interventions to manage their chronic diseases.

In particular, we advocate a patient-centered eHealth approach that integrates wellness, prevention, self-care education and chronic disease management. This approach requires that healthcare organizations change their perspective of patients from "end-users" to "front-seat drivers" and conduct a careful user analysis to design or select consumer eHealth applications that serve its intended purpose.

We suggest that healthcare organizations conduct user studies to understand the tasks, challenges, concerns, and specific health literacy needs of the targeted users. We will also address the importance of considering the fundamental literacy, language, and cultural barriers of the targeted users when designing or selecting consumer eHealth interventions. We will recommend a patient-centered, disease-specific, task-relevant, and contextualized health literacy approach that enables patients to make sense of their health records and understand how such data can help them make informed decisions such as better managing their medications and lifestyle changes that contribute to their treatment outcomes and overall health. To help consumers understand their health conditions and use their medical data to manage their health conditions effectively, specific requirements need to be met. These requirements are:

High-Quality, Up-to-Date Health Information From Reliable Sources

There is a general lack of health literacy integration in consumer eHealth interventions (Yamin et al., 2011). As a result, most users turn to the Internet to search for health information that they need. However, as the quality of health information on the Internet varies considerably, both physicians and patients are concerned about the credibility of the medical information that general search engines provide. There is a need to identify and provide high-quality health information from trusted sources and create a medical search engine that can provide high-quality medical information in the way that helps consumers understand and manage their health conditions (Chen & Decary, 2017), especially where patient education is concerned. Furthermore, it is vital to ensure that the information is aligned with the latest clinical guidelines, so that the information patients receive reflects the best practices in the field of medicine.

Disease-Specific and Task-Relevant Information Support

The scope of patient education content should cover the general health information related to preventive education and wellness promotion, as well as disease-specific and task-relevant information. The emphasis on disease-specificity and task relevance is significant because patients with different health conditions face a unique set of tasks and associated challenges. Therefore, the health information provided to patients needs to be relevant to their disease types, stages, and the specific tasks that patients need to perform in their self-management of the disease to improve their treatment outcomes. The information should help patients not only to understand their conditions, but to learn different ways to manage the multiple aspects of their conditions. This includes gaining the skills to make informed choices, effectively manage their medications and other treatments, modify unhealthy behaviors to improve treatment outcomes. In addition, patients need to have access to information that helps them deal with unforeseen challenges, complications, and concerns; they also need to know when, why, and how to make a lifestyle change or medication adjustment.

Contextualized Information Support and On-Demand Learning

Ideally, patients should follow a coherent education curriculum to learn everything they need to know about their health conditions and develop the ability to manage their conditions. However, the reality is that patients have to work, a family to care for, and many other responsibilities. Therefore, they do not have the time, energy and motivation to spend more time than they have to when dealing with their health conditions. Thus, providing contextualized, on-demand health literacy education while patients are performing the tasks related to their care might be the most efficient and practical way for them to learn. For instance, in the process of inspecting glucose monitoring data, hyperlinks can provide users with the crucial information that they need in order to make the connections between the levels of glucose and their diet and exercise. Information can also be provided on how their treatments should be adjusted based on the results.

Depending on the needs and preferences of the patients, such contextualized information support should enable the patients to learn everything they perceive as relevant, give them the opportunity to engage in on-demand learning. For instance, in the context of self-initiated care activities, the patients should be given access to relevant online courses about their conditions, and comprehensive information on a given topic if they request it.

Multiple Modes of Effective Presentations

Health information needs to be presented in a way that is understandable to the target patients to facilitate utilization of the information for their self-care (Skinner, 2002). There is a variety of knowledge and skills that patients need to learn, and some are conceptual in nature (disease definition, causes, development), and some are related to procedures and process (e.g., insulin injection, prosthetic fitting). To facilitate patient understanding, we recommend the use of multiple modes of presentation, adding audio and visuals to textual information whenever possible. Especially for demonstrating the procedures or processes, we recommend the use of graphic illustrations, animations, or videos in addition to descriptive text. This is especially useful for people who have low levels of general literacy, poor language competence and people with specific disabilities.

Accommodation to Diverse Population Needs

Most countries in North America and Europe are enriched by their cultural and language diversity. However, for eHealth technology developers, such diversity imposes one of the most significant challenges in application development. As a result, the vast majority of health websites, patient record systems, mobile apps and mobile self-care devices are created in one language only, mostly in English.

As the eHealth technology market grows, it is necessary to enable multi-language capacity to meet the diverse needs of users from different cultural and language background. Also, developers should pay particular attention to the needs of seniors because that population group is at high risk for chronic diseases.

Furthermore, the needs of people with lower levels of literacy need to be considered, because they are more likely to misunderstand medical directions, misuse medication and have more drug-related accidents. Therefore, it is essential to provide information in the way that they understand and can benefit from. There is no easy solution to accommodate the needs of diverse populations, however adding audio and visuals to textual information could help. In addition, even if some users lack the vocabulary to describe their symptoms while they search for health information, it is possible to use body images with body part indications and symptom descriptions so that users can point and click to find the information that is useful to them.

FUTURE DIRECTIONS OF RESEARCH AND DEVELOPMENT

Next Generation Health Literacy Interventions

An ideal model of patient education is one that can provide patients with high-quality medical information that is tailored to their specific diseases, challenges, preferences, and needs. The information should be provided in such a way that patients can truly understand it regardless of their general literacy level, language competence, and other limitations (Chen & Decary, 2017). With new technologies such as speech recognition, natural language processing, artificial intelligence, automatic translation, and augmented reality, this can become a reality.

For instance, imagine that an intelligent medical agent available on a smartphone can have conversations with patients and give them the health-related advice they need using speech recognition, natural language processing, and artificial intelligence technologies. Through language identification and automatic translation, an intelligent agent could also understand the language that patients speak, respond to them in their language of choice and even translate health information from one language to another in real time. Patients could see the organs inside of their bodies via augmented reality and get information on how to deal with different symptoms and diseases.

Through image recognition, a mobile device could scan the diseased skin of a patient then provide information about diagnosis, treatment options, and self-care. If the patient needs further advice or services, they could then consult a skin specialist via telemedicine without waiting or leaving their home. New technology developments can make these options possible in just a few years if countries have national strategies that leverage these resources and talents to develop such eHealth products that could benefit their citizens.

Intelligent, Integrated, and Connected Consumer eHealth Solutions

Some of the descriptions above might seem fictional; however, some companies have already been successfully working towards these solutions, which integrate patient education and eHealth interventions using emerging technologies. For instance, Visiomed Group, a French company specializing in next-generation medical electronics has developed an integrated consumer eHealth solution that consists of a variety of smart self-monitoring devices, an artificial intelligence diagnostic system that uses self-monitoring data from mobile devices to identify health problems and a telemedicine network linked to patient records and communication logs, as well as a health information library (Visiomed Group, 2017).

Another company, Cogilex R&D, a national language processing, artificial intelligence (AI) and consumer health information technology firm from Canada has been developing an AI-based patient self-care application. This application integrates (a) an AI conversation agent that understands health-related instruction and actions using speech recognition and natural language processing (b) comprehensive contextualized health information support and searches from high-quality medical sources on the Internet (c) access to patient data from mobile self-monitoring devices and electronic health records and (d) access to online health-related services such as e-booking, telemedicine and prescription renewal (Chen & Decary, 2017).

In addition, other technology companies and smart device makers are working towards this vision of intelligent, integrated and connected consumer eHealth solutions. With such high efforts in research and development, the future of consumer eHealth technology looks very promising.

CONCLUSION

In conclusion, we believe that only when patients have acquired the necessary health literacy for understanding their health conditions, can they make sense of their health data and achieve the desired outcomes. Patients will measure their health outcomes in terms of their perceived abilities to deal with unforeseen challenges, make informed choices, successfully manage their medications and other treatment interventions and form healthy behaviors. Patients will judge whether they will adopt and use a new eHealth application based on such perceptions. To increase the adoption and usage of consumer digital health interventions, health literacy/patient education must be an integral part of their development.

REFERENCES

Cammaerts, B. (Ed.). (2003). Beyond the digital divide: reducing exclusion, fostering inclusion. Brussels: University Press.

Chen, M., & Decary, M. (2017). Seenso Health – Medical Search Made Easier and Better, in Privacy. Medical Search Engine Exhibited at Consumer Electronics Show 2017 (CES 2017), Las Vegas, NV.

Chen, M., & Decary, M. (2017). *A Prototype of Seenso Self-care Hub*. Exhibition at The Canadian Conference on Medical Education 2017 (CCME 2017), Winnipeg, MA.

Curtis, J., Cheng, S., Rose, K., & Tsai, O. (2011). Promoting adoption, usability and research for personal health records in Canada: The MyChart experience. *Health Management Forum*, *24*(3), 149–154. doi:10.1016/j.hcmf.2011.07.004 PMID:22165576

Eng, T., Maxfield, A., Patrick, K., Deering, M. J., Ratzan, S. C., & Gustafson, D. H. (1998). Access to health information and support: A public highway or private road? *Journal of the American Medical Association*, *280*(15), 1371–1375. doi:10.1001/jama.280.15.1371 PMID:9794322

Gruman, J. (2014). *Self-Monitoring Health IT Falls Short of Providing the Information We Need*. Available from: http://www.cfah.org/blog/2014/self-monitoring-health-it-falls-short-of-providing-the-information-we-need

Institute of Medicine. (2004). *Health literacy: A prescription to end confusion*. Washington, DC: Institute of Medicine.

Kim, J. Y., Wineinger, N. E., Taitel, M., Radin, J. M., Akinbosoye, O., Jiang, J., ... Steinhubl, S. (2016). Self-Monitoring utilization patterns among individuals in an incentivized program for healthy behaviours. *Journal of Medical Internet Research*, *18*(11), e292. doi:10.2196/jmir.6371 PMID:27856407

Mancuso, J. M. (2009). Assessment and measurement of health literacy: An integrative review of the literature. *Nursing & Health Sciences*, *11*(1), 77–89. doi:10.1111/j.1442-2018.2008.00408.x PMID:19298313

McCray, A. T. (2005). Promoting Health Literacy. *Journal of the American Medical Informatics Association*, *12*(2), 152–163. doi:10.1197/jamia.M1687 PMID:15561782

Mukhopadhyay, S., & Postolache, O. (Ed.). (2013). *Pervasive and mobile sensing and computing for healthcare: technological and social issues*. Heidelberg, Germany: Springer.

Nielsen-Bohlman, L., Panzer, A. M., & Kindig, D. A. (2004). *Health Literacy, A Prescription to End Confusion*. Washington, DC: The National Academies Press.

Norman, C. D., & Skinner, H. A. (2006a). eHEALS: The eHealth Literacy Scale. *Journal of Medical Internet Research*, *4*(4), e27. doi:10.2196/jmir.8.4.e27 PMID:17213046

Norman, C. D., & Skinner, H. A. (2006b). eHealth literacy: Essential skills for consumer health in a networked world. *Journal of Medical Internet Research*, *8*(2), e9. doi:10.2196/jmir.8.2.e9 PMID:16867972

Nutbeam, D. (2000). Health literacy as a public health goal: A challenge for contemporary health education and communication strategies into the 21st century. *Health Promotion International*, *15*(3), 259–267. doi:10.1093/heapro/15.3.259

Parker, R. M., Baker, D. W., Williams, M. V., & Nurss, J. R. (1995). The test of functional health literacy in adults: A new instrument for measuring patients' literacy skills. *Journal of General Internal Medicine*, *10*(10), 537–541. doi:10.1007/BF02640361 PMID:8576769

Reeve, C. L., & Basalik, D. (2014). Is health literacy an example of construct proliferation? A conceptual and empirical evaluation of its redundancy with general cognitive ability. *Intelligence*, *44*(1), 93–102. doi:10.1016/j.intell.2014.03.004

Rootman, I. (2003). Literacy and health in Canada: Is it really a problem? *Canadian Journal of Public Health*, *94*(6), 405–406. PMID:14700236

Sarkar, U., Karter, A. J., Liu, J. Y., Adler, N. E., Nguyen, R., Lopez, A., & Schillinger, D. (2011). Social Disparities in Internet patient portal use in Diabetes: Evidence that the digital divide extends beyond access. *Journal of the American Medical Informatics Association*, *18*(3), 318–321. doi:10.1136/jamia.2010.006015 PMID:21262921

Schulz, P. J., & Nakamoto, K. (2013). Patient behavior and the benefits of artificial intelligence: The perils of "dangerous" literacy and illusory patient empowerment. *Patient Education and Counseling*, *92*(2), 223–228. doi:10.1016/j.pec.2013.05.002 PMID:23743214

Skinner, H. A. (2002). What motivates people to change? In H. A. Skinner (Ed.), *Promoting health through organizational change* (pp. 113–146). San Francisco, CA: Benjamin Cummings.

Smith, J. L., & Haggerty, J. (2003). Literacy in primary care: Is it a problem? *Canadian Journal of Public Health*, *94*(6), 408–412. PMID:14700237

Snowdown, A. (2015). Enhancing patient experience through personalization of health services. *Healthcare Management Forum*, *28*(5), 182–185. doi:10.1177/0840470415588656 PMID:26135292

Tieu, L. (2017). Online patient websites for electronic health record access among vulnerable populations: Portals to nowhere? *Journal of the American Medical Informatics Association*, *24*(e1), e47–e54. doi:10.1093/jamia/ocw098 PMID:27402138

Veenhof, B., Clermont, Y., & Sciadis, G. (2005). *Literacy and digital technologies: Linkages and outcomes*. Ottawa, Canada: Statistics Canada.

Visiomed Group. (2017). Bewell Connect Products. Products Exhibited at Consumer Electronics Show 2017 (CES 2017), Las Vegas, NV.

Wagner, E. H. (1998). Chronic disease management: What will it take to improve care for chronic illness? *Effective Clinical Practice*, *1*(1), 2–4. PMID:10345255

Wodchis, W., Dixon, A., & Anderson, G. (2015). Integrating care to older people and those with complex needs: Examining the lessons from international case studies. *International Journal of Integrated Care*, *15*(1), 1–15.

World Health Organization. (2017). *Chronic Diseases and Health Promotion*. Retrieved from: http://www.who.int/chp/en/

Yamin, C., Emani, S., Williams, D. H., Lipsitz, S. R., Karson, A. S., Wald, J. S., & Bates, D. W. (2011). The digital divide in adoption and use of a personal health record. *Archives of Internal Medicine*, *171*(6), 568–574. doi:10.1001/archinternmed.2011.34 PMID:21444847

Zelmer, J., & Hagens, S. (2014). Understanding the gap between the desire for and use of consumer health solutions. *Healthcare Papers*, *13*(4), 9–21. doi:10.12927/hcpap.2014.23871 PMID:25148119

Zhao, J., Freeman, B., & Li, M. (2016). Can mobile apps influence people's health behavior change? An evidence review. *Journal of Medical Internet Research*, *18*(11), e287. doi:10.2196/jmir.5692 PMID:27806926

KEY TERMS AND DEFINITIONS

Chronic Illnesses: Refers to diseases that last for three or more months and cannot be cured with medications or vaccines. They do not typically disappear.

Consumer E-Health Interventions: Refers to the utilization of digital tools to engage consumers/patients to complete an activity or make a change.

Cultural Competency: Refers to one's ability to understand, acknowledge, and display sensitivity to another person's culture, traditions, or language.

Digital Literacy: Refers to one's ability to effectively utilized technology or technology related devices to accomplish a goal.

Health Literacy: Refers to one's ability to comprehend complex health/medical information presented to them.

Linguistic Competency: Refers to one's ability to comprehend (understand, read, or write) and verbalize a concept or idea in a specified language, for example English or French.

Patient Empowerment: Refers to activities undertaken by healthcare providers or organizations to help patients gain confidence in completing an activity or making a change.

Patient Engagement: Refers to activities undertaken by healthcare providers or organizations to involve patients in their care. This can also involve providing patients with credible health/medical information.

Chapter 5
Uberization of Healthcare

Lizette Alvarez
University of Southern California (USC), USA

ABSTRACT

Over the years, health literacy has embodied various forms to aid healthcare decisions. For technology and health literacy to merge, the author examines and discusses how the following three elements can be applied to implement a type of technology and to what audience: 1) time, 2) cost, and 3) engagement. Through focused time, cost, and engagement efforts, healthcare can be optimized without reductions to the quality of information. Due to its rapid spread, information could to be fixed accordingly. This would positively impact the decision-making process for communities and public and private sectors. Benefits outweigh risks related to the implementation of technology and health literacy. Traditional medicine is known to have difficulties adapting to change. However, the risk is too high not to explore the use of technology and health literacy.

INTRODUCTION

Various forms of health literacy (i.e., graphic novels, comic books, brochures, and billboards) have aided in decisions related to healthcare, including health prevention (i.e., early pregnancy care, childhood immunization) and chronic illness (i.e., cancer and human immunodeficiency virus [HIV]). In the mid-1990s, healthcare researchers at the University of Southern California (USC) in Los Angeles studied health literacy. Inspired by the research, this chapter aims to creatively and unconventionally educate the public on disorders and diseases in the United States. Graphic novels and comic books served as tools to engage the target audience: monolingual, Spanish-speaking, low literate adults in Los Angeles, California. This population was being missed because of language, cultural, and educational barriers.

Evidenced-based evaluations at USC and an international collaboration with the University of Groningen, The Netherlands took place in 2017. The same concept produced positive significant results with outcomes suggesting that "a fotonovela may be a valuable health education format for adults with varying levels of literacy, even if it was developed for a target group with a different cultural background" (van Jagt et al., 2017, p. 284). This resulted in a Dutch audience that became engaged with the presentation and storytelling concept.

DOI: 10.4018/978-1-5225-4074-8.ch005

This chapter will examine the ability to merge technology and health literacy. The author will examine and discuss how the following elements can be applied to specific technology and audiences through: (1) time; (2) cost; and (3) engagement.

DEFINITION

According to the Collins English Dictionary, the technology and business concept definition of uberization is "to subject (an industry) to a business model in which services are offered on demand through direct contract between a customer and a supplier, usually via mobile technology" (https://www.collinsdictionary.com/us/dictionary/english/uberize). In this example, uberization conveys how the healthcare industry can benefit from a successful business model and innovative technology.

PROBLEM

Research in healthcare and technology has indicated a lack of innovation due to organizations' poor cooperation in building user applications. "Both public and private sector stakeholders, particularly government agencies and private corporations, will need to collaboratively reduce the gap between the health information 'haves' and 'have-nots'" (Eng et al., 1998, p. 1371). By fast forwarding to 2017, the aforementioned remains problematic.

Self-advocacy has become important as patients take healthcare into their own hands. Examples include social media groups for direct patient collaboration or applications developed by the private sector to manage health. Research has also noted that technology would be tailored by "developing applications for the growing diversity of users, funding research on access-related issues" (Eng et al., 1998, p. 1371). This mirrors how healthcare is being tailored through precision medicine and the human genome. Research is advancing at lightning speed.

However, it is important to address the lack of disseminated information. A study in the utilization of internet technology suggests that "significant advances in technology access and use could be sparked by developing technology interfaces that are accessible to individuals with limited literacy skills" (Jensen, King, Davis, & Guntziller, 2010, p. 804).

SOLUTION

It is widely recognized that technology and innovation regularly benefit society. These efforts improve speed and costs without compromising quality. Like most inventions, audiences and populations were left out during initial development (for example, radio and television platforms were readily accessible to higher socioeconomic groups).

Technology is already economically feasible and available. Yet, there are forgotten groups, including low literate audiences and certain cultures. To achieve potential solutions in electronic health (or e-health), we must "address disparities, several authorities have suggested the need for greater information technology research and investments" (Gibbons, 2005, para. 1). As organizations and individuals adopt technology and innovation in healthcare, they will continue to use creative ways to reach "potential benefits of e-health applications and possible contribution of the field to overcoming disparities in health and healthcare" (Gibbons, 2005, para. 1).

Opportunities exist to include populations that have been left out due to lack of time or high costs in research. As a recent study by Bickmore and Paasche-Orlow (2012, para. 1) in information technology and health literacy discovered:

... focused investment of time and energy, technology has the potential for reducing disparities through intelligent, usable, and accessible systems that tailor information, advice, counseling and behavioral support to an individuals need at a given time and place.

Time

Although the value of health literacy is steadily recognized around the world, it fails to efficiently reach its ultimate audiences. Uber, a global company, is a version of uberization. The rideshare transportation company leverages value with technology and on-demand service. Traditional taxis were unable to fill the on-demand niche. On-demand service is now achieved using a specific technology model (i.e., apps, mobile health, telehealth, sms/text, cloud services, or artificial and virtual intelligence).

Health literacy has the potential and opportunity to offer "healthcare at your fingertips" accessibility to audiences through an on-demand model. For example, an on-demand health model could deliver cancer information to people who must make immediate decisions on their health or the health of another individual.

Access to knowledge must be considered when developing high-quality technology for the dissemination of information. In an example addressing minority health and diabetes, a study investigated the use of "electronic, Web-enabled touch-screen information kiosks ... to provide culturally and linguistically appropriate diabetes information to Latino audiences" (Matthews, Darbisi, Sandmann, Galen, & Rubin, 2008, p. 520). Data found that, "users found the kiosks and their functions helpful and usable" (Matthews et al., 2008, p. 520). In regards to this group, prevention and management of diabetes is key at the right time. As in this example, information costs and time management must be considered for strategic dissemination (i.e., a general practitioner visit, classes, or pamphlets).

Another example of a time-saving platform and audience involves mobile health (or m-health) and children. m-Health is the practice of medicine and public health supported by mobile devices. Devices include mobile phones, tablet computers, and wearable devices (i.e., a smart watch). A U.S. study published in *Telemedicine and e-Health* found that "Cognitive behavioral therapy (CBT) for child anxiety, although efficacious, typically requires 16-20 weekly sessions with a therapist" (Pramana, Parmanto, Kendall, & Silk, 2014, p. 419). When targeted at the right population or audience, m-health can effectively deliver information (in vivo). According to Pramana et al. (2014, p. 419), "Integrating an m-health platform within BCBT for anxious children may facilitate involvement in treatment and dissemination of effective procedures."

Some have argued that creating or using the wrong technology platform is a waste of time and economically non-feasible. However, research discussed in this chapter identifies both successful and unsuccessful methods to redirect efforts and increase improvements.

Cost

While working on the fotonovela/graphic novel tool at USC, the author observed that costs remained high for traditional (i.e., print) dissemination methods. These methods also proved to be slow. Brochures, pamphlets, paper, ink, and delivery of the evidence-based research information were stored in cardboard boxes. Therefore, the information was exclusively available to organizations with funding to purchase, distribute, and share information with their targeted audiences. Exclusive availability of information would not exist with the use of technology (for example, an app). The information could be readily and virally spread in a cost-effective manner. Target audiences and communities could access the information at a fraction of traditional costs. Cost effective, accessible devices (i.e., smartphones, tablets, and mobile wearables such as Fitbits) would distribute information through a cost-effective platform.

An online article titled *Things Are Looking App* (2016, para. 9) discussed international healthcare systems and prescriptions:

When Britain's National Health service tested the cost-effectiveness of remote support for patients with chronic obstructive pulmonary disease, it found that an electronic tablet paired with sensors measuring vital signs could result in better care and enormous savings, by enabling early intervention.

"Reduced cost" is a dreadful term for the traditional healthcare field for fear of reduced quality. However, innovation has proven to be economically positive for the industry. m-Health and e-health generally use computers, patient monitors, communication satellites, etc. Apps, social media, and telemedicine would also be employed. m-Health has shown positive results in a costly population because "chronically sick are disproportionately costly in any health-care system." (2016, para. 7) One m-health service app, Diabetes+Me is "already showing that it can improve patient outcomes while reducing costs." (2016, para. 8) Diabetes+Me is a diabetes management tool on an electronic wearable watch for easy tracking of data. A patient or clinician can track, assess, and create a tailored plan for an individual patient's needs.

In the case of e-health, researchers in The Netherlands reconfirmed that "most articles show eHealth is effective/cost-effective or at least suggest evidence is promising, which is consistent with previous findings" (Elbert et al., 2014, para. 1). The study suggested that attention should be placed in the "development and evaluation of strategies to implement effective/cost-effective eHealth initiatives in daily practice" (Elbert et al., 2014, para. 1).

Apps are considered successful tools to both providers and health plans (Hostetter, 2011, para. 18):

... apps are shown to improve care and reduce costs—by avoiding complications and the need for in-person visits for instance—then they may be adapted by those who benefit from greater efficiency, including providers working in accountable care organization or undercapitalized reimbursement models.

It can be anticipated that health plans will help disseminate health literacy in a strategic, cost effective way to optimize health. According to Hostetter (2011, para. 18), "Health plans and integrated delivery systems that rely on such care management tools to reduce costs may also benefit."

As individuals and organizations seek to launch successful applications or high-quality platforms, they must consider the various parts and elements. Using the examples, they can implement a system to study users, identify populations to secure the technology, and determine what is it being applied to wellness, prevention, and chronic diseases.

Audience Engagement

Target audiences will benefit from technology while others choose to engage through traditional methods (i.e., paper copies, print, radio, and television). Rural communities without internet access would not use electronic platforms. However, much of the world would be able to readily make use of technology's on-demand and cost-efficient methods. The target audience would also help researchers, policymakers, and foundations make timely and quality-based decisions to aid patients and communities.

Organizations and individuals must assess the type of technology used to engage audiences. To realize successful outcomes, users must study prior examples and strategize how to reach and optimize their healthcare audiences. A 2006 Canadian study noted that in-depth discussions are required to identify the needs of populations using e-health platforms. Otherwise, "electronic health tools provide little value if the intended users lack the skills to effectively engage them" (Norman & Skinner, 2006).

A 2013 study in the *Journal of Cancer Education* found that (Pandey, Hasan, Dubey, & Sarangi, 2012, p. x):

There is an increased interest in smart phone applications as a tool for delivery of health-care information. There have been no studies which evaluated the availability and content of cancer-related smartphone applications.

In the author's health literacy study with fotonovelas/graphic novels, it was determined that displaying the printed tool on a technological platform would be timely, cost effective, and engaging to the audience. A 2017 study suggested that "health-related fotonovelas—booklets that portray a dramatic story using photograph and captions—may be effective health communication tools, especially for readers with a low level of literacy" (van Jagt et al., 2017, para. 1).

Based on work with fotonovela/graphic novels, the author recommends implementing a technology platform for additional, faster research. These efforts will assist in community-based recruitment efforts and evaluations. In addition, efforts will increase audience engagement and reported positive impacts. With creativity, strategy, and research on positive impact, the healthcare sector will be able to reach broader audiences.

CONCLUSION

Through focused time, cost, and engagement efforts, healthcare can be optimized without reductions to the quality of information. Due to its rapid spread, information could to be fixed accordingly. This would positively impact the decision-making process for communities and public and private sectors.

Benefits outweigh risks related to the implementation of technology and health literacy. Traditional medicine is known to have difficulties adapting to change. However, the risk is too high not to explore the use of technology and health literacy.

REFERENCES

Bickmore, T. W., & Paasche-Orlow, M. K. (2012). The role of information technology in health literacy research. *Journal of Health Communication, 17*(Sup3), 23-29. doi:10.1080/10810730.2012.712626

Elbert, N. J., Os-Medendorp, H. V., Renselaar, W. V., Ekeland, A. G., Roijen, L. H., Raat, H., ... Pasmans, S. G. (2014). Effectiveness and cost-effectiveness of eHealth interventions in somatic diseases: A systematic review of systematic reviews and meta-analyses. *Journal of Medical Internet Research, 16*(4), e110. doi:10.2196/jmir.2790 PMID:24739471

Eng, T. R., Maxfield, A., Patrick, K., Deering, M. J., Ratzan, S. C., & Gustafson, D. H. (1998). Access to health information and support: A public highway or private road? *Journal of the American Medical Association, 280*(15), 1371–1375. doi:10.1001/jama.280.15.1371 PMID:9794322

Gibbons, M. C. (2005). A historical overview of health disparities and the potential of eHealth solutions. *Journal of Medical Internet Research, 7*(5), e50. doi:10.2196/jmir.7.5.e50 PMID:16403714

Hostetter, M. (2011, October/November). Health care quality improvement: There's an app for that. *Quality Matters.* Retrieved from http://www.commonwealthfund.org/publications/newsletters/quality-matters/2011/october-november-2011/in-focus

Jensen, J. D., King, A. J., Davis, L. A., & Guntzviller, L. M. (2010). Utilization of internet technology by low-income adults: The role of health literacy, health numeracy, and computer assistance. *Journal of Aging and Health, 22*(6), 804–826. doi:10.1177/0898264310366161 PMID:20495159

Matthews, P. H., Darbisi, C., Sandmann, L., Galen, R., & Rubin, D. (2008). Disseminating health information and diabetes care for Latinos via electronic information kiosks. *Journal of Immigrant and Minority Health, 11*(6), 520–526. doi:10.100710903-008-9134-6 PMID:18392935

Norman, C. D., & Skinner, H. A. (2006). eHealth literacy: Essential skills for consumer health in a networked world. *Journal of Medical Internet Research, 8*(2), e9. doi:10.2196/jmir.8.2.e9 PMID:16867972

Pandey, A., Hasan, S., Dubey, D., & Sarangi, S. (2012). Smartphone apps as a source of cancer information: Changing trends in health information-seeking behavior. *Journal of Cancer Education, 28*(1), 138–142. doi:10.100713187-012-0446-9 PMID:23275239

Pramana, G., Parmanto, B., Kendall, P. C., & Silk, J. S. (2014). The SmartCAT: An m-health platform for ecological momentary intervention in child anxiety treatment. *Telemedicine Journal and e-Health, 20*(5), 419–427. doi:10.1089/tmj.2013.0214 PMID:24579913

Things Are Looking App. (2016, March 10). *The Economist.* Retrieved from https://www.economist.com/news/business/21694523-mobile-health-apps-are-becoming-more-capable-and-potentially-rather-useful-things-are-looking

van Jagt, R. K., Hoeks, J. C. J., Duizer, E., Baron, M., Molina, G. B., Unger, J. B., & Jansen, C. J. M. (2017). Sweet temptations: How does reading a fotonovela about diabetes affect Dutch adults with different levels of literacy? *Health Communication*, 284–290. Retrieved online http://www.tandfonline.com/doi/full/10.1080/10410236.2016.1258617 PMID:28094559

KEY TERMS AND DEFINITIONS

Audience Engagement: A metric used in technology and various industries to measure if audiences have an interest in topic and also how long their interest is in the topic.

Electronic Health (E-Health): A recent healthcare practice used to disseminate information and communicate through internet, computers and other devices.

Health Literacy: A way people understand health information to make appropriate healthcare decisions.

Mobile Health (m-Health): General term for use of mobile phone or wireless devices for medical care. Primarily used for health prevention.

On-Demand Technology Model: Primarily a business model used to fulfil consumer demand of a product or service immediately.

Patient Advocacy: An area of specialization in healthcare that is concerned primarily with one group of patients or disorders.

Patient Outcomes: A way to measure patient goals and improve healthcare access and delivery.

Technology: The science or knowledge put into practical use to solve problems or invent useful tools.

University of Southern California: A leading private research university located in Los Angeles that includes a world renowned medical school amongst other internationally recognized academic programs.

Chapter 6
Increasing Health Literacy to Improve Clinical Trial Recruitment

Saliha Akhtar
Seton Hall University, USA

ABSTRACT

Health literacy has been found to be linked to healthcare understanding and decision making. Therefore, it makes sense why individuals who do not understand clinical trials will be less likely to want to enroll in one. In fact, three major barriers found in the literature that prevent potential participants from enrolling in clinical trials include a distrust or negative perception, lack of understanding, and lack of accessible and affordable healthcare. Hence, there is a need to increase potential participants' healthcare understanding so that they can make the best healthcare decisions for themselves. Strategies suggested to help increase potential participants' health literacy include revising informed consent forms, utilizing culturally targeted statements, using a variety of material, and training investigative site personnel. These proposed strategies may help increase health literacy, which in turn could improve clinical trial recruitment. Furthermore, these strategies focus on different elements of health literacy and coupled together may bring the most improvement.

INTRODUCTION

Recruitment issues can be costly and lead to overall delays in the clinical trial process. In fact, "every month by which the development process can be shortened is worth US $25 million in additional income for the average drug" (Marks & Power, 2002, p.105). In addition, these delays can extend the time it takes to get needed medications or interventions to patients. Unfortunately, despite these factors, trials frequently discontinue even in late stage Phase III trials due to failure to accrue (Schroen et al., 2010). Current strategies for recruiting patients can no longer be viewed as the best practice and need to be revised. Health literacy should be considered a vital component to participant recruitment of clinical trials and there needs to be a closer look at its' role in the recruitment process. For example, if an individual does

DOI: 10.4018/978-1-5225-4074-8.ch006

not have sufficient healthcare understanding, they will most likely not enroll in a clinical trial. Therefore, improving health literacy could help in mitigating the gap in insufficient recruitment in clinical trials.

A study by Aetna found that only 18% of adults in the United States are proficient when it comes to health literacy (Aetna, n.d.). This considerably small number illustrates the lack of health literacy among Americans. According to Selden, Zorn, Ratzan, and Parker (2000), health literacy is "the degree to which individuals have the capacity to obtain, process, and understand basic health information and services needed to make appropriate health decisions" (p. vi). This is the ability of individuals to receive healthcare information and then comprehend it in order to make the best healthcare decisions. According to the Kindig, Panzer, and Nielsen-Bohlman (2004), patients who have low health literacy are less likely to have knowledge on how to take care of themselves such as disease management and health-promoting behaviors. Therefore, it makes sense that health literacy is "commonly defined as the skills and abilities needed to gain access to, understand, and use health-related information" (Rudd, 2010, p. 2283). This means that individuals need to be able to obtain the information, comprehend it, and then utilize it when it comes to their own health.

There is now more focus on the health literacy rate of Americans in the United States as it is found to be linked to healthcare understanding and decision-making. In fact, it is a vital component to improving the healthcare of underprivileged populations while at the same time mitigating inequalities related to healthcare (Coulter & Ellins, 2007). More specifically, research has shown that limited health literacy leads to inequalities including having less knowledge of disease management and of health-promoting behaviors, having poorer health status, being less likely to use preventive services, and a higher rate of hospitalization and use of emergency services which in turn will lead to higher healthcare costs (Kindig et al., 2004). Due to these reasons, there is a high need to educate the public and share information on healthcare. Not only does the information need to be shared with the general public, which will increase their healthcare knowledge, but it also needs to be targeted to specific populations such as different minority groups. If individuals do not understand clinical trials or research, they will be less likely to want to enroll in a clinical trial. In addition, with the lack of knowledge or information, they may have misconceptions of what a clinical trial actually entails and thus be less likely to want to enroll in one. More importantly, if patients do not understand healthcare, they will not be able to make the best healthcare decision for themselves.

BACKGROUND

As healthcare research expands, there has been an increase in the number of clinical trials that play an important role in the treatment of many conditions and diseases. As of September 2017, Clinicaltrials.gov noted having an outstanding 254,787 studies listed across 200 countries (Clinicaltrials.gov, 2017). Although they may be different in their disease-focus and study design, similar issues are generally experienced. From a patient perspective, common reasons for not enrolling in a clinical trial or research study include distrust or having a negative perception of research, lack of understanding, and lack of accessible and affordable healthcare, all which are further discussed below. It is important to highlight that the literature presented focus heavily on the lack of minority representation in clinical trials as this is a large contributing factor to the problem of insufficient recruitment. In addition, the literature presented focuses on research in the United States as it represents a significant portion of the literature on clinical trial recruitment; however, similar issues may be experienced globally.

Distrust/Negative Perception

Many common themes have emerged in attempts to explain why there continues to be insufficient recruitment in clinical trials. The most common theme from a patient perspective is related to trust. In fact, in a review of the literature performed on the topic by Ford et al. (2008), mistrust was the most frequently reported barrier. With good reason, individuals have a lack of trust in clinical research, especially minorities. They have concerns about receiving inadequate treatment or misdiagnosis due to their racial or ethnic background, or in other words, being discriminated (Mendoza, Williams, Chapman, & Powers, 2012). In a study that interviewed stakeholders of the recruitment process, all of the stakeholders felt that there was a level of skepticism by minorities when it came to participating in clinical trials (Durant et al., 2014). They felt that this reluctance was due to inherent uncertainty or negative connotations of clinical trials (Durant et al., 2014).

Past cases of discrimination have contributed to the mistrust. A well-known case that deals with the discrimination of minorities is the U.S. Public Health Tuskegee Syphilis Experiment. In this case, rural African American men who had syphilis were not diagnosed or treated properly by the U.S. government. As noted by Durant et al. (2014), this case and other past cases have led to the mistrust of clinical research perceived by African Americans and Native American. However, Durant et al. (2014) also feel that with other minorities such as Asians and Latinos, there is more of general fear of being mistreated in clinical research.

With the repeated mistakes that have been made in the past with specific minority populations such as African Americans, there continues to be a lack of trust in experimental research and the researchers. Minorities have raised concerns about the trustworthiness of the site personnel and during their time in a clinical trial (Roberson, 1994). Participants are skeptical about having similar experiences based on these cases. Specifically, research has shown that they have expressed mistrust about the investigators' motives (Corbie-Smith, Thomas, Williams, & Moody-Ayers, 1999). Participants want to either further healthcare research and knowledge or have access to potential treatments or interventions, but want to be fully informed about the research process and not be discriminated. Fouad et al. (2000) also found that minorities have distrust about the purpose of informed consent and incentives which they feel are inappropriate. Therefore, participants are wary of healthcare research and distrust researchers who conduct it. They want to be fully disclosed the benefits and risks of clinical trials and what they will entail.

Lack of Understanding

Another barrier for individuals that prevents them from enrolling in healthcare research is a lack of understanding of research. In the study surrounding African American perceptions of medical research, it was found that they have limited understanding of the informed consent process (Corbie-Smith et al., 1999). This is surprising as the informed consent process is required for experimental studies with the intent to ensure that participants are aware of the risks, benefits, and procedures associated with the trial. Furthermore, the informed consent process ensures that their consent is received, ensuring that they understand and agree to the care. However, in the study by Corbie-Smith et al. (1999), participants felt that the consent process was more for the legal protection of researchers rather than for their benefit and protection.

Linked with the process of informed consent and healthcare research in general is the lack of understanding of terminology. In the same study by Corbie-Smith et al. (1999), participants described the difficulty with understanding technical, medical, and legal terminology, along with other aspects of the research study such as the efficacy and safety profile. This has also been noted by other researchers. Ryan, Prictor, McLaughlin, and Hill (2008) recommend that additional research be performed to determine what interventions or tools could be used to explain complex concepts of clinical trials to ensure participants have a better understanding of the informed consent, and thereby, will potentially be more willing to participate.

Finally, there is a lack of understanding on the purpose of research studies. Sinclair et al. (2000) found that African Americans have a discomfort with participation because of their lack of knowledge about the research process and what is required. Without the basic knowledge of the research design, there will be a lack of understanding of the procedures associated with it. For example, in a study by Fouad et al. (2000), barriers to participation included factors such as whether or not blood would be drawn and whether radiation would be utilized. Without an understanding of the basic research purpose, treatment, or research design, potential participants will question participation to the study. Therefore, Fouad et al. (2000) recommend holding workshops in order to provide more information on clinical trials.

With the lack of knowledge about the informed consent process, research designs, and clinical research in general, potential participants will continue to not have an understanding about the potential benefits of participating. This means that these potential participants will make the decision to not enroll without having the adequate knowledge about what the research entails.

Lack of Accessible and Affordable Healthcare

Another common theme seen as a barrier is lack of accessible and affordable healthcare. In fact, as noted by Ma et al. (2014), in some studies, lack of accessible and affordable research were seen as common obstacles/barriers. More specifically, in a study performed by Durant et al. (2014), minorities felt that lack of insurance was a factor which made them less likely to be offered an opportunity to participate in clinical trials. These studies show that there is a perception that lack of insurance or access to research studies is linked to an inability to participate. Other studies have reported similar findings. In a study by researchers from California, it was found that patients who had non-government insurance were statistically less likely to participate in a clinical trial compared to those who had some type of government insurance (Lara et al., 2001). Other studies have also shown a link between participation and those who have insurance. In a study that interviewed community leaders, it was found that there was a perception that insurance will not cover participating in a clinical trial (Fouad et al., 2000). Moreover, socioeconomic factors such low income may be associated with lack of access to healthcare, and therefore, have an effect on the enrollment of trials. This was emphasized by Hussain-Gambles, Atkin, and Leese (2004), who found that "low ethnic minority accrual to clinical trials might be caused in part by 'racially' constructed socio-economic factors which allow less utilization of healthcare, and hence, a reduced opportunity to take part in trials" (p. 385).

Therefore, concerns with insurance issues, whether it's lack of insurance or issues with insurance coverage, limit participation in clinical trials. Potential participants feel that they do not have access to the opportunity of participating in a clinical trial because of the lack of access to affordable healthcare.

STRATEGIES FOR INCREASING HEALTH LITERACY IN CLINICAL TRIAL RECRUITMENT

In order to mitigate the problem of insufficient recruitment in clinical trials, changes need to be made with the way that healthcare professionals, including investigative site personnel, interact with potential participants. Furthermore, according to Michielutte, Alciati, and El Arculli (1999), health literacy may a strong predictor for the poor participation in clinical trial programs. Therefore, it makes sense to first begin with increasing the health literacy of potential participants. The next sections will delve into specific changes that can be implemented in the clinical trial process in order to increase health literacy.

Revising Informed Consent Forms

Informed consent forms are designed to ensure that potential participants for a clinical trial have the information they need in order to make the best decision. This means having a complete understanding of the benefits and risks of the new treatment in order to be able to appropriately make the decision of whether to enroll in the clinical trial. However, research has shown that low health literacy can impact an individual's understanding of the benefits (Davis, Williams, Marin, Parker, & Glass, 2002). Therefore, it is vital that clinical trial professionals re-evaluate the way that informed consent forms are written. If they are not written in a manner which is understandable to most individuals, then it defeats the purpose of them. In fact, in a study surrounding African American perceptions of medical research, it was found that they have limited understanding of the informed consent process (Corbie-Smith et al., 1999). This is surprising as the informed consent process is required for experimental studies with the intent to ensure that the participant is aware of all the risks, benefits, and procedures associated with the trial. Furthermore, the informed consent process ensures that their consent is received, ensuring that they understand and agree to the care. However, while potential participants may want to either further healthcare research and knowledge or have access to potential treatments or interventions, they want to be fully informed about the research process and have assurance that they will not be discriminated. Fouad et al. (2000) also found that minorities have distrust about the purpose of informed consent and incentives which they feel are inappropriate. Part of this mistrust could be due to the lack of understanding of what is written in them.

Therefore, informed consent forms should be written at a level which is understandable to most individuals. The benefits and risks in an informed consent form need to be revised to a format which would be understandable. Davis et al. (2002) noted that benefit and risk communication is a vital component of discussions about treatment options. Other studies have also supported this finding. For example, O'Connor and Jacobsen (2006) stressed the importance of an individual receiving information related to the potential outcomes of the options available, focusing on the benefits and risks of the potential outcomes (O'Connor & Jacobsen, 2006). However, Jacobson et al. (1999) were able to overcome this barrier. In a pneumococcal vaccine intervention project, health educators created a 1-page education tool, which was written at below the fifth-grade reading level and given to individuals who should potentially receive the pneumococcal vaccine. Those individuals who were given this 1-pager were more than five times likely to receive the pneumococcal vaccine. In addition, discussion was approximately four times more likely to occur between the patient and healthcare provider. This is a very important finding because research has shown that patient/healthcare professional discussion can be effective.

More importantly, Jacobson et al. (1999) noted that the 1-page tool appeared to empower patients to show a health-seeking behavior. In fact, self-efficacy and empowerment are important factors when it comes to recruitment. The self-efficacy theory which originated from the social cognitive theory is the "extent to which people believe they are capable of performing specific behaviors in order to attain certain goals" (Consumer Health Informatics Research Resource, 2012, paragraph 1). Efficacy is a major factor in determining the choice that individuals will make when it comes to taking an action (Bandura, Adams, & Beyer, 1977). This includes how much effort they will put in and for how long they will persist in making the effort (Bandura et al., 1977). This means that self-efficacy is an important element when one makes a decision, including whether they will take a certain action or make a change to a behavior, such as consenting to enroll in a clinical trial. As Bandura (1994) stated, "perceived self-efficacy is defined as people's beliefs about their capabilities to produce designated levels of performance that exercise influence over events that affect their lives" (p. 71). This means that perceived self-efficacy is the expectation that taking a certain action will lead to a desired outcome. For example, having confidence in making the decision to participate in a clinical trial will be an informed one. As Bandura et al. (1977) found, when individuals feel that they do not have the ability to deal with a situation, they will have fear or tend to avoid the uncomfortable situation. Individuals who do not have self-efficacy will be more likely to not deal with a situation or take any action. In fact, this low sense of efficacy means that they have low motivation or aspirations and a weak commitment to achieve a goal (Bandura, 1993). As further noted by Bandura (1993), individuals' beliefs in their capabilities will affect their level of motivation. When it comes to enrolling in a clinical trial, the application of the self-efficacy theory would be whether the potential participant has the power or ability to enroll in a clinical trial. Perceived self-efficacy would be the minority's perception of their ability to achieve the target of enrolling in a clinical trial. Therefore, minorities with low self-efficacy will tend to make the decision to not participate in the clinical trial because they may not feel confident or even motivated to participate. On the other hand, if they do have high self-efficacy, then they will be more likely to make an effort to make the best informed decision. It is the potential participant who has the power or ability to enroll in a clinical trial and through the utilization of the self-efficacy theory, it can be determined if they are even prepared to make the decision to enroll. Therefore, by providing them with information that they understand, they could have higher self-efficacy or empowerment to make the decision in the best interest of their health versus out of confusion or uncertainty. This is also emphasized by Kickbusch, Wait, and Maag (2005) who stated that health literacy is "a critical empowerment strategy to increase people's control over their health, their ability to seek out information and their ability to take responsibility" (p. 8).

In addition to ensuring that informed consent forms should be written at a level which is understandable to most individuals, it is important that informed consent forms along with related materials are an appropriate length. According to IRB regulations, sponsors such as pharmaceutical companies are required to ensure that the informed consent form for a clinical trial contain certain elements. These elements are to ensure that potential participants are given appropriate and balanced information to be able to make the best decision for themselves. In 1998, the Department of Health and Human Services (DHHS) created an informed consent checklist, which lists the elements that are required to be included in an informed consent form, along with additional items which should be included as appropriate (DHHS, 1998). As a result of the information that needs to be included, informed consent forms are long in length. In a study by Davis, Berkel, Holcombe, Pramanik, and Divers (1998), they found that expanding the length of the informed consent form did not lead to increased comprehension of the form. Instead, they found that, "participants preferred the shorter, easy-to-read material and found it less frightening.

Perhaps long forms written on a college level, though intended to provide complete information for the informed consent of a clinical trial, may inadvertently be frightening and overwhelming, especially for low-level readers" (p 672). Therefore, as suggested by David et al. (1998), consent forms should be brief and direct. The length of the consent form may impact the health literacy of an individual by making it more difficult for them to understand especially if it is longer.

Culturally-Tailoring Information

Although clinical trials may be different in their disease-focus and study design, similar issues are generally experienced. One set of challenges researchers face are those related to participant recruitment. Participant enrollment has proven to be difficult in all therapeutic and disease areas and especially difficult when it comes to the inclusion of minority populations. In fact, despite the increase in the number of clinical trials, minority enrollment continues to be an issue. Researchers have acknowledged this as an ongoing problem with effects seen throughout the clinical trial process. It is also known that despite the number of guidelines and mandates that have been implemented, more specific strategies are needed to enroll from the minority population. Utilizing culturally-targeted statements when conveying information about clinical trials may be a way to mitigate the gap that exists.

Ma et al. (2014) suggested that culturally tailoring educational interventions can effectively increase the understanding of clinical trials. More specifically, these types of interventions can increase the "knowledge about clinical trial randomization procedures, informed consent, participants' right, and benefits of clinical trials" (Ma et al., 2014, p.429). In the study by Ma et al. (2012), they intended to recruit Chinese individuals in a clinical trial education program. First of all, they used community-based organization community volunteers to help clarify information to participants such as reading the evaluation questions out loud to participants or interpreting the direct meaning of the specific question(s) if someone with low literacy level had difficulty in understanding them. More importantly, in the study Chinese community health educators used a variety of activities including linguistically appropriate printed materials to model and reinforce positive attitudes towards clinical trials. Chinese language handouts on clinical trials and some types of cancer were also provided. The study found that utilizing a culturally-tailored approach could be effective in sharing clinical trial information along with potentially increasing participation in clinical trials among Asian communities. In fact, an online Culturally Appropriate National Cancer Clinical Trial Education program was also launched for physicians who serve a large number of Asian American patients.

Another study that utilized a culturally-tailored approach is a study by Brown et al. (2012). In their behavioral weight management trial for obese women, they utilized ethnically-targeted statements in direct mail letters. Research has shown that using culturally targeting statements in direct mail is an effective strategy (Brown et al., 2012). This personalization allows the patient to have more trust in the communication. In the study, ethnically-targeted statements were used to convey ethnic-specific information about health risks of obesity. The letter included information on the trial's purpose/significance, benefits to recipients, recipients' importance, how recipients were selected, sender's appreciation, sender's importance, institution's importance, style, format/appearance, and brevity. The study found that women who were sent letters than contained ethnically-targeted statements were more likely to respond than those women were sent letters which only contained generic statements. Moreover, the researchers were able to recruit minorities from different minority groups. Therefore, utilizing culturally-tailored strategies could be effective in increasing health literacy among minority populations and lead to a higher enrollment of minorities in clinical trials.

Variety of Material

Some research has shown that patients who are presented with treatment options, such as whether to enroll in a clinical treatment, might experience uncertainty in the course of action to take. Decision support could be used as a way to help address the unresolved needs of the individual. The decision support can be in the form of clinical counselling, decision aids, and coaching (O'Connor & Jacobsen, 2006). This means that the healthcare professionals or the investigative site personnel would be the ones helping to clarify the different options, providing facts and probabilities, and moreover, being there to guide and support the individual (O'Connor & Jacobsen, 2006). They need to enable the participants to make an informed decision. This also means that they need to be ones to provide the potential participants with the information on each option and ensure that expectations are aligned. Guiding the potential participants through the steps in the decision-making can minimize the uncertainty.

A varied use of materials could help in providing this support and information to the patient. More specifically, besides the written information provided in informed consent forms, visual aids may be used to further support the discussion on whether to enroll in a clinical trial. In fact, international health experts agree that visual aids can help to communicate with non-literate persons (as cited in Williams et al., 2002). Pratt and Searles (2017) discuss the benefits of visuals aids which have the ability to go beyond the health literacy barriers from written communication and can be used to improve the effectiveness of communication while also being able to reach a wider patient pool. To support this notion, Pratt and Searles (2017) created a template to provide instructions for proper use and explanation of risks for adverse events which can be adapted for use in explaining any medication using universal pictograms. Although this type of aid cannot replace the information provided in an informed consent form, when used in conjunction, it can help facilitate the discussion and help increase the potential participant's understanding of the information relevant to the clinical trial, including the benefits and risks. In fact, Pratt and Searles (2017) noted that the use of visuals aids is simple and efficient, and not only does it increase health literacy, but it can also improve physician-patient relationships, allow for better health outcomes, and possibly reduce healthcare expenditures.

Research has also shown that some people have trouble comprehending numeracy information. Visual aids help overcome those obstacles by portraying the information in a manner which allows an individual to comprehend the benefits and risks in a quantitative manner. Garcia-Retamero and Galesic (2010) suggest using visual aids along with numerical information to allow individuals to make more accurate assessments such as of risk reduction. Finally, iconic arrays as visual aids may also be effective in increasing understanding. "Icon arrays are graphical representations consisting of a number of stick figures, faces, circles, or other icons symbolizing individuals who are affected by some risk" (Galesic, Garcia-Retamero, & Gigerenzer, 2009, p. 210). While the level of seriousness portrayed by icon arrays may be not clear, the visual display of the information can be more effective in attracting people's attention and affecting their judgment (Galesic et al., 2009). Therefore, they could also be used to help facilitate the sharing of information and during the discussion between the healthcare professional and potential participant.

Therefore, the use of visual aids when used in conjunction with informed consent forms may help increase the information on the clinical trial allowing an individual to be able to make a better assessment on whether enrolling in the clinical trial is the best decision for them. Research has found that healthcare professionals can use pictograms and iconic arrays to share important information on clinical trials. In addition, Davis et al. (2002) provided a wide variety of visual aids that can be used including pictures, videos and interactive computer programs, and stories and pictures. Williams et al. (2002) also summarized research, suggesting using videos, pictographs, cartoon illustrations, and interactive computer-based multimedia. Therefore, there are many options that can be taken when incorporating visual aids in the recruitment phase of a clinical trial.

Training Investigative Site Personnel

The opportunity for a potential participant to enroll in a clinical trial is largely contributed by investigators and their support team as they play a vital role in determining which trials are available and could be appropriate for their patients (i.e., underrepresented populations) (Howerton et al., 2007). However, Williams et al. (2002) noted that the language that healthcare professionals use to communicate with patients is a barrier for patients who have low health literacy. This means that the language that they use to communicate with patients may not be understandable. In consequence, it is necessary to understand what changes can be made to improve the way that healthcare professionals communicate clinical trial information and opportunities. The first step would be to provide appropriate training to investigative site personnel. As suggested by Sudore and Schillinger (2009), many of the skills needed in order to have clear healthcare communication could be offered as part of continuing medical education. In fact, there are many courses already available including through the Centers for Disease Control and Prevention (CDC) (CDC, 2016). Therefore, through training and courses already available, investigative site personnel may be able to change the manner in which they speak to potential participants to one which is understandable.

Davis et al. (2002) also advised that it may be easier to change the communication of healthcare providers than patients. Therefore, it should be the health providers' responsibility to ensure that they have the appropriate communication skills. Davis et al. (2002) further suggested specific strategies that could be used by healthcare professionals to increase health literacy including taking the time to speak with the patient, using language that the patient can understand, and repeating instructions and information. First of all, it is important for the healthcare professional to slow down and take the time to not only share the information in clear terms, but also take the time to allow the patient to voice his/her concerns. While research has shown that physicians have lack of time due to conflicting priorities, they need to make a change in the amount of time they allocate for discussing clinical trial opportunities. In fact, the literature has shown that patients who are given more time to make a decision on whether to participate in a trial are three times more likely to consent (Siminoff, Zhang, Colabianchi, Sturm, & Shen, 2000). In addition, as Davis et al. (2002) described, healthcare professionals need to use language also known as "living room language." "Perhaps by recruiting community members of the same culture as the patients to act as ombudsmen, physicians can be taught the appropriate language and style with which to communication. Additionally, these ombudsmen could serve as peer educators and resource guides for patients" (Davis et al., 2002, p. 145).

Finally, the teach-back method may be another way to ensure comprehension (Davis et al., 2002). After answering the patients' questions, the teach-back method, also known as the "teach-to-goal" or the "show me" method can be used to confirm patients' understanding. This method is where the healthcare professional asks patients to restate or demonstrate the information shared (Sudore & Schillinger, 2009). As explained by Schillinger et al. (2003), patients may have trouble recalling and comprehending what physicians convey to them, but at the same time, physicians rarely assess whether their patients recall or comprehend new information. By not taking this step to ensure understanding, it is considered a missed opportunity that may have major consequences. However, the teach-back method may help healthcare professionals determine whether the potential participants comprehend the information that has been shared and discussed. In addition, taking the extra time to implement the teach-back method has not found to extend the time of visits (Sudore & Schillinger, 2009). Hence, it is important to train investigative site personnel so that they have the proper skills and knowledge on how to interact with potential participants. By doing so, they are eliminating barriers that may otherwise exist unknowingly.

FUTURE RESEARCH DIRECTIONS

When it comes implementing different strategies for increasing health literacy, it would be useful to gauge the health literacy level of individuals in order to determine the type of strategy and communication that should be used. However, research has found that this is not easy to measure. For example, Davis et al. (2002) acknowledged the difficulty in identifying those individuals who have low health literacy. Therefore, it may be difficult to determine when an individual has lower health literacy compared to another individual. Furthermore, this means that there is a need for further research to determine ways in which it would be possible to determine the health literacy level of each individual, especially for both oral and written information. This information would be valuable, especially in determining how much time and effort is needed for each individual. More time and effort would most likely be needed for an individual with lower health literacy. In addition, investigative site personnel would know approximately how much time would be needed to spent with each individual. However, it should also be acknowledged that patients who have low health literacy may not be as open to admitting when they do not understand or have knowledge on a topic. A research study found that of patients who had low health literacy, many patients did not admit to it (Parikh, Parker, Nurss, Baker, & Williams, 1996). Therefore, future research will also have to determine how to overcome this barrier.

Future research should also look into the cost of each type of strategy and weigh the cost-benefit of each. With the high cost already associated with clinical trials, it is important that any new strategy that is implemented has a high value in the recruitment phase. Therefore, there is a need for future studies to draw conclusions about the true value of each intervention. At the same time, they need to analyze each intervention's impact on health outcomes such as a decrease in the uncertainty of whether to enroll in a clinical trial and the increase in the enrollment of clinical trials. Pignone, DeWalt, Sheridan, Berkman, and Lohr (2004) stated that intervention studies have mostly focused on short-term knowledge outcomes or health behaviors. However, they suggested future studies to focus more on important, longer-term health outcomes that are more meaningful to patients. In consequence, there is a need for future research to determine how long-term, positive changes can be made to healthcare rather than short gains. Therefore, there are several directions that future research can take to continue to improve health literacy in clinical trial recruitment.

CONCLUSION

Low health literacy has an impact on clinical trials, especially when it comes to the recruitment of participants. When patients have low health literacy, they are less likely to enroll in a clinical trial due to the lack of knowledge on what it entails. In turn, the lower than planned recruitment or slower recruitment of participants leads to higher costs and inability at times for patients to receive access to essential medications. Due to this, changes are needed with the recruitment process including the interaction between healthcare professionals and potential participants. Some strategies to increase health literacy of potential participants are revising informed consent forms so they are understandable to most individuals, culturally tailoring clinical trial information, using a variety of material when communicating clinical trial information, and training investigative site personnel to improve their communication with potential participants. These strategies focus on different elements on health literacy such as reading, listening, communication, and interaction skills. As per Coleman et al. (2011), health literacy skills include reading, writing, listening, speaking, numeracy, critical analysis, and communication and interaction skills. Therefore, the strategies coupled together may bring the most improvement with health literacy and recruitment.

Furthermore, addressing the gap of minority recruitment will require a great deal of support from all stakeholders. It is essential that investigative site personnel and sponsors such as pharmaceutical companies be invested in the improvement of health literacy. In addition, there needs to be a close relationship with the public as they can best share what terminology and communications are understandable and useful to them. For example, sharing with them a draft informed consent form and asking for their feedback in order to determine whether they understand it or if the wording needs to be revised. While this may extend the start-up period of a clinical trial, it may shorten the recruitment time period by being able to enroll patients faster in the clinical trial due to the increased health literacy. It is also important to note that there may need to be several iterations of the informed consent form until it is considered fully understandable to most individuals. However, taking these steps will help ensure that when healthcare professionals are communicating information or having a discussion with potential participants, the potential participants comprehend what is being said rather than being confused or having decisional conflict. Moreover, through these steps, there will be an increased chance of success for the trial while at the same time improving the health literacy of patients and skills of healthcare professionals.

REFERENCES

Aetna. (n.d.). *Survey finds Americans' health literacy lacking*. Retrieved from https://news.aetna.com/2015/04/survey-finds-americans-health-literacy-lacking/

Bandura, A. (1993). Perceived self-efficacy in cognitive development and functioning. *Educational Psychologist*, *28*(2), 117–148. doi:10.120715326985ep2802_3

Bandura, A. (1994). Self-efficacy. In V. S. Ramachaudran (Ed.), *Encyclopedia of Human Behavior* (Vol. 4, pp. 71–81). New York, NY: Academic Press.

Bandura, A., Adams, N. E., & Beyer, J. (1977). Cognitive processes mediating behavioral change. *Journal of Personality and Social Psychology*, *35*(3), 125–139. doi:10.1037/0022-3514.35.3.125 PMID:15093

Brown, D. R., & Topcu, M. (2003). Willingness to participate in clinical treatment research among older African Americans and Whites. *The Gerontologist*, *43*(1), 62–72. doi:10.1093/geront/43.1.62 PMID:12604747

Centers for Disease Control and Prevention. (2016). *Health literacy: Find training*. Retrieved from https://www.cdc.gov/healthliteracy/gettraining.html

Clinicaltrials.gov. (2017). *Trends, Charts, and Maps*. Retrieved from https://www.clinicaltrials.gov/ct2/resources/trends

Coleman, C., Kurtz-Rossi, S., McKinney, J., Pleasant, A., Rootman, I., & Shohet, L. (2008). *The Calgary Charter on health literacy: Rationale and core principles for the development of health literacy curricula*. Retrieved from http://www.centreforliteracy.qc.ca/sites/default/files/CFL_Calgary_Charter_2011.pdf

Consumer Health Informatics Research resource. (2012). *Variable: Self efficacy*. Retrieved from http://chirr.nlm.nih.gov/self-efficacy.php

Corbie-Smith, G., Thomas, S. B., Williams, M. V., & Moody-Ayers, S. (1999). Attitudes and beliefs of African Americans toward participation in medical research. *Journal of General Internal Medicine*, *14*(9), 537–546. doi:10.1046/j.1525-1497.1999.07048.x PMID:10491242

Coulter, A., & Ellins, J. (2007). Effectiveness of strategies for informing, educating, and involving patients. *BMJ (Clinical Research Ed.)*, *335*(7609), 24–27. doi:10.1136/bmj.39246.581169.80 PMID:17615222

Davis, T. C., Berkel, H. J., Holcombe, R. F., Pramanik, S., & Divers, S. G. (1998). Informed consent for clinical trials: A comparative study of standard versus simplified forms. *Journal of the National Cancer Institute*, *90*(9), 668–674. doi:10.1093/jnci/90.9.668 PMID:9586663

Davis, T. C., Williams, M. V., Marin, E., Parker, R. M., & Glass, J. (2002). Health literacy and cancer communication. *CA: a Cancer Journal for Clinicians*, *52*(3), 134–149. doi:10.3322/canjclin.52.3.134 PMID:12018928

Department of Health and Human Services. (1998). *Informed consent checklist (1998)*. Retrieved from https://www.hhs.gov/ohrp/regulations-and-policy/guidance/checklists/index.html

Durant, R. W., Wenzel, J. A., Scarinci, I. C., Paterniti, D. A., Fouad, M. N., Hurd, T. C., & Martin, M. Y. (2014). Perspectives on barriers and facilitators to minority recruitment for clinical trials among cancer center leaders, investigators, research staff, and referring clinicians: Enhancing minority participation in clinical trials EMPaCT). *Cancer*, *120*(S7), 1097–1105. doi:10.1002/cncr.28574 PMID:24643647

Ford, J. G., Howerton, M. W., Lai, G. Y., Gary, T. L., Bolen, S., Gibbons, M. C., ... Bass, E. B. (2008). Barriers to recruiting underrepresented populations to cancer clinical trials: A systematic review. *Cancer*, *112*(2), 228–242. doi:10.1002/cncr.23157 PMID:18008363

Fouad, M. N., Partridge, E., Green, B. L., Kohler, C., Wynn, T., Nagy, S., & Churchill, S. (2000). Minority recruitment in clinical trials: A conference at Tuskegee, researchers and the community. *Annals of Epidemiology*, *10*(8), S35–S40. doi:10.1016/S1047-2797(00)00199-X PMID:11189091

Galesic, M., Garcia-Retamero, R., & Gigerenzer, G. (2009). Using icon arrays to communicate medical risks: Overcoming low numeracy. *Health Psychology*, *28*(2), 210–216. doi:10.1037/a0014474 PMID:19290713

Garcia-Retamero, R., & Galesic, M. (2010). Who profits from visual aids: Overcoming challenges in people's understanding of risks. *Social Science & Medicine*, *70*(7), 1019–1025. doi:10.1016/j.socscimed.2009.11.031 PMID:20116159

Howerton, M. W., Gibbons, M. C., Baffi, C. R., Gary, T. L., Lai, G. Y., Bolen, S., ... Ford, J. G. (2007). Provider roles in the recruitment of underrepresented populations to cancer clinical trials. *Cancer*, *109*(3), 465–476. doi:10.1002/cncr.22436 PMID:17200964

Hussain-Gambles, M., Atkin, K., & Leese, B. (2004). Why ethnic minority groups are under-represented in clinical trials: A review of the literature. *Health & Social Care in the Community*, *12*(5), 382–388. doi:10.1111/j.1365-2524.2004.00507.x PMID:15373816

Jacobson, T. A., Thomas, D. M., Morton, F. J., Offutt, G., Shevlin, J., & Ray, S. (1999). Use of a low-literacy patient education tool to enhance pneumococcal vaccination rates: A randomized controlled trial. *Journal of the American Medical Association*, *282*(7), 646–650. doi:10.1001/jama.282.7.646 PMID:10517717

Kickbusch, I., Wait, S., & Maag, D. (2005). *Navigating health: The role of health literacy*. Retrieved from http://www.ilcuk.org.uk/index.php/publications/publication_details/ navigating_health_the_role_of_health_literacy

Kindig, D. A., Panzer, A. M., & Nielsen-Bohlman, L. (Eds.). (2004). *Health literacy: A prescription to end confusion*. Washington, DC: National Academies Press.

Lara, P. N. Jr, Higdon, R., Lim, N., Kwan, K., Tanaka, M., Lau, D. H., ... Lam, K. S. (2001). Prospective evaluation of cancer clinical trial accrual patterns: Identifying potential barriers to enrollment. *Journal of Clinical Oncology*, *19*(6), 1728–1733. doi:10.1200/JCO.2001.19.6.1728 PMID:11251003

Ma, G. X., Tan, Y., Blakeney, N. C., Seals, B. F., Ma, X. S., Zhai, S., ... Michaels, M. (2014). The impact of a community-based clinical trial educational intervention among underrepresented Chinese Americans. *Cancer Epidemiology, Biomarkers & Prevention*, *23*(3), 424–432. doi:10.1158/1055-9965.EPI-13-0773 PMID:24092627

Marks, L., & Power, E. (2002). Using technology to address recruitment issues in the clinical trial process. *Trends in Biotechnology*, *20*(3), 105–109. doi:10.1016/S0167-7799(02)01881-4 PMID:11841861

Mendoza, D. B., Williams, M. T., Chapman, L. K., & Powers, M. (2012). Minority inclusion in randomized clinical trials of panic disorder. *Journal of Anxiety Disorders*, *26*(5), 574–582. doi:10.1016/j.janxdis.2012.02.011 PMID:22445317

Michielutte, R., Alciati, M. H., & El Arculli, R. (1999). Cancer control research and literacy. *Journal of Health Care for the Poor and Underserved*, *10*(3), 281–297. doi:10.1353/hpu.2010.0585 PMID:10436728

O'Connor, A. M., & Jacobsen, M. J. (2006). *Decisional conflict: Supporting people experiencing uncertainty about options affecting their health.* Retrieved from http://careinaging.duke.edu/longtermcare/dynamic/resources/1027/Decisional_Conflict.pdf

Parikh, N. S., Parker, R. M., Nurss, J. R., Baker, D. W., & Williams, M. V. (1996). Shame and health literacy: The unspoken connection. *Patient Education and Counseling*, *27*(1), 33–39. doi:10.1016/0738-3991(95)00787-3 PMID:8788747

Pignone, M., DeWalt, D. A., Sheridan, S., Berkman, N., & Lohr, K. N. (2005). Interventions to improve health outcomes for patients with low literacy. *Journal of General Internal Medicine*, *20*(2), 185–192. doi:10.1111/j.1525-1497.2005.40208.x PMID:15836553

Pratt, M., & Searles, G. E. (2017). Using visual aids to enhance physician-patient discussions and increase health literacy. *Journal of Cutaneous Medicine and Surgery*, *21*(6), 497–501. doi:10.1177/1203475417715208 PMID:28614954

Roberson, N. L. (1994). Clinical trial participation: Viewpoints from racial/ethnic groups. *Cancer*, *74*(S9), 2687–2691. doi:10.1002/1097-0142(19941101)74:9+<2687::AID-CNCR28207418173.0.CO;2-B PMID:7954287

Rudd, R. E. (2010). Improving Americans' health literacy. *The New England Journal of Medicine*, *363*(24), 2283–2285. doi:10.1056/NEJMp1008755 PMID:21142532

Ryan, R., Prictor, M., McLaughlin, K. J., & Hill, S. (2008). Audio-visual presentation of information for informed consent for participation in clinical trials. *The Cochrane Library*, 1. PMID:18254029

Schillinger, D., Piette, J., Grumbach, K., Wang, F., Wilson, C., Daher, C., ... Bindman, A. B. (2003). Closing the loop: Physician communication with diabetic patients who have low health literacy. *Archives of Internal Medicine*, *163*(1), 83–90. doi:10.1001/archinte.163.1.83 PMID:12523921

Schroen, A. T., Petroni, G. R., Wang, H., Gray, R., Wang, X. F., Cronin, W., & ... . (2010). Preliminary evaluation of factors associated with premature trial closure and feasibility of accrual benchmarks in phase III oncology trials. *Clinical Trials*, *7*(4), 312–321. doi:10.1177/1740774510374973 PMID:20595245

Selden, C. R., Zorn, M., Ratzan, S., & Parker, R. M. (2000). *National Library of Medicine current bibliographies in medicine: Health literacy*. Retrieved from https://www.researchgate.net/profile/Marcia_Zorn/publication/230877250_National_Library_of_Medicine_Current_Bibliographies_in_Medicine_Health_Literacy/links/56794b7408ae6041cb49f348/National-Library-of-Medicine-Current-Bibliographies-in-Medicine-Health-Literacy.pdf

Siminoff, L. A., Zhang, A., Colabianchi, N., Sturm, C. M. S., & Shen, Q. (2000). Factors that predict the referral of breast cancer patients onto clinical trials by their surgeons and medical oncologists. *Journal of Clinical Oncology*, *18*(6), 1203–1211. doi:10.1200/JCO.2000.18.6.1203 PMID:10715289

Sinclair, S., Hayes-Reams, P., Myers, H. F., Allen, W., Hawes-Dawson, J., & Kington, R. (2000). Recruitment African Americans for health studies: Lessons From the Drew-Rand Center on Health and Aging. *Journal of Mental Health and Aging*, *6*(1), 39.

Sudore, R. L., & Schillinger, D. (2009). Interventions to improve care for patients with limited health literacy. *Journal of Clinical Outcomes Management: Journal of Clinical Outcomes*, *16*(1), 20. PMID:20046798

Williams, M. V., Davis, T., Parker, R. M., & Weiss, B. D. (2002). The role of health literacy in patient-physician communication. *Family Medicine-Kansas City*, *34*(5), 383–389. PMID:12038721

Chapter 7
Health Literacy and Patient -Reported Outcomes

Maria Irene Bellini
Imperial College London, UK

Andre Kubler
Imperial College London, UK

ABSTRACT

Modern healthcare needs to identify parameters for high-quality care. Quality improvement is the key for advancing in healthcare, and the new assessment tool shifts from a disease-centered outcome to a patient-centered outcome. Clinical outcome such as morbidity and mortality are directly connected and interdependent from patient-reported outcomes: well-informed patients who decide with their healthcare provider what treatment is best for them have better outcomes and higher patient satisfaction rates. These subjective data collected by rigorous, meaningful, and scientific methods and presented in a utilizable format can be used to create care objectives towards which both the surgeon and their patient can travel. Time has come to carry patient-centered outcomes from research into decision making and daily care plans. This chapter outlines a focus beyond life-prolonging therapy, aiming to minimize the negative effects of treatment, optimize quality of life, and align medical decisions with patient expectations.

INTRODUCTION

The physician should not treat the disease but the patient who is suffering from it — Maimonides 1134-1204

The goal of medicine is to improve the quality and duration of life through the treatment or prevention of disease. How do we measure this impact? Quantity of life is easily calculated, but quality of life is subjective and difficult to measure. Objective health measures do not necessarily correlate with patient values (Contopoulos-Ioannidis, Karvouni, Kouri, & Ioannidis, 2009). By allowing patients to report their opinions on quality of life, through patient reported outcomes (PROs), quantitative data of meaning can drive medical progress. PROs are now widely accepted as valid outcome measures, and this is reflected in the utilisation of PRO data in approval pathways for medical interventions.

DOI: 10.4018/978-1-5225-4074-8.ch007

PROs are self-reported assessments that quantify symptoms, physical function or emotional well-being; related either to a specific condition, or to general quality of life (Higgins, Green, & The Cochrane Collaboration, 2011). Typically, a PRO instrument consists of several items (questions or statements) to which a Likert scale or binary response is recorded. Individual statements can be scored and sometimes an overall score is calculated. Some scores also include a generic overall scale which can be compared to the contributing individual item scores. PROs can also contain temporal data; asking about experiences either at a singular moment in time, or over a period of time. This subjectivity is the value of the derived data, but utilisation of data comes with some caveats.

PROs are at risk of bias from the researchers that generate them, the populations in which they were generated, and the cultures in which they are accepted. For example, the Nottingham Health Profile (NHP), was derived from statements made by individuals seeking healthcare in Nottingham, UK, and reflects the overall culture of this area at the time it was generated. From 2,200 statements made by patients, 88 were picked by researchers to represent quality of life, reflecting the values of the researchers. The NHP became a widely-accepted measure of 'quality of life'; reflecting the culture of health research at the time. It has fallen from favour due to the lack of validation studies, which reflects the current more rigorous academic culture. Such flux is a reason for reticence in accepting PRO data, but with appropriate methodological development, objectivity and validity can be measured, and such hurdles overcome.

Although the quality of PRO data is improving, the variety of PRO instruments and poor data reporting causes a challenge in synthesising PRO data (King et al., 2017). The importance of PRO data for policy makers, researchers and clinicians has seen the development of initiatives to try and increase their use, and improve the quality of PRO data collection (Table 1). PROs are often confused with patient reported experience measures (PREMs) which measure patients attitudes towards healthcare. Such confusion can also drive inappropriate responses to PRO data and can confound PRO studies (Black, Varaganum, & Hutchings, 2014). The health community must become more literate in PRO methodology if they are to collaborate with patients to generate the weight of evidence required to change clinical practice in a way that is meaningful to patients. This chapter describes the fundamental aspects of PROs; how they are collected, utilised and analysed, before proceeding to speculate how they might, in future, be integrated into clinical practice.

INTRINSIC QUALITIES OF PRO DATA

The clinician must be careful when they collect and use PRO data. Several strategies exist for making judgements on the utility, relevance and interpretation of collected PRO data (McLeod, Coon, Martin, Fehnel, & Hays, 2011; Mokkink et al., 2010). Accurate use of PRO data requires an understanding of the qualities of PROs; and this requires an understanding of some basic psychometric theory. PRO data analysis is based on two psychometric theories, Classical Test Theory (CTT) and Item Response Theory (IRT); which are discussed in the latter part of this chapter. The understanding of these theories requires comprehension of the terms that underpin them.

Table 1. Large scale initiatives aiming to collect, validate and standardise PROs

Initiative	Website	Summary
Patient Reported Outcomes Measurement Information System (PROMIS)	http://www.nihpromis.com	A collection of PRO compiled by the NIH which are integrated into a computer based reporting system.
The International Consortium for Health Outcomes Measurement (ICHOM)	http://www.ichom.org	A collaboration aiming to produce outcome measures combining PROs with physiologic and health economy data, with a view to creating a global standard for health outcome reporting.
Patient-Centred Outcomes Research Institute (PCORI)	http://www.pcori.org	Funding organisation aiming to enhance patient-directed research and care through delivery of patient centred health information
European Organisation for the Research and Treatment of Cancer (EORTC)	http://www.eortc.org	Organisation that provides cancer related quality of life questionnaires (EORTC QLQ)
EuroQol	https://euroqol.org	Developers of the most widely used quality of life questionnaire the EQ-5D, which aims to be a globally standardised measure of health outcomes
Mapi Research Trust: Patient-Reported Outcome and Quality of Life Instruments Database (PROQOLID)	http://mapi-trust.org	Extensive database of quality of life measures in a searchable format
Cochrane Patient Reported Outcome Methods Group	http://methods.cochrane.org/pro/welcome	A subgroup of the Cochrane collaborative with a special interest in standardising and reporting meta-analysis of PRO data
Consensus-based Standards for the selection of health Measurement Instruments (COSMIN)	http://www.cosmin.nl	Institute aiming to improve selection of health outcome measures. Provides peer-reviewed checklists useful for both PRO selection and critical review
Medical Outcomes Trust (Lohr et al., 1996)	http://www.outcomes-trust.org	Database of outcome measures, appears to no longer be updated
Registry of Outcome Measures	http://www.researchrom.com	Neurology and general quality of life questionnaires database
The On-Line Guide to Quality of Life assessment (OLGA)	http://www.olga-qol.com	Membership only database of quality of life assessments
Core Outcome Measures in Effectiveness Trials Initiative (COMET)	http://www.comet-initiative.org	Organisation aimed at standardising development and application of quality of life measurements
International Society for Quality of Life Research (ISOQOL)	http://www.isoqol.org	Non-profit membership based organisation promoting quality of life research aiming to establish standards of practice
Centres for Disease Control, Health related quality of Life (CDC-HRQOL)	https://www.cdc.gov/hrqol/index.htm	The CDC website provides tools and education related to quality of life assessment
Rehabilitation Measures Database	http://www.rehabmeasures.org	A database which includes some PRO measures as well as data on traditional rehab measures; usefully includes reference literature on metrics of many of the scales.

Construct and Content

A construct is a theoretical (and subjective) model that the PRO aims to measure. For example, 'quality of life' is a construct that has no single definition. Instead it is derived from a subjective interpretation of a number of components. A PRO can explore the construct of 'quality of life' by asking for quantitative answers about these components of quality of life. These questions about these components are the content of a PRO, and the theoretical link between these components and the overall measure is the construct. A PRO instrument may be unimodal (containing a singular question), or multimodal (containing multiple questions or question areas), or a combination of both. A unimodal construct allows a respondent to bring their own opinion to a measure; for example, a patient may report an overall change in quality of life in a unimodal instrument, despite reporting no significant change across a multimodal response. If this occurs it suggests the content of the multimodal construct does not reflect the patient's own construct of 'quality of life'. The best PROs use evidence-based constructs; which require input from the target population through qualitative methodologies (Patrick et al., 2011).

For complex constructs such as quality of life, subdivisions of the construct can be used to understand how an intervention impacts overall quality of life. For example, the multimodal EQ-5D includes questions about mobility, self-care, usual activities, pain/discomfort and anxiety/depression (EuroQol-Group, 1990). This means that overall changes in quality of life can be attributed to individual components of the PRO measure; which may help to increase the validity of an observed effect. For example, an intervention that aims to reduce pain would be hypothesised to influence overall quality of life, with specific effects in pain/discomfort, and lesser effects in the remaining areas. Condition specific PRO instruments also exist – allowing for investigation of effects on specific symptoms of interest, for example, nausea in chemotherapeutic trials (Lindley et al., 1992). It is essential to remember that although often assumed that these condition specific PROs measure quality of life, they are only surrogate markers and in isolation of little significance to patients.

Validity

Validity describes how well the measurements correlate with changes in the construct being measured. The simplest assessment is face-validity; in which the interpreter relies on their own understanding of a construct to decide whether the questions included in a PRO reflect the construct accurately. More formal measures of validity exist. It is key to remember that constructs are evolving, and influenced by each set of data collected about them – either strengthening the theory of the relations within the construct or weakening them. This philosophical nature of psychometric measures leads to debate about their value, to engage in this debate some accepted definitions must be understood:

Content Validity

This metric describes the degree to which the PRO instrument examines the components of the construct. This can be formalised using a Delphi method, ideally involving patients, to decide on what really are important measureable components of a construct; but is often derived from a consensus of experts with little formal development.

Construct Validity

The definition of construct validity is the degree to which a test measures what it claims to be measuring. Cronbach and Meehl proposed a widely accepted process underling construct validity: First, the construct needs to exist within a set of 'laws' which are in some way measureable, and interconnected (a nomological network). Second, these elements of the construct or the construct itself need to be evaluated. Finally, the degree of agreement between them need to tested in an appropriate sample (Cronbach & Meehl, 1955). Construct validity can also be strengthened by contrasting opposite concepts within the construct (i.e. divergent); for example, when exploring the construct of mobility one would expect the degree of pain to decrease as the amount of mobility increased. A correlation co-efficient can be calculated which suggests the degree to which the content within a construct are related to each other; validating the existence of the proposed nomological network. There may also be correlation with objective, non-PRO data, which may further validate the construct. Depending on whether IRT or CCT are used, quantitative measures of construct validity can be used (Mokkink et al., 2010).

Structural Validity

The degree to which the weighting of the components (either number, or contribution to an overall score) within a PRO reflect their effect on the overall outcome of a construct (Mokkink et al., 2010).

Cross-Cultural Validity

Constructs may exist cross-culturally. PROs will be affected to a varying degree by translation to new cultures, exhibiting either a high or low degree of cultural validity (Mokkink et al., 2010).

Criterion Validity

On certain occasions, there may be a gold standard to which the PRO data can be compared; the agreement with this gold-standard is known as criterion validity (Mokkink et al., 2010).

Reliability

Reliability is the degree to which a measurement reflects the actual value of what it measures. This can be interpreted as the degree of freedom from measurement error. The COSMIN extended definition is 'The extent to which scores for patients who have not changed are the same for repeated measurement under several conditions: e.g. using different sets of items from the same health related-patient reported outcomes (HR- PRO) (internal consistency); over time (test-retest); by different persons on the same occasion (inter-rater); or by the same persons (i.e. raters or responders) on different occasions (intra-rater). In contrast to reliability, a measurement error can be quantified, and reflects the systematic and random error not attributed to true change' (Mokkink et al., 2010). Reliability is a description of the PRO instrument, and should not be confused with the reliability of data from a study.

Responsiveness/Sensitivity

Responsiveness of an instrument is the ability to detect a change in a construct. This can be defined at the overall level; but also, whether each item may be responsive to change. There are published methods for determining the responsiveness of an instrument (Dennis Revicki, Ron D. Hays, David Cella, & Jeff Sloan, 2008). Responsiveness may vary across a given scale (de Vet et al., 2015).

Psychometric Theories

In general, two psychometric concepts are used to develop PRO instruments: classical test theory and item response theory. A numerical degree of validity, reliability and responsiveness can be defined in relation to these psychometric frameworks.

Classical Test Theory (CTT)

In CTT, an assumption is made that a tool's outcome is the consequence of the true score for the construct and some error. CTT then seeks to assess the probable values of the error and utilise the observed value to understand the true value. Crucially, it evaluates the entire tool based upon presumed equal contribution of each item within the construct, as oppose to IRT which considers the contribution of individual items to the overall error and validity. In CTT the degree of agreement is quantified using Cronbach's alpha.

Item Response Theory (IRT)

IRT is more complex than CTT. It assumes that the construct is a unidimensional trait, the items of the test are locally independent (i.e. although items may be related to each other, their relationship is not causal), and that a person's response can be modelled using an item response function. As oppose to assuming error for the overall tool to predict outcome, item response theory uses individual item response validity to generate numerical data about reliability, validity and responsiveness. In IRT the degree of agreement is quantified using a goodness of fit statistic.

USING PRO INSTRUMENTS

Once a researcher has gained an understanding of PRO instruments, they can consider utilising them. In addition to assuring the quality of the instrument to be used, researchers utilising PRO instruments must also consider some more practical elements prior to initiating a study. What is the respondent and administrative burden? Is it applicable to the target population? (for example; can it be adapted for the visually impaired or are there valid translations?) Large databases of PROs facilitating the identification and selection of robust tools (table 1).

PRESENTING PRO DATA

Consolidated Standards of Reporting Patient Trials (CONSORT) have developed guidelines for the presentation of PRO data (Calvert et al., 2013). They recommend inclusion of what type of outcome the PRO is (primary or secondary) – a suggestion which implies that this decision must be pre-defined during planning. CONSORT also recommend the provision of evidence of validity and reliability of the PRO. Finally, they suggest the statistical approaches to missing data, as well as the limitations of the PRO data be discussed. A checklist is provided on their website (www.consort-statement.org).

INTERPRETING PRO DATA

COSMIN provide a comprehensive manual and checklist for evaluating the quality of PRO studies (available at www.cosmin.nl) based on a rigorous development process (Mokkink et al., 2010). Alternative options for day-to-day interpretation of PRO studies exist (Alrubaiy, Hutchings, & Williams, 2014; Lohr et al., 1996; Terwee et al.; Valderas et al., 2008). Cochrane group authors have also published advice on PRO meta-analysis (Johnston et al., 2013). Whichever strategy is used to appraise PRO data, some simple concepts are vital to understand:

Minimally Important Difference

Perhaps most important for clinical interpretation is the concept of the minimally important difference (MID) or minimally important change. MID is the change in value that corresponds to a perceivable difference in health as related to the construct. Methods for calculating MID are available (D. Revicki, R. D. Hays, D. Cella, & J. Sloan, 2008). MID is context specific and can also be influenced by the average baseline of the subject (de Vet et al., 2015; Olsen et al., 2017).

Floor and Ceiling Effect

Certain scales may exhibit end of spectrum effects. This occurs when a score cannot detect improvements above or below a certain level, understanding where a population sits with relation to the floor or ceiling of scale is important before lack of effect (or in particular non-inferiority) is applied (Terwee et al., 2007).

Standardised Mean Differences

Meta-analysis leads to a challenge in understanding change particularly when different instruments have been used. By basing pooled calculations on the effect of change in the standard deviations of the experimental and control groups an overall estimate can be made. This is known as the standardised mean difference and is the most accepted outcome for pooling meta-analysis data. This references contains an extensive discussion regarding meta-analysis of patient reported outcomes (Johnston et al., 2013).

PRO INFLUENCE ON CLINICAL PRACTICE

Although there is a vast number of PROs, it is worth being aware of some of the most common instruments:

EQ-5D

The most commonly utilised PRO instrument is the EQ-5D, which assesses health-related quality of life across 5 domains – mobility, self-care, usual activities, pain/discomfort and anxiety/depression and also includes a generic 100 point visual analogue scale (VAS) (EuroQol-Group, 1990). The minimally important difference in specific conditions is between 0.07-0.12 (over a range of 0-1) on the EQ-5D and 8-12 on the 100 point VAS (Pickard, Neary, & Cella, 2007). It is the recommended PRO for calculating quality adjusted life-years (QALYs), which is used by the National Institute for Health and Care Excellence (NICE) when calculating the cost-benefit of health interventions (NICE, 2013).

Sickness Impact Profile

Another commonly used quality of life scale is the Sickness Impact Profile (SIP) which has 136 items in 12 domains: sleep and rest, eating, work, home management, recreation and pastimes, ambulation, mobility, body care and movement, social interaction, alertness behaviour, emotional behaviour, and communication (Bergner, Bobbitt, Carter, & Gilson, 1981). A shorter 68 question (SIP-68) version of this questionnaire exists (Nanda, McLendon, Andresen, & Armbrecht, 2003).

Health Utilities Index

The health utilities index (HUI) now in its third form is, as the name suggests, utilitarian. The domains it extends across include vision, hearing, speech, ambulation, dexterity, emotion, cognition & pain (Furlong W, Feeny D, Torrance G, & Barr R T, 2001); and responses in the HUI-3 are scored on a 6-point scale. The HUI has an estimated MID of 0.02-0.04 (Samsa et al., 1999).

Medical Outcomes Study and Short Forms

The Medical Outcomes Study (MOS) recorded 1,014 patient experiences health related outcomes, from English speakers in 3 US cities at 2 time-points (Tarlov et al., 1989). From this data, which included physician reported medical and psychological conditions, various short-form surveys were derived (Brazier, Usherwood, Harper, & Thomas, 1998). Validity was assessed by the ability of the surveys components to distinguish mental from physical illness effects on domains related to activity and mental-health (Ware & Sherbourne, 1992). The MID of the commonly used SF-6D is estimated to be between 0.03-0.04 across 0-1 range (Khanna et al., 2007).

Nottingham Health Profile

The Nottingham health profile was developed from patient statements collected in general practice in the 1970s. A series of studies led to a 45-item questionnaire that was validated in multiple patient groups. 38 of these statements cover 6 descriptors of symptoms, with various weightings depending on the number of questions per category (energy levels, pain, emotional reaction, sleep, social isolation, physical abilities), with the remaining 7 questions relating to affected life areas (Work, Home life, Social life, Looking after the home, Sex life, Interests and Hobbies, Vacations) (Martini & McDowell, 1976). Despite it's relatively common use, little quality data on MID and responsiveness is available.

World Health Organization Quality of Life

The World Health Organization Quality of Life (WHOQOL) includes 100 statements which cover the following domains: 1. Physical health, 2. Psychological, 3. Level of independence, 4. Social relationships, 5. Environment. It can be extended to include 'spiritual, religious and personal beliefs' by including a further 32 statements, covering; spiritual connection, meaning and purpose in life, experience of awe and wonder, wholeness and integration, spiritual strength, inner peace, hope and optimism, and faith. It was generated in 14 different centres using only 300 people – 250 without disease and 50 with disease, and answers are given on a 1-5 Likert scale; 1 (not at all), 2 (a little) 3 (a moderate amount), 4 (very much) and 5 (an extreme amount) as to the degree of the subjects agreement with a given statement (WHOQOL-Group, 1998b). An estimated MID of 1 across the 100 point scale has been proposed (Den Oudsten, Zijlstra, & De Vries, 2013). A short form (WHOQOL-BREF) version also exists (WHOQOL-Group, 1998a).

PROMIS® (Patient-Reported Outcomes Measurement Information System)

Promis is a National Institutes of Health (NIH) funded attempt to collect and validate paper and computer-assisted PROs, in both clinical and research settings. Based in the biopsychosocial model of health, it divides scales into physical, mental and social health. PROMIS reviews measures through a rigorous process: First, constructs are defined from published literature. Next, they are reviewed by experts, patients, clinicians, and end-users through accepted qualitative methodologies. The characteristics of the included items are then interrogated thoroughly, and validity and reliability of the instruments assessed. Finally, the guidelines for interpretation of the instrument are assessed and the appropriateness of translations are reviewed. Only after completing this process are the items are included within the database. At the time of writing 332 items are included in the database, which are available through a searchable online database (Cella et al., 2007).

PRO DATA IN PRACTICE

The use of PRO data is now common across medical and surgical practice and has improved our understanding of therapeutic interventions. This is especially important for surgical interventions where immediate impacts may have rapidly measurable clinical effects, but long term sustained benefits of physiological markers might not be so apparent; for example, Mathus-Vliegen and colleagues demonstrated that weight loss surgery led not only to effective persistent weight loss, but also improvements in quality of life beyond the initial period of weight loss (Mathus-Vliegen & de Wit, 2007). In orthopaedic surgery PROs have been used to demonstrate the negative effect of waiting times on patient well-being – data that can be used to drive delivery of care (Ackerman, Bennell, & Osborne, 2011).

We are reaching a period in research history where long term studies have collected quality of life data over extended periods using validated instruments. The ProtecT study demonstrated a practice changing benefit of disease monitoring over both surgical intervention and radiotherapy in prostate cancer (Donovan et al., 2016). It's validity confirmed by correlating improved sexual function, bowel function and quality of life in the 10-years from randomisation (Donovan et al., 2016). Unfortunately, influential articles still use surrogate disease specific markers and fail to present overall quality of life changes (Labrie et al., 2013). This risks the failure to identify non-disease specific consequences of interventions. PROs also can help answer controversial questions, where physiologic data may be misleading. For example in subclinical hypothyroidism, where physiologic changes can be observed, and patients often claim symptomatic consequences, there is demonstrably no identifiable patient reported benefit (Stott et al., 2017). It is important to remember that PROs need not be confined to quality of life criteria; for example, by adapting the National Cancer Institute's Common Terminology Criteria for Adverse Events (CTCAE) for tablet usage, patients were empowered to accurately self-report adverse events (Basch, Dueck, Rogak, & et al., 2017).

PROs in the Consulting Room

There has been a move to collecting routine patient reported outcome measures in clinical practice, and even encouragement of patients to collect and interpret their own data to guide individualised treatment (Nelson et al., 2015). There is limited data to suggest that in general this improves patient-satisfaction, but not patient-outcomes (Holmes, Lewith, Newell, Field, & Bishop, 2017). Common sense would suggest that PROs might help focus a consultation, and in certain conditions, for example depression, it is routine and advised practice (NICE, 2015). However, we would advise caution in widely adopting this strategy as it risks check-listing the patient-physician relationship, and there is not evidence to support patient outcomes at present.

Creating Comprehensive PRO Inclusive Outcome Measures

Moving towards the future, we are beginning to see a move towards the unification of data through meta-analysis and combination of outcomes. Whilst PROs form one arm of assessing clinical outcomes, the relative cost and impact of providing this health intervention, as well as the measurable effects on disease measures need to be combined. The ICHOM is an institution aiming to provide validated PROs and integrate these with physiological, and health care-system relevant measures to provide implementable trial data (Porter, Larsson, & Lee, 2016).

THE FUTURE OF PRO: CHALLENGES AND HOPES

In a world where everything is becoming virtual, we have to use new tools for patient-centred healthcare. Science is rapidly evolving and patients must have a central role in directing their care and also pushing the frontiers of their care. Information technology is a powerful tool to achieve this and industry and academia should work alongside patients if they want to build patient-centred health care systems. Is there a future where instead of waiting months for appointments, an electronic platform integrated into the electronic health record can provide real time PROs that prioritise patient needs and simultaneously avoid unnecessary consultations?

Despite progress, challenges remain for widespread implementation of PRO collection platforms. There is a lack of consensus on which PRO is best for many conditions, but there is hope. Groups such as PROMIS provide free, concise, valid PROs, and the International Consortium for Health Outcomes Measurement (ICHOM) are encouraging coalescence around a single set of measures for particular diagnoses. If PROs are to be used as a quality measure for reimbursement programs, health care professionals must determine how to risk-adjust for clinical and sociodemographic patient characteristics. Data interoperability will also be essential. Finally, as PRO collection becomes more widespread, we must be cautious of overwhelming patients with constant surveys, factoring in convenience and privacy.

CONCLUSIONS: PATIENT REPORTED OUTCOMES AS A SHARED LANGUAGE IN HEALTH LITERACY

Modern health care needs to identify parameters for high-quality care. Quality improvement is the key to advancing health care, and our assessment of quality must shift from disease-centred to patient-centred outcomes. PROs represent an evolving shared language between the care-receiver, care-giver and health researcher. The consequence of this evolution is a new form of health literacy bridging the gap between an individual patient, their personal values and the clinician's knowledge of physiologically and objectively perceivable outcomes. This shared language can be derived from a unified source which factors in patient specific values as they relate to physiological data and information on the cost and implementation of health care resources. Patient reported outcomes are linked to health literacy by elevating the patient experience to a quantifiable, measurable format, integrated into the scientific method rather than simply applied *ad hoc* at the bed side. Clinicians and patients sharing PRO information can discuss patient choices as supported by rigorous and factual information. Health professionals would benefit from PRO as tools to monitor patients, better understand their symptoms, and determine practical action to improve patient health. PRO integration will put data behind the patient's ability to guide their own care; the data having started in the language the patient speaks.

The surgical community has a golden opportunity to take the lead in bringing PRO data to the bedside and integrating it into practice. There is no area of clinical care where we ask patients to participate in such significant risk-based decisions, and at present we often only communicate in a language of percentages of risks and mortality. Most people want to know the impact of morbidity relating to an intervention, not just the rate at which it happens. Achieving this goal is only feasible if we start to understand what the patient's experience of care is. Utilising PROs can convert treatment impact on subjective experiences into data which when presented in a utilisable format can be used to create care objectives towards which both the surgeon and their patient can travel. Time has come to carry patient-centred outcomes from research into decision-making and daily care plans. PROs are the source of the lexicon we need to build patient-clinician relationships that minimise the negative effects of treatment, optimise quality of life, and align medical decisions with patient expectations.

REFERENCES

Ackerman, I. N., Bennell, K. L., & Osborne, R. H. (2011). Decline in Health-Related Quality of Life reported by more than half of those waiting for joint replacement surgery: A prospective cohort study. *BMC Musculoskeletal Disorders*, *12*(1), 108–108. doi:10.1186/1471-2474-12-108 PMID:21605398

Alrubaiy, L., Hutchings, H. A., & Williams, J. G. (2014). Assessing patient reported outcome measures: A practical guide for gastroenterologists. *United European Gastroenterology Journal*, *2*(6), 463–470. doi:10.1177/2050640614558345 PMID:25452841

Basch, E., Dueck, A. C., Rogak, L. J., Minasian, L. M., Kelly, W. K., O'Mara, A. M., ... Schrag, D. (2017). Feasibility assessment of patient reporting of symptomatic adverse events in multicenter cancer clinical trials. *JAMA Oncology*, *3*(8), 1043. doi:10.1001/jamaoncol.2016.6749 PMID:28208174

Bergner, M., Bobbitt, R. A., Carter, W. B., & Gilson, B. S. (1981). The Sickness Impact Profile: Development and final revision of a health status measure. *Medical Care*, *19*(8), 787–805. doi:10.1097/00005650-198108000-00001 PMID:7278416

Black, N., Varaganum, M., & Hutchings, A. (2014). *Relationship between patient reported experience (PREMs) and patient reported outcomes (PROMs) in elective surgery. BMJ Quality & Safety.*

Brazier, J., Usherwood, T., Harper, R., & Thomas, K. (1998). Deriving a preference-based single index from the UK SF-36 Health Survey. *Journal of Clinical Epidemiology*, *51*(11), 1115–1128. doi:10.1016/S0895-4356(98)00103-6 PMID:9817129

Calvert, M., Blazeby, J., Altman, D. G., Revicki, D. A., Moher, D., Brundage, M. D., & CONSORT PRO Group. (2013). Reporting of patient-reported outcomes in randomized trials: The CONSORT PRO extension. *Journal of the American Medical Association*, *309*(8), 814–822. doi:10.1001/jama.2013.879 PMID:23443445

Cella, D., Yount, S., Rothrock, N., Gershon, R., Cook, K., Reeve, B., ... Rose, M. (2007). The Patient-Reported Outcomes Measurement Information System (PROMIS): Progress of an NIH Roadmap cooperative group during its first two years. *Medical Care*, *45*(5Suppl 1), S3–s11. doi:10.1097/01.mlr.0000258615.42478.55 PMID:17443116

Contopoulos-Ioannidis, D. G., Karvouni, A., Kouri, I., & Ioannidis, J. P. A. (2009). Reporting and interpretation of SF-36 outcomes in randomised trials: Systematic review. *BMJ (Clinical Research Ed.)*, *338*(jan12 1), a3006. doi:10.1136/bmj.a3006 PMID:19139138

Cronbach, L. J., & Meehl, P. E. (1955). Construct validity in psychological tests. *Psychological Bulletin*, *52*(4), 281–302. doi:10.1037/h0040957 PMID:13245896

de Vet, H. C., Foumani, M., Scholten, M. A., Jacobs, W. C., Stiggelbout, A. M., Knol, D. L., & Peul, W. C. (2015). Minimally important change values of a measurement instrument depend more on baseline values than on the type of intervention. *Journal of Clinical Epidemiology*, *68*(5), 518–524. doi:10.1016/j.jclinepi.2014.07.008 PMID:25544741

Den Oudsten, B. L., Zijlstra, W. P., & De Vries, J. (2013). The minimal clinical important difference in the World Health Organization Quality of Life instrument--100. *Supportive Care in Cancer*, *21*(5), 1295–1301. doi:10.100700520-012-1664-8 PMID:23203652

Donovan, J. L., Hamdy, F. C., Lane, J. A., Mason, M., Metcalfe, C., Walsh, E., ... Neal, D. E. (2016). Patient-Reported Outcomes after Monitoring, Surgery, or Radiotherapy for Prostate Cancer. *The New England Journal of Medicine*, *375*(15), 1425–1437. doi:10.1056/NEJMoa1606221 PMID:27626365

EuroQol-Group. (1990). EuroQol--a new facility for the measurement of health-related quality of life. *Health Policy (Amsterdam)*, *16*(3), 199–208. doi:10.1016/0168-8510(90)90421-9

Furlong, W., Feeny, D., Torrance, G., & Barr, R. T. (2001). *The Health Utilities Index (HUI) System for Assessing Health-Related Quality of Life in Clinical Studies*. Academic Press.

Higgins, J. P. T., & Green, S. (2011). *Cochrane handbook for systematic reviews of interventions Version 5.1.0*. Chichester, UK: Wiley-Blackwell.

Holmes, M. M., Lewith, G., Newell, D., Field, J., & Bishop, F. L. (2017). The impact of patient-reported outcome measures in clinical practice for pain: A systematic review. *Quality of Life Research: An International Journal of Quality of Life Aspects of Treatment, Care and Rehabilitation*, *26*(2), 245–257. doi:10.100711136-016-1449-5 PMID:27815820

Johnston, B. C., Patrick, D. L., Busse, J. W., Schünemann, H. J., Agarwal, A., & Guyatt, G. H. (2013). Patient-reported outcomes in meta-analyses – Part 1: Assessing risk of bias and combining outcomes. *Health and Quality of Life Outcomes*, *11*(1), 109–109. doi:10.1186/1477-7525-11-109 PMID:23815754

Khanna, D., Furst, D. E., Wong, W. K., Tsevat, J., Clements, P. J., Park, G. S., ... Hays, R. D. (2007). Reliability, validity, and minimally important differences of the SF-6D in systemic sclerosis. *Quality of Life Research: An International Journal of Quality of Life Aspects of Treatment, Care and Rehabilitation*, *16*(6), 1083–1092. doi:10.100711136-007-9207-3 PMID:17404896

King, M. T., Winters, Z. E., Olivotto, I. A., Spillane, A. J., Chua, B. H., Saunders, C., ... Rutherford, C. (2017). Patient-reported outcomes in ductal carcinoma in situ: A systematic review. *European Journal of Cancer (Oxford, England)*, *71*, 95–108. doi:10.1016/j.ejca.2016.09.035 PMID:27987454

Labrie, J., Berghmans, B. L. C. M., Fischer, K., Milani, A. L., van der Wijk, I., Smalbraak, D. J. C., ... van der Vaart, C. H. (2013). Surgery versus Physiotherapy for Stress Urinary Incontinence. *The New England Journal of Medicine*, *369*(12), 1124–1133. doi:10.1056/NEJMoa1210627 PMID:24047061

Lindley, C. M., Hirsch, J. D., O'Neill, C. V., Transau, M. C., Gilbert, C. S., & Osterhaus, J. T. (1992). Quality of life consequences of chemotherapy-induced emesis. *Quality of Life Research: An International Journal of Quality of Life Aspects of Treatment, Care and Rehabilitation*, *1*(5), 331–340. doi:10.1007/BF00434947 PMID:1299465

Lohr, K. N., Aaronson, N. K., Alonso, J., Burnam, M. A., Patrick, D. L., Perrin, E. B., & Roberts, J. S. (1996). Evaluating quality-of-life and health status instruments: Development of scientific review criteria. *Clinical Therapeutics*, *18*(5), 979–992. doi:10.1016/S0149-2918(96)80054-3 PMID:8930436

Martini, C. J., & McDowell, I. (1976). Health status: Patient and physician judgments. *Health Services Research, 11*(4), 508–515. PMID:1025054

Mathus-Vliegen, E. M., & de Wit, L. T. (2007). Health-related quality of life after gastric banding. *British Journal of Surgery, 94*(4), 457–465. doi:10.1002/bjs.5607 PMID:17310505

McLeod, L. D., Coon, C. D., Martin, S. A., Fehnel, S. E., & Hays, R. D. (2011). Interpreting patient-reported outcome results: US FDA guidance and emerging methods. *Expert Review of Pharmacoeconomics & Outcomes Research, 11*(2), 163–169. doi:10.1586/erp.11.12 PMID:21476818

Mokkink, L. B., Terwee, C. B., Patrick, D. L., Alonso, J., Stratford, P. W., Knol, D. L., ... de Vet, H. C. (2010). The COSMIN checklist for assessing the methodological quality of studies on measurement properties of health status measurement instruments: An international Delphi study. *Quality of Life Research: An International Journal of Quality of Life Aspects of Treatment, Care and Rehabilitation, 19*(4), 539–549. doi:10.100711136-010-9606-8 PMID:20169472

Nanda, U., McLendon, P. M., Andresen, E. M., & Armbrecht, E. (2003). The SIP68: An abbreviated sickness impact profile for disability outcomes research. *Quality of Life Research: An International Journal of Quality of Life Aspects of Treatment, Care and Rehabilitation, 12*(5), 583–595. doi:10.1023/A:1025036325886 PMID:13677503

Nelson, E. C., Eftimovska, E., Lind, C., Hager, A., Wasson, J. H., & Lindblad, S. (2015). Patient reported outcome measures in practice. *BMJ: British Medical Journal, 350.*

NICE. (2013). *Guide to the methods of technology appraisal 2013 (PMG9).* Retrieved from nice.org.uk/process/pmg9

NICE. (2015). *NICE Clinical Knowledge Summary: Depression.* Retrieved from https://cks.nice.org.uk/depression

Olsen, M. F., Bjerre, E., Hansen, M. D., Hilden, J., Landler, N. E., Tendal, B., & Hrobjartsson, A. (2017). Pain relief that matters to patients: Systematic review of empirical studies assessing the minimum clinically important difference in acute pain. *BMC Medicine, 15*(1), 35. doi:10.118612916-016-0775-3 PMID:28215182

Patrick, D. L., Burke, L. B., Gwaltney, C. J., Leidy, N. K., Martin, M. L., Molsen, E., & Ring, L. (2011). Content validity--establishing and reporting the evidence in newly developed patient-reported outcomes (PRO) instruments for medical product evaluation: ISPOR PRO Good Research Practices Task Force report: part 2--assessing respondent understanding. *Value in Health, 14*(8), 978–988. doi:10.1016/j.jval.2011.06.013 PMID:22152166

Pickard, A. S., Neary, M. P., & Cella, D. (2007). Estimation of minimally important differences in EQ-5D utility and VAS scores in cancer. *Health and Quality of Life Outcomes, 5*(1), 70–70. doi:10.1186/1477-7525-5-70 PMID:18154669

Porter, M. E., Larsson, S., & Lee, T. H. (2016). Standardizing Patient Outcomes Measurement. *The New England Journal of Medicine, 374*(6), 504–506. doi:10.1056/NEJMp1511701 PMID:26863351

Revicki, D., Hays, R. D., Cella, D., & Sloan, J. (2008). Recommended methods for determining responsiveness and minimally important differences for patient-reported outcomes. *Journal of Clinical Epidemiology*, *61*(2), 102–109. doi:10.1016/j.jclinepi.2007.03.012 PMID:18177782

Revicki, D., Hays, R. D., Cella, D., & Sloan, J. (2008). Recommended methods for determining responsiveness and minimally important differences for patient-reported outcomes. *Journal of Clinical Epidemiology*, *61*(2), 102–109. doi:10.1016/j.jclinepi.2007.03.012 PMID:18177782

Samsa, G., Edelman, D., Rothman, M. L., Williams, G. R., Lipscomb, J., & Matchar, D. (1999). Determining clinically important differences in health status measures: A general approach with illustration to the Health Utilities Index Mark II. *PharmacoEconomics*, *15*(2), 141–155. doi:10.2165/00019053-199915020-00003 PMID:10351188

Stott, D. J., Rodondi, N., Kearney, P. M., Ford, I., Westendorp, R. G., Mooijaart, S. P., ... Bauer, D. C. (2017). Thyroid hormone therapy for older adults with subclinical hypothyroidism. *The New England Journal of Medicine*, *376*(26), 2534–2544. doi:10.1056/NEJMoa1603825

Tarlov, A. R., Ware, J. E. Jr, Greenfield, S., Nelson, E. C., Perrin, E., & Zubkoff, M. (1989). The Medical Outcomes Study. An application of methods for monitoring the results of medical care. *Journal of the American Medical Association*, *262*(7), 925–930. doi:10.1001/jama.1989.03430070073033 PMID:2754793

Terwee, C. B., Bot, S. D. M., de Boer, M. R., van der Windt, D. A. W. M., Knol, D. L., Dekker, J., ... de Vet, H. C. W. (2007). Quality criteria were proposed for measurement properties of health status questionnaires. *Journal of Clinical Epidemiology*, *60*(1), 34–42. doi:10.1016/j.jclinepi.2006.03.012 PMID:17161752

Valderas, J. M., Ferrer, M., Mendivil, J., Garin, O., Rajmil, L., Herdman, M., & Alonso, J. (2008). Development of EMPRO: A tool for the standardized assessment of patient-reported outcome measures. *Value in Health*, *11*(4), 700–708. doi:10.1111/j.1524-4733.2007.00309.x PMID:18194398

Ware, J. E., & Sherbourne, C. D. (1992). The MOS 36-Item Short-Form Health Survey (SF-36): I. Conceptual Framework and Item Selection. *Medical Care*, *30*(6), 473–483. doi:10.1097/00005650-199206000-00002 PMID:1593914

WHOQOL-Group. (1998a). Development of the World Health Organization WHOQOL-BREF quality of life assessment. The WHOQOL Group. *Psychological Medicine*, *28*(3), 551–558. doi:10.1017/S0033291798006667 PMID:9626712

WHOQOL-Group. (1998b). The World Health Organization quality of life assessment (WHOQOL): Development and general psychometric properties1. *Social Science & Medicine*, *46*(12), 1569–1585. doi:10.1016/S0277-9536(98)00009-4 PMID:9672396

Chapter 8
Healthy Thanks to Communication:
A Model of Communication Competences to Optimize Health Literacy – Assertiveness, Clear Language, and Positivity

Célia Belim
University of Lisbon, Portugal

Cristina Vaz de Almeida
University of Lisbon, Portugal

ABSTRACT

This chapter focuses on the contribution of communication competences, used by healthcare professionals in the clinical relationship with patients, to improve therapeutic adherence through a better understanding of health instructions and, hence, higher competences in health literacy. It is a main and specific goal to construct a model of communication competences that includes the interdependent use of assertiveness, clear language, and positivity by the healthcare professional, validated by a focus group of specialists. The participants of focus group validate the model and most punctuate, in assertiveness, active behavior, ability to listen, and ability to openly speak; in clarity, the simple language, utilization of verbs; and in positivity, orientation to a positive behavior of the patient. The results confirm that the assertiveness, clear language, and positivity are pivotal and strategic elements to the optimization of health literacy and clinical practices, recognized in the literature and by the participants in the focus group.

DOI: 10.4018/978-1-5225-4074-8.ch008

INTRODUCTION

Communication is a *sine qua non* for human life and social order (Watzlawick, Beavin & Jackson, 1967) and all communication affects human behavior (Watzlawick et al., 1967), including health one.

Communication competences are vital to the optimization of the therapeutic relationship (e.g. Silverman, Krutz & Draper, 2013; Van't Jagt, de Winter, Reijneveld, Hoeks & Jansen, 2016) and of the health literacy due to better health results based on the ability to communicate with patients (e.g. Benson, 2014, p. S55). It is pertinent to study health literacy due to the importance of being correctly enlightened about the good health behaviours and decisions due to improved clinical practices and given the findings of statistical data. The therapeutic relationship is the interaction where health literacy can be nurtured and stimulated: enlightenment, empowerment, understanding, confidence, decision-making, and pro-activity of the patient can be motivated and optimized through the communication competences of the health professional. Studies show that the relationship between limited health literacy and poor health is due to poor communication quality within health care delivery organizations (e.g. Wynia & Osborn, 2010). In the Wynia and Osborn's study (2010), after communicational adjustment for patient demographic characteristics and health care organization type, patients with limited health literacy were 28-79% less likely than those with adequate health literacy to report their health care organization "always" provides patient-centered communication across seven communication items.

Limited health literacy (LHL) impacts negatively in the doctor–patient communication within the clinical encounter (e.g. Agency for Healthcare Research and Quality, 2010). Patients with LHL have greater difficulty understanding clinicians' verbal explanations of medical conditions and instructions about medication changes, and they report poor satisfaction with patient–physician communication (Baker et al., 1996; Schillinger et al., 2003; Schillinger, Bindman, Wang, Stewart & Piette, 2004). Therefore, the communication requirements with these patients must be doubled and communication should have specific features so that it can increase health literacy. There is a dependent relationship that needs to be explored and which is object of our research commitment.

The health context in terms of communication is both problematic and challenging: a) the Europeans have low levels of health literacy (HLS-EU, 2012); b) in current medical practice, the human communication is often poorly utilized (Kreps, 1996, p. 43); c) the research has identified that nurses overestimate their patients' health literacy (Johnson, 2014, p. 43), and that overestimation of a patient's health literacy by nurses may contribute to the widespread problem of poor health outcomes and hospital readmission rates and increased costs to the health system (Dickens, Lambert, Cromwell & Piano, 2013); d) it has been exposed that, even in non-stressful clinical encounters, patients are still reluctant to admit to any lack of understanding and feel compelled to follow the recommendations as they understand them, rather than ask for clarity (Baker et al., 1996; Dickens et al., 2013; Martin et al., 2011; Parikh, Parker, Nurss, Baker & Williams, 1996); e) the studies on communication/interaction and health literacy remain limited (e.g. Ishikawa & Kiuchi, 2010).

Detecting and fulfilling this gap and opportunity, this proposal aims to evaluate the contribution of communication competences, used by healthcare professionals in the clinical relationship with patients, to improve therapeutic adherence through a better understanding of health instructions and, hence, higher competences in health literacy. And at a more proactive level and in an attempt to solve the problem of fragile communication, with failures in patient understanding, it is a main goal to construct a model of communication competences that includes the interdependent use of assertiveness, plain language and positivity by the healthcare professional, to which we will designate "ACP model and technique".

Although these components of the therapeutic relationship are listed in the bibliography consulted (e.g. Keller, Sarkar and Schillinger, 2014, p. 23) refer to the "plain language" as "a means of effectively communicating information to patients"), they are not yet systematized and organized as an interdependent contribution to improve the therapeutic relationship, reflected in optimized outcomes in health literacy and in clinical practices. In order to confirm its value and utility, the empirical research was conducted to validate by specialists this 3-factor model of communication competences.

BACKGROUND

Communication is an essential dimension of human life and of social spheres, such as health sphere, and concretely of therapeutic relations. Health decides the human well-being. However, Europeans face an urging problem related with low levels of health literacy (HLS-EU, 2012) and human communication in doctor-patient relationship has not concentrated in an effective comprehension, indispensable to the health treatment (e.g. Ishikawa & Kiuchi, 2010). There are several studies on the need to use communication competences as better health outcomes are based on the ability to communicate with patients (e.g. Benson, 2014, p. S55; Silverman, Krutz & Draper, 2013; Van't Jagt, de Winter, Reijneveld, Hoeks & Jansen, 2016). Studies show that a fragile communication quality within health professional influences the relationship between low health literacy and a deficient health (e.g. Wynia & Osborn, 2010).

To Be or Not to Be Healthy: A Communicational Question? The Health Communication

Human communication reveals the essence of Man (Onjefu & Olalekan, 2016). And in the health field, the type and quality of communication used reveals and anticipates the expected results. However, a pressing problem is overshadowing the health results since in current practice human communication is often poorly utilized (Kreps, 1996, p. 43), which weakens the efficiency of therapeutic relationship.

Originating in the Latin *communicare,* "communication" means sharing, being in relation with the other, in common (Cobley & Schulz, 2013). It is the basis of interpersonal relations and of communities.

In the *Health Promotion Glossary* (1998), health communication is described as: "interpersonal or mass communication activities which are directed towards improving the health status of individuals and populations" (Nutbeam, 1998, p. 355). The Center for Disease Control and Prevention (CDC) (2011) defines the concept of "health communication" and adds "the study and use of communication strategies to inform and influence individual decisions that enhance health". Communication is a core clinical skill, at the heart of health, and an essential component of clinical competence (e.g. Silverman et al., 2013, p. 7) because every clinical action is shaped by the information available (Coiera & Ong, 2014, p. 156). The field of health communication, and its ideal reliance on strong, trusting, coactive relationships, presents essential requirements that are aspired to attain (Ratzan, 1996, p. 324). We assume as bases of health communication: a) healthcare professionals depend upon communication to provide their patients information on prescribed treatment strategies; b) the human communication is the primary tool that patients have for gathering relevant information (Jones, Kreps & Phillips, 1995; Kreps, 1988a); c) the quality of communication between healthcare providers and patients strongly influences the effectiveness of modern healthcare (Kreps & O'Hair, 1995; Kreps, 1988b). Admitting these premises, *How is the most efficient model of communication in health? Which are the communication competences required to the health professional?*

Competence is defined by the presence or absence of specific behaviors as well as verbal and non-verbal behaviors within the context of individual interactions with patients or families (Schirmer et al., 2005). Communication competences are the behavioral repertories or set of behaviors that support the attainment of organizational goals (Gregory, 2008, p. 216) and allow the successful accomplishment of tasks and responsibilities over time and in a stable way (Tench & Konczos, 2013). The concept means the "perceived tendency to seek out meaningful interaction with others" (Query, Jr. & Kreps, 1996, p. 339) and integrates along three dimensions of cognitive (information interpretation, exchanges skills of individuals across contexts), behavioral (skills which individuals employ to select and implement goal-oriented strategies while maintaining the integrity of other interactants) and affective skills (influence of locus of control orientations upon interpersonal interaction) (Kreps & Query, 1990).

Health communication becomes an increasingly important element to achieving greater empowerment of individuals and communities (Nutbeam, 1998, p. 355) has its origin at one institutional level (laws from government) and can come from the people as a form of advocacy for health as well (Nutbeam, 1998, p. 356) (see Figure 1).

In the complex interpersonal relation, where the words can have a sort of positive or negative consequences in human life, each individual needs to communicate effectively with another (e.g. Chant, Jenkinson, Randle & Russell, 2002; Hargie and Dickson, 2004; Rungapadiachy, 1999, p. 193), and this matrix is transposed to the therapeutic relationship. There are some authors that divide verbal interaction in "care" talk, as an affective or socio-emotional interaction, and "cure" talk which is instrumental or task-focused interaction (e.g. Greenhalgh & Heath, 2010, p. 16).

The use of health information depends on four factors: 1) information must be available, 2) patients must have knowledge of it, 3) have time to access information, and 4) understand this information (Longo & Patrick, 2001). Research and evidence confirm that mere provision of information is insufficient to enhance active and informed health behavior (e.g. Faber, Bosch, Wollersheim, Leatherman & Grol, 2009; Hibbard, Peters, Dixon & Tusler, 2007; Nijman, Hendriks, Brabers, Jong & Rademakers, 2014). "Building health literacy is more than providing health information" (Kickbush, Wait & Maag, 2005, p. 9).

There are preconditions in health communication for it to be effective, that is, to produce the desired results. It is a communication made to measure. For this, it must be clear, comprehensible, meaningful, credible, consistent over time, based on the evidence, personalized, tailored to the user's information needs at that time, adapted to his/her cultural level and cognitive style (Teixeira 1999, p. 617), "a practice that adapts messages to individuals" (Noar, Harrington, Van Stee & Aldrich, 2011, p. 113). The persuasion theory (e.g. Hovland, Janis & Kelley, 1953) advocates that persuasive communication, transmitting the *why*, is pivotal when communicating a message to ignite behavior. Hovland group confirmed that communicators high in expertise and trustworthiness tend to be more persuasive (Ajzen, 1992, p. 5). In this theoretical anchorage in the field of communication, it is of note that Hall's concepts of "hegemony" and "preferred reading", which allude to the symmetry and perfect fit between the encoding (of the health professional) and the decoding (patient) (Hall, 1973; 1980). It means that the receiver's decoding strategies proceed along the same logic as the producer's encoding strategies. Without conflict, the meaning is secured hegemonically, i.e., correctly perceived.

The right to know about his/her state of health (even if there may be patients who do not want to know about their condition, as they believe this could bring them more anxiety) allows a value-based person-centered approach and negotiation of understanding between the professional and the patient, therefore, tends to improve health outcomes. Therapeutic communication produces more rewarding social relations (Lucena & Goes, 1999, p. 41).

It is necessary for the patient to understand the medical information and have the self-efficacy and motivation to make sound health decisions. Education, governments and schools can help health professionals develop their own health literacy, and a key component of this construct is communication and listening (Kickbush, Wait & Maag, 2005) to wake up patients from their latent attitude.

The activation of the patient makes them more satisfied, with a greater perception of their health, thus provoking a greater therapeutic adherence (Katz, Jacobson, Veledar & Kripalani, 2007).

Do Communication Competences Influence Health Literacy?

Communication competences are essential for health literacy, enabling the understanding of the health process to make sound decisions (Gastein Health Declaration, 2005), so it is evident a dependency. These competences are particularly acute mainly because people with low literacy have difficulty in accessing, using, applying and understanding information and the health system (e.g. Kickbusch, 2001; Nutbeam, 2000; Rootman, 2002).

The World Health Organization (WHO) (1998) defines "health literacy" as the set of "cognitive and social skills which determine the motivation and the ability of individuals to gain access to, understand and use information in ways which promote and maintain good health". The concept can be perceived as the awareness of the learning and acting person in the development of his or her capacities of understanding, management and investment, favorable to the promotion of health (Saboga-Nunes, Sørensen & Pelikan, 2014, p. 95). The main competences of a person considered to be health literate are very coincident with general communicative competences. The first ones revolve around the competences to (Sørensen et al., 2012): (1) access (the ability to seek, find and obtain health information), (2) understand (to comprehend health information), (3) appraise (interpret), (4) apply, means to communicate and use the information to maintain and improve health. Within the literature on health literacy, awareness, motivation, ability to understand and use information, promotion of health are the keywords.

In order for these results to be efficient, the information contents, made available by the sender, the health professional (through verbal and non-verbal language), must be clearly understood by the recipient, the patient (Silverman et al., 2013, p. 20). There is data showing that, after leaving the consultation, the patient remembers less than 50% of the information given to him (Dowell, Jones & Snadden, 2002). On the other hand, the reduced time in which the interaction of the relationship occurs (Clochesy et al., 2015) also requires the learning and the development of techniques (see Table 1) to improve the understanding of patients, especially those who have lower health literacy, in that period of the consultation.

There are several problematic consequences, when health communication is not understood by patients. Lack of understanding, especially due to low health literacy, leads to more hospitalizations (e.g. Baker, Parker, Williams & Clark, 1998; Baker et al., 2002; Espanha, Avila & Mendes, 2016), to premature deaths and poorer health outcomes (HLS-EU, 2012).

Having general communication skills is not enough for effective communication in health. It needs particular models and techniques in order to achieve the best outcomes, i.e. to be a guarantee that the patient will adhere to the treatment, understand and have efficacy in the received health instructions that contribute to positive health outcomes and self-care. Understanding what health communication can or cannot do, i.e., the potential of communication is decisive for the health professional to successfully communicate.

Table 1. Steps to increase understanding in patients with low health literacy

Check, with time and observation, the patient's health literacy skills
Use plain, simple, clear and accessible language to communicate, and when use technical jargon translate the sense
Show or draw, to increase patient's understanding and recall
Limit the amount of information to each interaction
Repeat the health instructions and encourage the patient to repeat by their own words (teach-back)
Be respectful, careful with the patient's language and feelings
Do not interrupt the patient before he/she explains what he/she feels and what his/her problems are
Encourage the patient to participate through open-ended questions (such as: What is worrying you? What can I do for you?
Accept the patient's feelings, without reacting defensively, offensively or with fear

Source: (Own elaboration. Based on The Joint Commission, 2016)

After the consultation and the inherent interpersonal relationship, the patient should be able to return to his/her environment and context, effectively informed and precisely instructed of what he/she has to do to be healthier. In the triangle of the therapeutic relationship, where the health professional, the patient and the specific contents that lead to this encounter are positioned, the communicational component is the determinant for the integral understanding by the patient of the steps to be taken after leaving this clinical setting. Thus, for the improvement of the health literacy, it is crucial that health professionals perceive the risk of patients not understanding the information that is transmitted to them and that is relevant to health maintenance (Koh, Brach, Harris & Parchman, 2013). In this scenario, some assumptions of the symbolic interaction theory (e.g. Blumer, 1969; Mead, 1934; Reynolds & Herman-Kinney, 2003) bring enlightenment to the importance of the communication (and comprehension) in the therapeutic relationship: humans act towards others on the basis of meanings, the meaning is created in an interaction, meanings are modified through an interpretative process, and finally individuals develop self-concept through interaction with others.

Having this awareness and sensibilization and being endowed with the necessary communication competences, the health results appear. So, health communication is one tool for promoting or improving health, and public health professionals should use the full range of health communication strategies in the effort to eliminate health disparities (Freimuth & Quinn, 2004).

Effective communication in health helps to reinforce positive and decisive attitudes in the prevention and treatment of diseases (Elbina et al., 2010). Communication can, also, increase the audience's knowledge and awareness of a health issue, problem, or solution, influence perceptions, beliefs, and attitudes that may change social norms. It can also reinforce knowledge, attitudes or behavior, refute myths and misconceptions and show benefits (e.g. "Pink Book"), but the evaluation of the degree of patient's health literacy and understanding of health instructions has to be done. It should be emphasized that communicating health, without environmental supports, is not effective at sustaining behavior changes at the individual level (Freimuth & Quinn, 2004).

The degree of health literacy of the participants in the therapeutic relationship is an essential competence and a public health imperative (Kickbusch & Maag, 2008). Communication can act on health literacy, being a key variable in the quality of Public Health (WHO Health Promotion Glossary, 1998, p. 10). So, a model of the best communication practices to improve health literacy and clinical practices is needed.

ASSERTIVENESS, CLARITY AND POSITIVITY (ACP): A 3-FACTOR MODEL OF COMMUNICATION TO OPTIMIZE HEALTH LITERACY

Presentation of the Model

Health literacy critically affects health communication between health professional and patient (e.g. Williams, Davis, Parker & Weiss, 2002). Knowledge, health promoting behaviors, and understanding of health instruction make the individual stronger, more active, and more participatory in his/her health decisions. This training through communication increases the health literacy of patients, achieving better health outcomes.

To exercise control over their health, people need comprehensible health messages that are accessible and appropriate to their individual needs and cultural and social backgrounds (International Encyclopedia of Public Health, 2008, pp. 204-211), respecting the meanings of words with which they are familiarized (symbolic interaction theory and Hall's concepts of "hegemony" and "preferred reading").

The steps to increase the understanding of patients with low health literacy go through an effective communication in health, assumed by the "stronger" side of this relationship that is the health professional and where assertiveness, clarity of language and positivity are interdependent keys to achieve positive outcomes.

An assertive personality has the ability to self-analyze in order to evaluate one's own feelings and to control one's personal impulses (Stein & Book, 2006, pp. 73-93) and recognizes one's rights and the others' rights and does not violate them (e.g. Alberti & Emmons, 2008; Smith, 1985). The assertiveness can be understood as certainty (e.g. Salter, Wolpe) and capacity to openly speak (e.g. Lazarus, 1973; Salter, 2002; Wolpe, 1990) about desires and needs, to tell "no", and to begin, maintain and conclude a conversation (Lazarus, 1973). Assertiveness is linked to self-esteem, assuming "a form of behavior characterized by a confident declaration or affirmation of a statement without need of proof" (Dorland's Medical Dictionary, 2014). Assertive posture is a social competence (Lazarus, 1971) and a virtue in the sense it remains in the middle between two inappropriate extremes, one for excess (aggression), another for lack (submission). The implementation of an assertive behavior conducts to self and mutual respect, benevolent perseverance, and politeness (Smith, 1985). Assertiveness is also a component of the patient participation, within the utterances, in which the patient expresses an opinion, states a preference, offers a suggestion/recommendation, expresses a disagreement or some other challenge to the health professional, or issues a request (Cegala, 2011, p. 428).

A patient focused communication, based on assertiveness of the health professional, increases the patient involvement, trust and confidence, and improves health outcomes, specially patient's satisfaction (Ahmed & Bates, 2016). The assertive outreach is based on the responsibility of the health professional or team to deliver patient-centered care (Ryan & Morgan, 2004, p. 12), understood as an approach to care and perceived as the right thing to do or a quality of personal, professional, and organizational relationships (Epstein & Street, Jr., 2011). Including all these attributes/indicators, the assertiveness presents itself as a pivotal resource in the clinical relationship.

People need information to make decisions about their health. However, a lot of health information is not easy to understand. Plain language makes health information more accessible and is a necessary requirement in healthcare professionals' daily practice when communicating with patients (Bittner et al., 2015, p. 1137).

Clarity (of language) is immediately understandable (Kripalani & Weiss, 2006) and, in this sense, is based on short, simple, nonmedical words that are easily comprehensible (Williams et al., 2002). Real-life analogies or stories relevant to patients' experiences are also helpful (Mayeaux et al., 1996). Patients misunderstand health communications more often than clinicians might think (Brega et al., 2015, p. 16). Therefore to ensure the understanding, it is of the utmost necessity to confirm the exact decoding of the transmitted information. Using clear oral communication strategies can help the patients to better understand health information, and communicating clearly also helps patients to feel more involved in their health care and increases their likelihood of following through on their treatment plans (Brega et al., 2015, p. 16).

Clear or plain language presupposes the use of the active voice, the use of second person of the verb (you), that the technical jargon must be limited, the sentences should only be up to 15 words or less and 8th grade reading level, and data should be easy to understand (Wittenberg, Goldsmith & Ferrel & Platt, 2015). Some strategies for communicating clearly are: greet patients warmly, make eye contact, listen carefully, use plain, non-medical language, use the patient's words, slow down, limit and repeat content, be specific and concrete, show graphics, demonstrate how it is done, invite patient participation, encourage questions and apply teach-back (Brega et al., 2015, pp. 16-17). The recommendations state that professionals should provide non-technical explanations, or explain carefully the technical terms, including making use of written instructions, so that the patient can remember health instructions more easily (Jackson, 1992).

Most health literacy experts emphasize several important behaviors to foster clear communication. Plain language is a logical and flexible response and refers to communications that engage and are accessible to the intended audience (Stableford & Mettger, 2007, p. 75). Plain language communication is part of the solution to major public health and health delivery problems (Stableford & Mettger, 2007, p. 76). Plain language is not about transmitting ''dumbing down'' information, in a condescending tone, or neglecting the need for accuracy: it is about communicating for clarity and meaning (p. 79). Good plain language is creative, vibrant, and emotionally resonant (p. 80). The process of developing plain language contents requires knowledge and skills, a clear understanding of the target audience, and the use of an evidence-based approach (p. 81).

Positive language is associated with approach goals instead of avoidance goals. The use of positive language has a compelling effect on the patients (Joseph, 2015, p. 652).

The positive language can literally change the brain and contributes to have good mental and physical health. The recommendations consist in avoiding the use of negative words and phrases, such as "I cannot", "never", "I do not", "always" and "I will not", and in constructing a framing to ideas through positive sentences, such as "I choose", "I can", "I will" (Corbin, McConnell, Le Masurier, Corbin & Farrar, 2014). People influence each other. Eventual negative acts and speeches of the healthcare professional tend to influence negatively the patient (Corbin et al., 2014). Similarly, when the healthcare professional is positive, optimistic and hopeful, the influence over the patient will be more often hopeful (Corbin et al., 2014). The health care providers can affect some sources of self-efficacy. Specifically, the health care provider can manipulate self-efficacy by using positive language, which can, in turn, improve patient adherence with health care instructions (Stemple & Hapner, 2014, p. 489).

The positive subject (Luthans, Youssef & Avolio, 2007, p. 3) is characterized by: (1) having confidence (self-efficacy) to take on and put in the necessary effort to succeed at challenging tasks; (2) making a positive attribution (optimism) about succeeding now and in the future; (3) persevering toward goals and, when necessary, redirecting paths to goals (hope) in order to succeed; and (4) when beset by problems and adversity, sustaining and bouncing back and even beyond (resilience) to attain success.

The figure 1 summarizes the 3-factor model of communication competences that we identify and propose based on the contributions from the literature review. The focus group will be used to validate this model.

Methodological Options

The research is subordinated to the starting question: *What is the contribution of communication competences to optimizing the results of the therapeutic relationship and health literacy?* More specifically, *What is the contribution of the model of communication competences, composed of assertiveness, clarity and positivity?* Based on the literature, one operational hypothesis can be formulated: *The 3-factor model of communication competences, composed of assertiveness, clarity and positivity, contributes to the improvement of the medical relation and to the better results of health literacy.*

In this sense, an exploratory study was conducted, on 28 March 2017, comprising one focus group with key health professionals (N = 9) to explore the health professionals' perception of communication to increase health literacy on patients. Data (the focus group participants' discourse) was analyzed using qualitative techniques, namely the qualitative content analysis. Qualitative content analysis is "the most prevalent approach to the qualitative analysis of documents" (Bryman, 2012, p. 557). It comprises a searching-out of underlying themes and a generation of categories (therapeutic relationship, communication competences, assertiveness, clarity and positivity) that guide the collection of data. The sections of text (quotations and ideas exposed by participants) concerning the themes of interest were identified and retrieved.

Figure 1. Communication competences in the context of therapeutic relationship and health literacy
Source: (Own elaboration. Based on CDC, 2011; Greenhalgh & Heath, 2010; Nutbeam, 1998; Ratzan, 1996; Silverman et al., 2013; Vaz de Almeida, 2011)

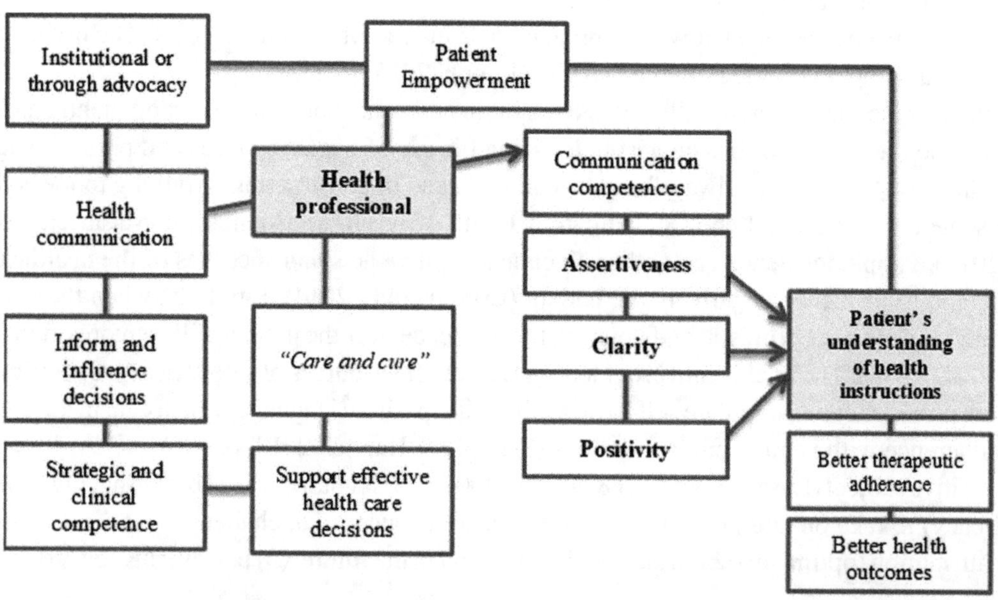

The focus group was based on a semi-structured script (see Appendix 1), with five areas focusing on the importance of communication competences and the communicational process within the therapeutic relationship. Based on a 40 items list, the whole group was encouraged to discuss and select (either by concordance or discordance) the items included or associated with communication competencies in the therapeutic relationship (see Appendix 2).

The participants were selected through the database of health professionals who attended post-graduate training in Communication and Health Literacy, and due to their active intervention in the fields of Health Literacy. After being identified, they were invited by e-mail and by telephone, having all answered affirmatively and participated in the focus group.

In sociodemographic terms, the group includes three male specialists and six female specialists. Eight of these experts perform active professional duties and one (female) specialist who is already retired, nevertheless she remains active in research and academic intervention.

Five specialists perform academic functions, however they have already had extensive experience in the field and direct contact with patients and within this group three had nursing experience. The group has also one surgeon, one retired nurse, one hospital nurse and one whose background includes Traditional Chinese Medicine. The average age is around 46.1 years. Professional activities are related to the various health areas, namely: oncology, dental medicine, rehabilitation nursing, pediatric rehabilitation, sterilization, and traditional Chinese medicine. Table 2 presents the participants' demographic and socioeconomic characteristics.

The contribution of communication competences for the success of the therapeutic relationship and for the increase in health literacy was discussed. The evaluation and obtained results express the perception of these experts.

Given the need to validate the ACP (Assertiveness, Clarity and Positivity) model and technique to improve results in the therapeutic relationship, the issues related to the definition of assertiveness, clear or plain language and positivity in the context of the therapeutic relationship were addressed. In the scope of the therapeutic relationship, the experts were asked to define and comment on what they understood by these elements of communication.

Table 2. List of participants and of their demographic and socioeconomic characteristics

Participant	Gender	Age	Education	Professional activity
A	M	50-59	Medicine	Surgeon at the IPO
B	M	40-49	PhD in Dental Medicine	Professor
C	M	40-49	PhD in Dental Medicine	Professor
D	F	50-59	PhD in Nursing	Professor
E	F	50-59	PhD student in Nursing	Professor
F	F	30-39	PhD student in Nursing	Professor
G	F	30-39	M.Sc. in Nursery	Nurse in HFF
H	F	50-59	M.Sc. in Nursery	Retired nurse
I	F	30-39	M.Sc. in Chinese Medicine	Professor in ESMTC

Source: (Own elaboration)

Findings

Specificities of an Effective Therapeutic Relationship: The Decisive Weight of Communication

The group of experts is unanimous in affirming that an effective therapeutic relationship is dynamic, symmetrical and trustworthy, built daily and in a specific context (the patient looks for the doctor and recognizes that the professional has the authority to accompany him therapeutically). The therapeutic relationship is fueled by empathy and availability between health professional and patient. Health professionals must possess both technical and communicational competences.

In this process, the group unanimously postulates that, no matter how competent the healthcare professional is and how active the patient is, an easy communication, with fluidity, clarity and simplicity to be understood by the patient, must exist. A well-structured therapeutic relationship can be established, generating effective results to the health literacy. In addition to the technical competences of the professional, the communication competences consolidate trust and stimulate the individual into the decision making process for better therapeutic adherence and health instruction.

Being a "dynamic process", the therapeutic relationship can both increase and decrease, advocates the group of experts. It depends on the balance state of those who seek the health professional. One expert (C) points out that the biopsychosocial state of the patient influences his/her degree of confidence in the professional. "If a person is in a weakened situation, he or she will place greater confidence in the professional. If the person is in a situation of control, sometimes may not have as much need to have a relationship of trust with the professional".

Symmetry requires balance between the parts. However some studies prove that there is an imbalance in the therapeutic relationship. According to the opinion of most experts of this focus group, the part considered "stronger" is on the side of the health professional. But one expert explains that "I also have to recognize the patient with his/her competences, the patient is expert in his/her life".

Patients, especially "those with low health literacy, come in search of authority, and often do not even question what is being transmitted to them by health professionals. They are often embarrassed to ask and often they do not even know what to ask and want to be told what to do". The focus group also reinforce and question a very recurring issue: "There is much talk today about empowerment. But how do we empower people? How do we require the person's training when he/she has very low ability to understand?"

Space and time influence the therapeutic relationship, which is built step by step, in a process based on the trust in the other (D). In this dialogical relationship, it is the need for interaction, where communication is pivotal (H and A, with the agreement of the whole group). It is necessary to understand what another wants to explain. During a genuine empathic process, the patient must believe in what the professional says with a biopsychosocial and also a spiritual alignment. C exposed that: "We teach our students that when we go to see the patient we may be on the worst day of our life, but the patient is not guilty. We should smile and serve the patient the best we can. We know that the patient's situation is very specific and delicate. The professional must open this "door of communication". When the professional does not make this effort to communicate, there is the abandonment of therapy. Inherently, what do we have to invest? The answer is: in the [communicational] capacitation of the health professional". All agreed and verbalized their agreement.

To Invest in What? Qualification vs. Time and Space

In these critical times of low literacy in health, the group agrees that "we must invest on the qualification of the health professional". Counterbalancing immediately, A and G emphasize that this process is important, but, currently, "health organizations generally do not give time and space". Everyone nods with this statement.

C underlines that the quality assurances, required by the health system, increasingly guarantee the quality of the service itself, in particular by reduced interaction times, with consequences in the relationship. C strengthens that "when a professional has only 10 minutes", instead of 40 minutes, to interact with the patient (the patient and the relation may need that time), "the professional cannot perform miracles". Specialist A stresses, in the same sense, that, "although the time of consultation is easy to measure, it is difficult to evaluate the results of adherence to therapy, cure or non-cure, recurrent visits to emergencies, and patient satisfaction. It is not only the time that influences". There are other contributive elements, such as the physical and organic structure of the health service and all the social determinants of health.

The group converges to the need for clarification and prior information to the patient, to enable him/her to make sound health decisions, in a complex process involving a set of interrelated competences.

The group agrees that early explanations of health issues can reduce patients' doubts. "The previous interview, to clarify doubts, allows a first reflection by the patient", underlines A, confirmed by C, who says that the previous interviews allow uncertainties to dissipate and, consequently, to facilitate the therapeutic relationship.

ACP Model and Technique: Searching Validation by Specialists

The participants in the focus group most punctuate, in assertiveness, active behavior, ability to listen and ability to openly speak; in clarity, the simple language, utilization of verbs; and, in positivity, orientation to a positive behavior of the patient.

Assertiveness

The group of experts agrees that the concept of assertiveness "has to do with the concept of participation" and depends on the cultural context in which it is used. There are people (such as the Eastern civilizations) whose feelings, attitudes or actions are not considered positive. But assertiveness must contain something straightforward and should not confuse the other part. "If a person tells me various symptoms and if the message is not direct, it can lead to some confusion. The professional must know how to refocus the question". Assertiveness is when the person makes himself understandable. It is also direct and positive language and it can be measured, because assertiveness is also guiding patient behaviors.

Assertiveness can be related to clarity and objectivity that reinforce the essential information that the patient must know and understand, to the adequacy that they may assert their rights. All agree that assertiveness is very useful in the therapeutic relationship.

According to these experts, the opposite of assertiveness is aggression, manipulation, confusion and insecurity. *Does the assertiveness always depend on the health professional?* Most of the group confirms this dependent relation because health professional is the "stronger part" and has more information and capacity to coordinate the therapeutic relationship and therefore to influence the results. It is mainly the lack of assertiveness on the professional side that can lead to poor diagnosis, although other factors such as low levels of literacy level, culture, language skills, and socioeconomic characteristics can predict poor health outcomes.

But a patient with some cognitive ability and higher health literacy should also argue and assert his/her opinion. Although it is important that the physician guide the patient to the questions he/she should ask, the patient should ask for clarification.

The group of experts emphasizes that the health professionals are the ones who have the responsibility to improve the individual's level of literacy. A person with greater literacy will know how to take good care of his/her health and his/her life. The focus group agrees that there must be investment in patient's self-efficacy through the intervention of the professional, as the specialists of the focus group often find that patients have some knowledge but it is not effective, as they do not know how to use it to improve their health.

Clarity

The group agrees that being "clear" also means focusing on essential and using an assertive language, which everybody understands at first time. Clear language is simple and can be enunciated in a technical way as long as an explanation of meaning is immediately made (professional jargon). The group also emphasizes that simple and clear language does not mean simplistic or infantilized one, which they consider a mistake. "One thing is the simplification of language, another is the infatilization of language", says a specialist.

Positivity

The experts consider that this concept is critical and dispersed in literature. Positivity is focused on the action that the patient performs, which should have effectiveness. Thus, when the patient is focused on a positive aspect related to his/her behavior, he/she becomes more available for the action he/she must take in order to achieve the best health results. For example, a patient may have most of his teeth poorly washed or sanitized, but there is one in good state. "We must start there by valuing what people already do effectively and with positive results", says one of the experts.

Motivation should be triggered by the communicational process, where the form and content of the language used influence the patient as an interpreter. In this sense, the patient's motivation should be done without using the word "no", such as "do not do this, do not do that". It is preferable to enunciate the positive behavior that the individual is supposed to have: "To heal your wound you must have your arm dry" instead of "You cannot dip your arm in water".

One participant defends that the medical professional should not constrain the patient, arguing that the self-efficacy and the trust of both actors in the relationship are significant. If the professional believes in the results and in the capacity of the patient to be able to operationalize the action, this trust factor in the other has an impact on the increase of his self-esteem and his effectiveness to do the action that leads to a greater therapeutic adherence.

The group recognizes that it is also possible to speak in collective positivity, which includes group therapies, legislation promoting, better health and healthy lifestyles, among others. Motivation and contagion by the presence and sharing of positive emotions and actions can be stimulated in a group, inducing the patient to a role of agent of action. The group acts as a stimulator of behavior by sharing experiences, creating expectations of action towards their members (psychological pressure), and doing certain healthy activities together (for example, sports, balanced and complete nutrition). The power of the group on action is a factor to be considered in the context of positivity.

DISCUSSION

The communication is a pivotal dimension in the therapeutic relationship (e.g. Silverman et al., 2013, p. 7). The technical competences required for clinical practice are enriched by the professional's communication competences. The literature on the subject also confirms that the patients' judgment about the professionals' competences, that is, the confidence the patients have in them, is not usually based on a technical nature, but mainly based on the socio-emotional dimension of the relationship, which includes interpersonal communication (e.g. DiMatteo, Prince & Taranta, 1979, p. 280).

The focus group refers to the importance and difficulties of empowering the patients, becoming possible thanks to communication (Ishikawa & Kiuchi, 2010). It is still necessary to give hypotheses to the person, and to know what this person can do, according to his/her illness situation. People having more or less therapeutic adherence are influenced by various social, economic, cultural determinants of health (Wilkinson & Marmot, 2003). There are recommendations to strengthen communication skills among patients with low health literacy (The Institute of Medicine, 2004) and to consider health literacy not only in terms of the characteristics of individuals, but also in terms of the interactional processes (Ishikawa & Kiuchi, 2010).

The focus group and literature emphasize the problem of the lack of time devoted to the patient in the medical encounter. For example, a recent study (HealthDay News, 2017) reveals that physicians spend roughly as many hours on computer work as they do meeting with patients. On average, they clocked about 3 hours with patients and around 3 hours on so-called "desktop medicine".

The therapeutic relationship has to be endowed with certain requirements that will optimize the health outcomes: trust, empathy, understanding, firmness, determination. These requirements can be condensed into a communication model composed of three components: assertiveness, clarity and positivity.

An assertive affirmation or response can include empathy, where the person demonstrates understanding with the situation or position of his/her interlocutor (Rego, 2016, p. 313). Clinical and care competences are required. There are studies that affirm that the patient has more therapeutic adherence, if there is a better communication relationship and a doctor-patient eye contact. Looking directly into the patient's eyes, giving him attention, show that the doctor cares with him (e.g. Eisenberg, 1992; Gerteis, Edman-Levitan, Daley & Del Blanco, 1993). In practice, good eye contact suggests confidence and honesty, also a more meaningful therapeutic relationship, and a doctor creates a positive atmosphere with their patients by simply looking at them (Eisenberg, 1992). Communication research suggests that a doctor's message will be decoded as being more favorable when associated with more eye contact than with less eye contact. Experts speculate that it is almost impossible for an individual to disguise eye meaning from someone who is a member of the same culture.

Salter (1949) and Wolpe in the 1950s were the first experts, referring to the concept of assertiveness applied to patients with mental diseases. The meaning of assertiveness was associated to certainty, related to ways of treating or reducing the neurotic influence. "Where the patient has neurotic fears in interpersonal interchanges (…) is encouraged to express what he really wants. This is what is meant by assertive behavior" (Wolpe, 1968, pp. 235-236). In opposition, the lack of assertiveness is linked to uncertainty, concretely linked to the formation of "inhibitory" behaviors that inhibit individuals from openly and spontaneously expressing their feelings, desires and needs. They were limited in their self-realization and inherently experienced problems in social connections. Similarly, in the focus group, the proposed opposite of assertiveness is aggression, manipulation, confusion and insecurity.

The participants of the focus group highlight that the patients are often embarrassed to ask and often do not even know what to question. Alike, previous research has identified that, for example, nurses overestimate their patients' health literacy (Johnson, 2014, p. 43), and that overestimation of a patient's health literacy may contribute to the widespread problem of poor health outcomes (e.g. Dickens et al., 2013). In summary, a trustful and open relation, a non-inhibitory environment, the confirmation of the patient's understanding of message and the motivation of the patient to question are crucial.

Assertiveness is linked to the control of one's personal impulses (Stein & Book, 2006, pp. 73-93), the recognition of one's own rights and the others' rights (respect) (e.g. Alberti & Emmons, 2008; Smith, 1985), certainty (e.g. Salter, Wolpe), capacity to openly speak (e.g. Lazarus, 1973; Salter, 2002; Wolpe, 1990), self-confidence (of both professional and patient) (Ahmed & Bates, 2016) and generates the mutual respect, benevolent perseverance and politeness (Smith, 1985). The credibility of the health professional can reinforce the assertiveness (Hovland's orientations) and the explanation of *why* is crucial to assume the medical instructions (persuasion theory).

Clear language is immediately understandable (Kripalani & Wieiss, 2006) and the health professionals should use strategies for confirming that the instructions that are being transmitted are accurately understood. There is a basic principle in this component: the comprehension. Referring Hall, for the necessary for decoding of the message by the recipient – the patient –, it was pointed out that the responsibility for the content should be to the sender – the health professional – who must ensure that the message is perceived and understood by the recipient. At the level of the receiver's understanding, Hall (1973; 1996) reflects that, before the message has an effect or satisfies a need, it must have a meaningful discourse. It is the decoding of the message, which will have a degree of influence over the receiver, with cognitive, emotional, ideological, and behavioral consequences. In this sense, the whole group agrees that language must be clear, accessible and simple in order to contribute to a better health literacy. The decoding and apprehension of the right meanings are pivotal due to the efficacy of communication and the premises of the symbolic interaction theory: humans act towards others on the basis of meanings, the meaning is created in an interaction, meanings are modified through an interpretative process, individuals develop self-concept through interaction with others.

Positive language is associated with approach goals instead of avoidance goals. The use of positive language has a compelling effect on the patients (Joseph, 2015, p. 652). So, the motivation is important to reinforce Bandura's (1999) position on the "agent" as one who intentionally makes things happen by his/her action. Being motivated then means moving to do something (Ryan & Deci, 2000). The concept of self-efficacy, which consists in the person's confidence to practice certain action (Bandura, 1986), should be stimulated in the patient.

For all the exposed reasons and theoretical foundation, the training of health professionals on the ACP (assertiveness, clarity and positivity) model and technique can be an efficient path to optimize the therapeutic relationship and to combat the more than 50% inadequate or problematic health literacy (HLS-EU, 2012).

SOLUTIONS AND RECOMMENDATIONS

The 3-factor model constructed and inspired by the literature analyzed and validated and enriched by the specialists of the focus group constitutes a solution and a recommendation for medical or health practice. This 2 in 1 solution (both model and technique) can be a communicational practice that contributes to improve clinical practices, since, based on quality communication and based on specific assumptions, the patient's understanding of the message is ensured and, thus, the therapeutic adherence and health literacy increase.

There are also some recommendations or indicators within each of the competencies that the health professional must comply with (see Table 3).

FUTURE RESEARCH DIRECTIONS

Given the empirical evidence and awareness of the importance of communication for health and the poor indicators on health literacy, the intersection seems to be inevitable between the paths of investigation of health literacy with those of communication. The research gap of the scarcity of the studies on articulation between communication/interaction and health literacy (e.g. Ishikawa & Kiuchi, 2010) seems to be bridged. This chapter is an effort in this sense.

This chapter provides a useful contribution to improve the therapeutic relationship and adherence and health literacy by proposing a model and technique for health professionals with interdependent competencies and respective elements to be applied in the health professional-patient relation. Although the three communication competences approached in this chapter are listed in the bibliography consulted, it is the first effort to systematize and organize them as an interdependent contribution to improve the therapeutic relationship, reflected in best outcomes in health literacy and in clinical practices.

The theoretical assumptions of the approach of symbolic interactionism, of the theory of persuasion/Yale attitude change approach and of encoding-decoding model of communication (Hall) adequately frame the thematic investigations on communication in interactional context, on persuasive aims within the health system, and on codification and understanding of the message.

Possible future research paths are to test the model presented here in an experimental context (social experiment) and to apply questionnaire surveys to patients in order to ascertain their opinion and experience in therapeutic relationships, concretely about communication tools and competences used by health professionals, and to test the influence of these tools and competences on the health literacy of patients. The social experiment will allow to test and evaluate, in a real context (in a medical consultation environment), the effectiveness of the proposed communication model. In measuring the impact of the referred model, the researcher can assess what the outcomes of the relevant population would have been in the absence of the model.

CONCLUSION

Both literature and the focus group are in harmony on the importance of health professionals developing communication competences, specially the assertiveness, the clarity and the positivity, to enhance patient health literacy level – the hypothesis formulated was confirmed. These communication competences include verbal and non-verbal forms, attitudes and behavior able to generate patients' confidence and heighten therapeutic adherence, as well as the positive consolidation of the therapeutic relationship. Therefore, our objectives are achieved: we assess the importance and contributions of communication competences for the health relationship and health literacy and construct a model, which was discussed and validated by a panel of experts within a focus group.

Table 3. Recommendations or indicators of the 3-factor model of communication competences: assertiveness, clarity and positivity

Assertiveness
Approach to care; The right thing to do; Be balanced; Confirm the understanding of the interlocutor; Guide the patient to the questions he/she should ask; Initiate, maintain and conclude a conversation; Openly speak about desires and needs; Practice benevolent perseverance and politeness; Practice the certainty, a form of behavior characterized by a confident declaration of a statement without need of proof; Recognize self and hetero rights and do not violate them; Reveal self-esteem; Revel self and mutual respect; Self-analyze, e.g., evaluate one's own feeling and control one's personal impulses; Tell "no"; Use clarity and objectivity that reinforce the essential information.
Clarity (of language)
Apply teach-back; Avoid technical jargon; Be creative, vibrant, and emotionally resonant; Be immediately understandable; Be specific and concrete; Communicate for clarity and meaning; Demonstrate how it is done; Encourage questions; Greet patients warmly; Invite patient participation; Limit and repeat content; Listen carefully; Make eye contact; Match patients' vocabulary; Offer concrete advice and recommendations; Show graphics; Slow down; The level of reading should be in the 8th grade; The sentences should only be up to 15 words or less; Understand the target audience; Use of a "living room" language; Use of active voice, the use of second person of the verb (you); Use of an evidence-based approach; Use the patient's words; Use written instructions to facilitate the memory.
Positivity
Avoid the use of negative words and phrases, such as "I cannot", "never", "I do not", "always" and "I will not"; Be positive, optimistic, hopeful, and confident (self-efficacy); Believe (and exteriorize this believe) in the results and in the capacity of the patient to be able to operationalize the action; Motivate the patient for the construction of positive sentences, such as "I choose", "I can", "I will" (empowerment and self-efficacy); Make a positive attribution (optimism) about succeeding now and in the future; Motivate; Persevere toward goals and, when necessary, redirect paths to goals (hope) in order to succeed; Take on and put in the necessary effort to succeed at challenging tasks; Use positive language; When beset by problems and adversity, sustain and bounce back and even beyond (resilience) to attain success.

Source: (Own elaboration)

A person with greater literacy will know how to take better care of his/her health and life, but the reality presents us a rate of more than 50% with problematic or inadequate literacy. Reinforcing with literature, Tu and Hargraves (2003) say that education is the key to explain the differences in information demand. Concretely, in the therapeutic relationship, the health professionals assume a pivotal function, in which the communication competences can make the difference. The investment must be centralized specially on communication competences of healthcare professionals.

Clinical competences should be combined and enriched with communication competences. It will be useful to explore variables based on health communication domains that can positively influence the therapeutic relationship and therapeutic adherence.

In order to understand the importance of communicational interaction for the strengthening of therapeutic relationship and consecutively for better adherence and health outcomes, it has to be considered that human interaction is based on cognitive, emotional and social issues. Assertive, plain and positive language, attitude and behavior are determinants and the key in this health process and inherent health communication, where the persons and their interactions are the focus. In sum, the proposed model is a contribution to be "healthy thanks to communication".

REFERENCES

Agency for Healthcare Research and Quality. (2010). *Health Literacy Universal Precautions Toolkit*. Rockville, MD: US Department of Health and Human Services. Retrieved June 10, 2017, from http://www.ahrq.gov/qual/literacy/

Ahmed, R., & Bates, B. R. (2016). To accommodate, or not to accommodate: Exploring patient satisfaction with doctors accommodative behaviour during clinical encounter. *Journal of Communication in Healthcare*, *9*(1), 22–32. doi:10.1080/17538068.2015.1126936

Ajzen, I. (1992). *Persuasive communication theory in social psychology: A historical perspective*. Amherst, MA: University of Massachusetts.

Alberti, R. E., & Emmons, M. L. (2008). *Your perfect right: Assertiveness and equality in your life and relationships*. Atascadero, CA: Impact Publishers.

Baker, D. W., Gazmararian, J. A., Williams, M. V., Scott, T., Parker, R. M., Green, D., ... Peel, J. (2002). Functional health literacy and the risk of hospital admission among Medicare managed care enrollees. *American Journal of Public Health*, *92*(8), 1278–1283. doi:10.2105/AJPH.92.8.1278 PMID:12144984

Baker, D. W., Parker, R. M., Williams, M. V., & Clark, W. S. (1998). Health literacy and the risk of hospital admission. *Journal of General Internal Medicine*, *13*(12), 791–798. doi:10.1046/j.1525-1497.1998.00242.x PMID:9844076

Baker, D. W., Parker, R. M., Williams, M. V., Pitkin, K., Parikh, N., Coates, W., & Imara, M. (1996). The health care experience of patients with low literacy. *Archives of Family Medicine*, *5*(6), 329–334. doi:10.1001/archfami.5.6.329 PMID:8640322

Baker, D. W., Parker, R. M., Williams, M. V., Pitkin, K., Parikh, N. S., Coates, W., & Imara, M. (1996). The health care experience of patients with low literacy. *Archives of Family Medicine*, *5*(6), 329–334. doi:10.1001/archfami.5.6.329 PMID:8640322

Bandura, A. (1986). *Social foundations of thought and action: A social cognitive theory*. Englewood Cliffs, NJ: Prentice Hall.

Bandura, A. (1999). Social cognitive theory of personality. In L. A. Pervin & O. P. John (Eds.), *Handbook of personality: Theory and research* (pp. 154–196). New York: The Guilford Press.

Benson, B. J. (2014). Domain of competence: Interpersonal and communication skills. *Academic Pediatrics*, *14*(2S), S55–S65. PMID:24602649

Bittner, A., Jonietz, A., Bittner, J., Beickert, L., & Harendza, S. (2015). Translating medical documents into plain language enhances communication skills in medical students: A pilot study. *Patient Education and Counseling*, *98*(9), 1137–1141. doi:10.1016/j.pec.2015.05.024 PMID:26095344

Blumer, H. (1969). *Symbolic interactionism: Perspective and method*. Englewood Cliffs, NJ: Prentice-Hall.

Brega, A. G., Barnard, J., Mabachi, N. M., Weiss, B. D., DeWalt, D. A., Brach, C., . . . West, D. R. (2015). AHRQ Health Literacy Universal Precautions Toolkit. Prepared by Colorado Health Outcomes Program, University of Colorado Anschutz Medical Campus. AHRQ Publication No. 15-0023-EF. Rockville, MD: Agency for Healthcare Research and Quality.

Bryman, A. (2012). *Social Research methods*. Oxford, UK: Oxford University Press.

Cegala, D. J. (2011). An exploration of factors promoting patient participation in Primary Care Medical Interviews. *Health Communication*, *26*(5), 427–436. doi:10.1080/10410236.2011.552482 PMID:21416422

Centers for Disease Control and Prevention. (2011). *Health communication basics*. Atlanta: Division of Public Affairs (DPA), Office of the Associate Director for Communication (OADC). Retrieved June 10, 2017, from http://www.cdc.gov/healthcommunication/healthbasics/whatishc.html

Chant, S., Jenkinson, T., Randle, J., & Russell, G. (2002). Communication skills: Some problems in nursing education and practice. *Journal of Clinical Nursing*, *11*(1), 12–21. doi:10.1046/j.1365-2702.2002.00553.x PMID:11845748

Clochesy, J. M. (2015). Wait, won't! Want: Barriers to health care as perceived by medically and socially disenfranchised communities. *Journal of Health and Human Services Administration*, *38*(2), 174–214. PMID:26442361

Cobley, P., & Schulz, P. J. (2013). *Theories and models of communication. Handbook of Communication Science* (Vol. 1). De Gruyer Mouton. doi:10.1515/9783110240450

Coeira, E., & Ong, M.-S. (2014). Systemwide communication. In L. R. Martin & M. R. DiMatteo (Eds.), *The Oxford handbook of health communication, behavior change, and treatment adherence* (pp. 155–176). Oxford, UK: Oxford University Press.

Corbin, C. B., McConnell, K., Le Masurier, G., Corbin, D., & Farrar, T. (2014). *Health opportunities through physical education*. Springfield, IL: Human Kinetics.

Dickens, C., Lambert, B., Cromwell, T., & Piano, M. (2013). Nurse overestimation of patients' health literacy. *Journal of Health Communication, 18*(sup1), 62–69. doi:10.1080/10810730.2013.825670 PMID:24093346

DiMatteo, M. R., Prince, L. M., & Taranta, A. (1979). Patients' perceptions of physicians' behavior: Determinants of patient commitment to the therapeutic relationship. *Journal of Community Health, 4*, 280–290. PMID:469038

Dorland's. (2014). *Dorland's medical dictionary*. Retrieved June 10, 2017, from https://www.dorlands.com/

Dowell, J., Jones, A., & Snadden, D. (2002). Exploring medication use to seek concordance with 'non-adherent' patients: A qualitative study. *The British Journal of General Practice, 52*, 24–32. PMID:11791812

Eisenberg, A. (1992). Doctor-patient eye contact. *Dynamic Chiropractic, 10*(1). Retrieved June 10, 2017, from http://www.dynamicchiropractic.com/mpacms/dc/article.php?id=43000

Elbina, R., Kawasaki, F., Taniguchi, I., Togari, T., Yamasaki, Y., & Sparks, M. (2010). The effectiveness of Health Communication strategies in health education in Kushima, Japan. *Global Health Promotion, 17*(1), 5–15. doi:10.1177/1757975909356628 PMID:20357347

Epstein, R. M., & Street, R. L. Jr. (2011). The values and value of patient-centered care. *Annals of Family Medicine, 9*(2), 100–103. doi:10.1370/afm.1239 PMID:21403134

Espanha, R., Ávila, P., & Mendes, R. M. (2016). *A literacia em saúde em Portugal*. Lisboa: Fundação Calouste Gulbenkian.

European Health Forum Gastein. (2005). *Gastein health declaration 2005*. Partnerships for Health. Retrieved from June 10, 2017, http://www.ehfg.org/

Faber, M., Bosch, M., Wollersheim, H., Leatherman, S., & Grol, R. (2009). Public reporting in health care: How do consumers use quality-of-care information? A systematic review. *Medical Care, 47*(1), 1–8. doi:10.1097/MLR.0b013e3181808bb5 PMID:19106724

Freimuth, V. S., & Quinn, S. C. (2004). The contributions of health communication to eliminating health disparities. *American Journal of Public Health, 94*(12), 2053–2055. doi:10.2105/AJPH.94.12.2053 PMID:15569949

Gerteis, M., Edgman-Levitan, S., Daley, J., & Delblanco, T. L. (Eds.). (1993). *Through the patient's eyes. Understanding and promoting patient-centered care*. San Francisco, CA: Jossey-Bass.

Greenhalgh, T., & Heath, I. (2010). *Measuring quality in the therapeutic relationship: An inquiry into the quality of general practice in England*. London: The King's Fund.

Gregory, A. (2008). Competencies of senior communication practitioners in the UK: An initial study. *Public Relations Review, 34*(3), 215–223. doi:10.1016/j.pubrev.2008.04.005

Hall, S. (1973). *Encoding and decoding in the media discourse. Stencilled Paper 7*. Birmingham: CCCS.

Hall, S. (1980). Encoding/decoding. In D. Hobson, A. Lowe, & P. Willis (Eds.), *Culture, Media, Language* (pp. 128–138). London: Hutchinson.

Hall, S. (1996). Cultural studies and its theoretical legacies. In *D. Morley & K.-H. Chen, Critical dialogues in cultural studies* (pp. 261–274). London, New York: Routledge.

Hargie, O., & Dickson, D. (2004). *Skilled interpersonal communication: Research, theory, and practice.* London: Routledge.

HealthDay News. (2017, April 11). Is 'desktop medicine' chipping away at patient care? *MedlinePlus.* Retrieved June 10, 2017, from https://medlineplus.gov/news/fullstory_164571.html

Hibbard, J. H., Peters, E., Dixon, A., & Tusler, M. (2007). Consumer competencies and the use of comparative quality information: It isn't just about literacy. *Medical Care Research and Review: MCRR, 64*(4), 379–394. doi:10.1177/1077558707301630 PMID:17684108

HLS-EU Consortium. (2012). *Comparative report of health literacy in eight EU member states. The European health literacy survey HLS-EU* (second revised and extended version, July 22th, 2014). Retrieved June 10, 2017, from HTTP://WWW.HEALTH-LITERACY.EU

Hovland, C. I., Janis, I. L., & Kelley, H. H. (1953). *Communication and Persuasion: Psychological studies of opinion change. Yale.* Yale University Press.

Howard, T., Jacobson, K. L., & Kripalani, S. (2013). Doctor talk: Physicians' use of clear verbal communication. *Journal of Health Communication, 18*(8), 991–1001. doi:10.1080/10810730.2012.757398 PMID:23577746

Institute of Medicine. (2004). *Health literacy: A prescription to end confusion.* Washington, DC: National Academies.

Ishikawa, H., & Kiuchi, T. (2010). Health literacy and health communication. *BioPsychoSocial Medicine, 4*(1), 1–5. doi:10.1186/1751-0759-4-18 PMID:21054840

Jackson, L. D. (1992). Information complexity and medical communication: The effects of technical language and amount of information in a medical message. *Health Communication, 4*(3), 197–210. doi:10.120715327027hc0403_3

Johnson, A. (2014). Health literacy, does it make a difference? *The Australian Journal of Advanced Nursing, 31*(3), 39–45.

Jones, J. A., Kreps, G. L., & Phillips, G. M. (1995). *Communicating with your doctor: Getting the most out of health care.* Cresskill, NJ: Hampton Press.

Joseph, S. (Ed.). (2015). Positive psychology in practice: Promoting human flourishing in work, health, education, and everyday life. Hoboken, NJ: John Wiley & Sons.

Katz, M. G., Jacobson, T. A., Veledar, E., & Kripalani, S. (2007). Asking questions in the medical encounter. *General Internal Medicine, 22*, 782–786. doi:10.100711606-007-0184-6

Keller, D. B., Sarkar, U., & Schillinger, D. (2014). Health literacy and information exchange in medical settings. In L. R. Martin & M. R. DiMatteo (Eds.), *The Oxford handbook of health communication, behavior change, and treatment adherence* (pp. 23–37). Oxford, UK: Oxford University Press.

Kickbusch, I., & Maag, D. (2008). Health literacy. In K. Heggenhougen & S. Quah (Eds.), *International Encyclopedia of Public Health* (Vol. 3, pp. 204–211). San Diego: Academic Press. doi:10.1016/B978-012373960-5.00584-0

Kickbusch, I. S. (2001). Health literacy: Addressing the health and education divide. *Health Promotion International*, *16*(3), 289–297. doi:10.1093/heapro/16.3.289 PMID:11509466

Kickbush, I., Wait, S., & Maag, D. (2005). Navigating health: The role of health literacy. London: Alliance for Health and the Future. International Longevity Centre.

Koh, H. K., Brach, C., Harris, L. M., & Parchman, M. L. (2013). A proposed 'health literate care model' would constitute a systems approach to improving patients' engagement in care. *Health Affairs (Project Hope)*, *32*(2), 357–367. doi:10.1377/hlthaff.2012.1205 PMID:23381529

Kreps, G. L. (1988a). The pervasive role of information in health and health care: Implications for health communication policy. In J. Anderson (Ed.), *Communication yearbook 11* (pp. 238–276). Newbury Park, CA: Sage.

Kreps, G. L. (1988b). Relational communication in health care. *Southern Speech Communication Journal*, *53*(4), 344–359. doi:10.1080/10417948809372736

Kreps, G. L. (1996). Promoting a consumer orientation to health care and health promotion. *Journal of Health Psychology*, *1*(1), 41–48. doi:10.1177/135910539600100104 PMID:22011519

Kreps, G. L., & O'Hair, D. (Eds.). (1995). *Communication and health outcomes*. Cresskill, New Jersey: Hampton Press.

Kreps, G. L., & Query, J. L. (1990). Health communication and interpersonal competence. In G. M. Phillips & J. T. Wood (Eds.), *Speech communication: Essays to commemorate the 75th anniversary of the Speech Communication Association* (pp. 292–323). Carbondale, IL: Southern Illinois University Press.

Kripalani, S., & Weiss, B. D. (2006). Teaching about health literacy and clear communication. *Journal of General Internal Medicine*, *21*(8), 888–890. doi:10.1111/j.1525-1497.2006.00543.x PMID:16881953

Lazarus, A. A. (1971). *Behavior therapy and beyond*. New York: McGraw-Hill.

Lazarus, A. A. (1973). On assertive behavior: A brief note. *Behavior Therapy*, *4*(5), 697–699. doi:10.1016/S0005-7894(73)80161-3

Longo, D. R., & Patrick, T. B. (2001). Consumer reports and health care information: A call for research. *Journal of Health Care Finance*, *28*, 92–96. PMID:11669296

Lucena, A. de F., & de Góes, M. O. (1999). O processo de comunicação no cuidado do paciente submetido ao eco-stress: Algumas reflexões. *Revista Gaúcha de Enfermagem*, *20*, 37–48.

Luthans, F., Youssef, C. M., & Avolio, B. J. (2007). *Psychological capital*. New York: Oxford University Press.

Martin, L., Schonlau, M., Hass, A., Derose, K., Rosenfeld, L., Buka, S., & Rudd, R. (2011). Patient activation and advocacy: Which literacy skills mater most? *Journal of Health Communication*, *16*(3), 177–190. doi:10.1080/10810730.2011.604705 PMID:21951251

Martin, L. R., & Di Matteo, M. R. (Ed.). (2014). The Oxford handbook of Health Communication, behavieoural change and Treatment Adherence. New York: Oxford.

Mayeaux, E. J. Jr, Murphy, P. W., Arnold, C., Davis, T. C., Jackson, R. H., & Sentell, T. (1996). Improving patient education for patients with low literacy skills. *American Family Physician, 53*(1), 205–211. PMID:8546047

Mead, G. H. (1934). *Mind, self, and society*. Chicago: University of Chicago Press.

Nijman, J., Hendriks, M., Brabers, A., de Jong, J., & Rademakers, J. (2014). Patient activation and health literacy as predictors of health information use in a general sample of Dutch health care consumers. *Journal of Health Communication: International Perspectives, 19*(8), 955–969. doi:10.1080/10810730.2013.837561 PMID:24397280

Noar, S. M., Harrington, N. G., Van Stee, S. V., & Aldrich, R. S. (2011). Tailored health communication to change lifestyle behaviours. *American Journal of Lifestyle Medicine, 5*(5), 112–122. doi:10.1177/1559827610387255

Nutbeam, D. (1998). Health promotion glossary. *Health Promotion International, 13*(4), 349–364. doi:10.1093/heapro/13.4.349

Nutbeam, D. (2000). Health literacy as a public health goal: A challenge for contemporary health education and communication strategies into the 21st century. *Health Promotion International, 15*(3), 259–267. doi:10.1093/heapro/15.3.259

Onjefu, O., & Olalekan, A. G. (2016). Human communication as a correlate of the essence of Man: A Philosophical perspective. *Arts and Social Sciences Journal, 7*(1), 1–4.

Parikh, N., Parker, R., Nurss, J., Baker, D., & Williams, M. (1996). Shame and health literacy: The unspoken connection. *Patient Education and Counseling, 27*(1), 33–39. doi:10.1016/0738-3991(95)00787-3 PMID:8788747

Query, J. L. Jr, & Kreps, G. L. (1996). Testing a relational model for health communication competence among caregivers for individuals with Alzheimer's disease. *Journal of Health Psychology, 1*(3), 335–351. doi:10.1177/135910539600100307 PMID:22011996

Ratzan, S. C. (2016). Effective decision-making: A negotiation perspective for Health Psychology and Health Communication. *Journal of Health Psychology, 1*(3), 323–333. doi:10.1177/135910539600100306 PMID:22011995

Rego, A. (2016). *Comunicação pessoal e organizacional*. Lisboa: Sílabo.

Reynolds, L. T., & Herman-Kinney, N. J. (2003). *Handbook of symbolic interactionism*. Walnut Creek, CA: AltaMira.

Rootman, I. (2002). *Health literacy and health promotion*. Ontario: Ontario Health Promotion E-Bulletin.

Rungapadiachy, D. M. (1999). *Interpersonal communication and psychology for health care professionals: Theory and practice*. Edinburgh, UK: Butterworth-Heinemann.

Ryan, P., & Morgan, S. (2004). *Assertive outreach: A strengths approach to policy and practice*. London: Churchill Livingstone.

Ryan, R. R., & Deci, E. L. (2000). Intrinsic and extrinsic motivations: Classic definitions and new directions. *Contemporary Educational Psychology*, *25*(1), 54–67. doi:10.1006/ceps.1999.1020 PMID:10620381

Saboga-Nunes, L., Sørensen, K., & Pelikan, J. M. (2014). *Hermenêutica da literacia em saúde e sua avaliação em Portugal (HLS-EU-PT)*. Paper presented at the VIII Congresso Português de Sociologia, Évora, Portugal. Retrieved June 10, 2017, from http://www.aps.pt/viii_congresso/VIII_ACTAS/VIII_COM0526.pdf

Salter, A. (1949). *Conditioned reflex theory*. New York: Creative Age Press.

Salter, A. (2002). *Conditioned reflex therapy: The classic book on assertiveness that began behavior therapy*. Gretna, LA: Wellness Institute.

Schillinger, D., Bindman, A., Wang, F., Stewart, A., & Piette, J. (2004). Functional health literacy and the quality of physician-patient communication among diabetes patients. *Patient Education and Counseling*, *52*(3), 315–323. doi:10.1016/S0738-3991(03)00107-1 PMID:14998602

Schillinger, D., Piette, J., Grumbach, K., Wang, F., Wilson, C., Daher, C., ... Bindman, A. B. (2003). Closing the loop: Physician communication with diabetic patients who have low health literacy. *Archives of Internal Medicine*, *163*(1), 83–90. doi:10.1001/archinte.163.1.83 PMID:12523921

Schirmer, M., Mauksch, L., Lang, F., Marvel, K., Zoppi, K., Epstein, R. M., ... Pryzbylski, M. (2005). Assessing communication competence: A review of current tools. *Family Medicine*, *37*(3), 184–192. PMID:15739134

Silverman, J., Krutz, S., & Draper, J. (2013). *Skills for communicating with patients*. Boca Raton, FL: Taylor & Francis Group.

Smith, M. J. (1985). *When I say no, I feel guilty*. New York: Bantam Books.

Sorensen, K., Van den Broucke, S., Fullam, J., Douyle, G., Pelikan, J., Slonska, Z., & Brand, H. (2012). Health literacy and Public health: A systematic review and integration of definitions and models. *BMC Public Health*, *12*(1), 80. doi:10.1186/1471-2458-12-80 PMID:22276600

Stableford, S., & Mettger, W. (2007). Plain Language: A Strategic Response to the Health Literacy Challenge. *Journal of Public Health Policy*, *28*(1), 71–93. doi:10.1057/palgrave.jphp.3200102 PMID:17363939

Stein, S., & Book, H. (2006). *The EQ edge: Emotional intelligence and your success*. Toronto: Jossey-Bass.

Stemple, J. C., & Hapner, E. R. (2014). *Voice therapy: Clinical case studies*. San Diego, CA: Plural Publishing.

Teixeira, J. A. C. (2004). *Comunicação em saúde: Relação técnicos de saúde – utentes*. Lisboa: Instituto Superior de Psicologia Aplicada.

Tench, R., & Konczos, M. (2013). Mapping European communication practitioners competencies: A review of the European communication professionals skills and innovation programme. *ECOPSI*, 35-64.

The Joint Commission, Division of Health Care Improvement (2016, November). Advancing patient-provider communication and activating patients. *Quick Safety*, (29).

Tu, H. T., & Hargraves, J. L. (2003). Seeking health care information: Most consumers still on the sidelines. *Center for Studying Health System Change*, (61). Retrieved June 10, 2017, from http://www.hschange.org/CONTENT/537/?words=Tu%20&%20Hargraves%20200344

Van't Jagt, K., de Winter, A. F., Reijneveld, S. A., Hoeks, J. C., & Jansen, C. J. (2016). Development of a communication intervention for older adults with limited health literacy: Photo stories to support doctor-patient communication. *Journal of Health Communication*, *21*(sup2), 69–82. doi:10.1080/10810730.2016.1193918 PMID:27662265

Vaz de Almeida, C. (2011). Communication and Literacy in e-Health. In *V SEMiME Exclusão Digital na Sociedade da Informação*. FMH-Universidade Técnica de Lisboa.

Watzlawick, P., Beavin, J. H., & Jackson, D. D. (1967). *Pragmática da comunicação humana: Um estudo dos padrões, patologias e paradoxo da interação* (S. Paulo, Ed.). Cultrix.

Wilkinson, R., & Marmot, M. (Eds.). (2003). *Social Determinants of Health. The solid facts*. Geneva: WHO Europe International Centre for Health and Society.

Williams, M. V., Davis, T., Parker, R. M., & Weiss, B. D. (2002). The role of health literacy in patient-physician communication. *Family Medicine*, *34*(5), 383–389. PMID:12038721

Wittenberg, E., Goldsmith, J., Ferrell, B., & Platt, C. S. (2015). Enhancing communication related to symptom management through plain language: A brief report. *Journal of Pain and Symptom Management*, *50*(5), 707–711. doi:10.1016/j.jpainsymman.2015.06.007 PMID:26162506

Wolpe, J. (1968). Psychotherapy by Reciprocal Inhibition. *Conditional Reflex: A Pavlovian Journal of Research & Therapy*, *3*(4), 234-240.

Wolpe, J. (1990). *The practice of behavior therapy*. New York: Pergamon.

World Health Organization. (1998). *Health Promotion Glossary*. Geneva: WHO.

Wynia, M. K., & Osborn, C. Y. (2010). Health literacy and communication in health care organizations. *Journal of Health Communication*, *15*(sup2), 102–115. doi:10.1080/10810730.2010.499981 PMID:20845197

KEY TERMS AND DEFINITIONS

Communication Competences: The mobilization of appropriate communication behaviors, which include cognitive, affective and behavioral components, to a concrete situation, which is only possible through reflection and action; or a combination of communication resources (knowledge, know-how and professional behavior) needed to respond to evolving professional situations, structured in action, and, when interacting with others, also in a social and symbolic dimension.

Health: Dynamic state of well-being characterized by the physical, mental and social potential that meets the vital needs according to age, culture and personal responsibility.

Health Communication: Use of communication strategies and interpersonal or media communication activities to inform and influence individual decisions that enhance health.

Health Literacy: Informed decisions and health management by the individual, through a conscious, active and permanent process of access, use and understanding of health information, which generates health outcomes.

Health Prevention: Previous actions that prevent the onset and evolution of diseases and, at the same time, decrease their incidence and prevalence in societies.

Health Professionals: Professionals in the health field, including doctors, physicians, nurses, therapists, psychologists, social workers, auxiliaries, among others who move in the area of health care and who may not be exclusively health professionals.

Health Promotion: Measure to increase health and general well-being of individuals and groups.

Patients: Users of a health service, such as primary health care or health centers, hospital services, secondary health care or rehabilitation services (tertiary care).

Therapeutic Relationship: A communicative and collaborative interpersonal relationship between professional and patient, in a certain space and time, that aims at enhancing and empowering the patient, so that he/she understands and can independently adhere to health instructions, with best results in health.

APPENDIX 1

Script for Focus Group

Set of guiding questions for the implementation of the Focus Group on 28 March 2017: Proposal of the ACP Model and Technique

1. Therapeutic relationship
   a. How do you define the therapeutic relationship?
   b. Do you have another suggestion for the classification of the relationship between the health professional and the patient? Why?
2. Contribution of communication competences to the success of the therapeutic relationship and to the increase of health literacy
   a. What importance do you give to the contribution of communication competences for the success of the therapeutic relationship? And for the increase of health literacy?
   b. Which communication competences do you consider most crucial to the success of the therapeutic relationship? Why? And for the increase of health literacy? Why?
3. Assertiveness in the context of the therapeutic relationship and health literacy
   a. What do you consider to be assertiveness?
   b. What are the contributions of assertiveness to the therapeutic relationship and health literacy?
4. larity in the context of the therapeutic relationship and health literacy
   a. What do you understand about clarity?
   b. What are the contributions of clarity to the therapeutic relationship and health literacy?
5. Positivity in the context of the therapeutic relationship and health literacy
   a. What do you understand about positivity?
   b. What are the contributions of positivity to the therapeutic relationship and health literacy?

APPENDIX 2

Elements Present in the Therapeutic Relationship That I Consider Included/Associated (Either by Agreement or Opposition) to Assertiveness, Clarity, and Positivity

1. Recognition of one's rights and the rights of others
2. Commitment in relation
3. Control of individual pulses
4. Non-aggressiveness
5. Use of verbs
6. Uncertainty
7. Simple language
8. Use of technical jargon
9. Intonation or tone
10. Knowing how to say "no"
11. Trust
12. Guidance for positive patient behavior
13. Silences of the professional
14. Direct language
15. Courage
16. Guidance for action
17. Simple words
18. Teach-back method (confirmation of correct perception)
19. Respect for others
20. Contact control
21. Personal attributes
22. Encouragement of cooperation
23. Guilt and shame
24. Conflict management
25. Empathy
26. Understanding for the others' mistakes
27. Acceptance of criticism
28. Aggressiveness and imposition
29. Clear instructions
30. Leadership
31. Affirmation without the need for proof
32. Understanding the mistakes of others
33. Active behavior
34. Ability to listen
35. Ability to openly speak

36. Strengthening of attitudes towards the disease prevention and treatment
37. Motivation
38. Use of the first person "I" in the speech
39. Specific action leading to better health
40. Certainty

Chapter 9
Reflections and Understanding of Quality Management in Healthcare

T. Ray Ruffin
University of Phoenix, USA

ABSTRACT

Healthcare organizations (HCOs) leadership must be involved with patient safety inventiveness and healthcare strategy. Leadership is essential to implementing and sustaining continuous performance quality improvement for patient-centered care. Quality management is of extreme significance to the United States (U.S.) healthcare industry and patients. Included are an introduction and background of the U.S. healthcare systems as well as the joint commission and government mandates. One of the primary focuses of the chapter is to enhance health literacy by developing a robust lexicon of fundamental healthcare terms and concepts. Healthcare reforms such as Patient Protection and Affordable Care Act (PPACA) are explored. The quality of healthcare delivery, involuntary reporting, patient safety indicators (PSIs), prevention quality indicators (PQIs), and inpatient quality indicators (IQIs) are explained. The chapter culminates with a discussion focusing on transformational leadership and the strategies for quality management implementation, along with a conclusion.

INTRODUCTION

The health care systems are an assortment of a set of public and private information gathering systems (Agency for Healthcare Research and Quality [AHRQ], 2014). A health care system includes other administrative registration such as medical billing, and non-medical billing, and medical records. Different organizations and Health Care Organizations (HCOs) use health care systems. The chapter focuses on United States (U.S.) HCOs which are normally comprised of hospitals, Community Health Centers (CHCs), general practitioners, clinics, specialty physicians and health plans (AHRQ, 2014). An additional focus of the chapter centers on enhancing health literacy by developing a robust lexicon of fundamental health care terms and concepts. Conflicting views exist around the decision-making processes of health

DOI: 10.4018/978-1-5225-4074-8.ch009

care provider leadership in U.S. HCOs (Hinami, Whelan, Konetzka, & Meltzer, 2012). Based on the Avedis Donabedian Model, high quality of care requires observing the structure of the HCO, evaluating the care processes, and measuring patients' care outcomes (Haj, Lamrini, & Rais, 2013). The structure of the HCO denotes the features HCO give to the care of the patient. Assessing the characteristics of U.S. HCOs could include:

- Health care providers specialty
- Type of individuals hired
- The proprietorship of the health organization
- Regulations/Policies related provisions of care, and
- Patient safety.

Change management strategies and employee engagement are effective ways to reinforce the foundation for patient-centered care and patient safety (Frampton, Guastello, Brady, Hale, Horowitz, Smith, & Stone, 2008). The change process is the result of patients receiving care based on industry standard or evidence based on the systems implemented. Patient-centered care and patient safety are based on all the interactions between the patient and the health care provider, and leaders in HCOs. The strategies include involving patients in the decision process and making patients feel comfortable and anodyne. The procedure helps patients to consider their thoughts and ideas, interpersonal processes, as well as providing emotional and informational support. The Donabedian Model related to testing results and to order the correct test such as mammograms, preventive ultrasounds, Electrocardiograms (ECG or EKG), and cancer screenings (E-Source, n.d.).

Outcomes are the change in the status of the patient resulting from the care and treatment provided by the health care provider. Improvements could be in the patient condition, as well as improvements from complications of the symptoms diagnosed. Outcomes included measurements like blood work levels for patients with varying conditions such as high triglyceride levels and associated with other health risk outcomes (E-Source, n.d.). Ruffin (2015) proposed one of the most widely discussed areas is improving the quality of patient-centered care with the use of Health Information Technology (HIT). Operational inefficiencies exist in the utilization of HIT and documentation of individual health care information throughout HCOs (Ruffin, 2015). Operational inefficiency neglects the right people, processes, and technology impacting the ability to enhance productivity and worth of HCO operations (Operations Research, 2007). The neglect could create an increased cost in routine operations for HCOs. There is a direct relation to having the right structures, processes, and outcomes in place for HCOs to operate successfully.

Health Care practitioners in the U.S. have the tools to create a multifaceted overview to include medical terminology, administration, ethical, legal, and standard requirements. Transforming health care systems through consumers participating in health self-management through their health records will be beneficial (Operations Research, 2007). Hopefully, the transformation will lead to improved outcomes, reduced medical errors, and eliminating complications. HCOs are confronted with new challenges and the ability to seize new alternatives day-to-day. Technology in the form of software and hardware has given the health care industry the opportunity to transform services.

The practice types could have immediate and long-term benefits for HCOs and patients. HCOs can standardize practices and requirements consistent with efficiency and effectiveness to avoid high cost (Operations Research, 2007). Health Care providers attempting to improve quality of care and reduce costs are progressively more turning to Information Technology (IT) -enabled business strategies. Business Intelligence (BI) in the health care provider market is roughly 25 years old and traces back to the mid-1980s. With the start of the Diagnosis-Related Group (DRG) based reimbursement models, there was enlightened interest in tools designed to analyze cost and profitability by clinical product lines (Health Industry Insights, an IDC Company, 2009).

BACKGROUND

The connection between Health Technology Assessment (HTA) and Health Information Technology (HIT) is essential because the HIT was the forefather to HTA. HTA was a form of policy research studying short and long-term consequences of the application of health-care technology (O'Donnell, Pham, Pashos, Miller, & Smith, 2009). During the 1960's computer vendors wanted to handle many hospital medical issues by installing a 96-button punch pad throughout the hospital to handle physician orders (Cantrill, 2010). However, restriction in the 1960's and 1970's hardware limited Central Processing Unit (CPU) speed connectivity between workstations (Cantrill, 2010). During this time, the mass storage limit would only support 144 patients.

In 1965, the Congressional Committee on Science and Astronautics perceived the need to assist in evaluating the legal impact of technology (US Congress House of Representatives, 1967). The U.S. Office of Technology Assessment (OTA) spawned an agency delivering independent evaluations of technologies in medicine to Congress. As well as distributing telecommunications, agriculture, materials, and transportation information. The OTA became the foundation of numerous public policies in the latter part of the 20th century (O'Donnell, et al., 2009). In 1987, an early model of the HTA was Sweden's 'Statens beredning för medicinsk utvärdering' (SBU) (Institute for Quality and Efficiency in Health Care, 2004).

In 1999, the United Kingdom (UK) announced the National Institute for Clinical Excellence (NICE). Later in the century, NICE was renamed the National Institute for Health and Clinical Excellence (NICE), the accoym stayed the same (O'Donnell et al., 2009). To deliver direction on new technologies and treatment of diseases, NICE expressively contributed to the globalization of HTA century (O'Donnell et al., 2009). The U.S. has experimented with the HTA since the 1990's, and around the same time, the Federal Government recognized a necessity for disease-specific Patient Outcomes Research Teams (PORTs). One of the earlier HTA models was introduced by Germany during its 2004 health care reform and focused on the independent health care body the Institute for Quality and Efficiency in Health Care (Institut für Qualität und Wirtschaftlichkeit im Gesund-heitswesen [IQWiG] (Institute for Quality and Efficiency in Health Care, 2004).

The initial system evolved into the contemporary Electronic Health Record (EHR) (Cantrill, 2010). Cantrill (2010) posited computer systems have progressed over time from a single central CPU with dumb workstations to networks with increased processing capabilities at each workstation. In 2006, the Portland Informatics Center (PIC) and the Portland Veterans Affairs Medical Center (PVAMC) developed a medication history collection technology that interfaced with the legacy EHR systems (Lesselroth, Felder, Adams, Cauthers, Dorr, Wong, & Douglas, 2009). Cantrill (2010) posited there had been little called-for response to the need for an overall system. The systems left HCOs with the creation of computer systems that do not integrate efficiently with each other.

Patients' expectations have made an impact on health care and have proved to be harder than projected. A study at Private Primary Health-Care Center in a semi-rural area in New Delhi was designed to ascertain elements of patient experience to access, staff care, and physician care. The purpose of the study was to determine which traits of each attribute are of utmost importance in patients' response to the services received (Ardey & Ardey, 2015). Investigation outcomes showed among the three attributes physician care was the most significant, closely followed by the staff care, with access having the least impact (Ardey & Ardey, 2015). In a comparative study of patient satisfaction noted there are five determinants of patient satisfaction.

1. Reliability: The capacity to accomplish the guaranteed service consistently and precisely.
2. Responsiveness: The preparedness to assist the patients and deliver quick service.
3. Assurance: The awareness and civility of employees and their talent to deliver trust and confidence.
4. Empathy: The establishment of caring and personalized attention to patients.
5. Tangibles: The presence of physical facilities, equipment, personal, and communiqué resources (Otani, Kurz, & Harris, 2005).

A significant reason for the difficulty in meeting patient expectations is reduced funding. HCOs are discovering old-style methodologies to quality management returns presented in economic terms, and are no longer passable (James, n.d.). The result was supporting the suggestion of a system to achieve high-quality care to be a front-runner to lower health care costs (Operations Research, 2007). Furthermore, connecting efficiency and quality has historically gone down the path of the old-style approach. The old-style approach accepts a negative rate of adjustment concerning efficiency and quality (Operations Research, 2007). Exploring how quality management returns presented in economics is imperative to understand the Joint Commission requirements and the readmissions reductions initiatives (James, n.d.).

Joint Commission

The Joint Commission authority established by the Centers for Medicare and Medicaid Services (CMS) became operative July 15, 2010. The Joint Commission mandate was to certify health plans, and hospitals in agreement with their CMS' Certification Number (CCN), identified as the Medicare Provider Number (The Joint Commission, 2010). Translated, an individual counterpart between a Joint Commission accreditation award and a hospital's CCN. A single accreditation award means one single CCN for one accreditation decision (The Joint Commission, 2010). A hospital's CMS CCN is the hospital's identification number connected to its Medicare provider agreement. However, the health plans are ranked by CMS using a number from one to six, depending on their compliance status (National Committee Quality Assurance [NCQA], 2016).

The National Committee Quality Assurance (NCQA) ranked approximately 1400 health plans and nearly 1000 of the HCOs based on the health plan and HCO clinical practices, patient satisfaction, and outcomes from NCQA previous surveys. Therefore, patient quality of care, safety, and satisfaction are crucial factors in the health care industry (NCQA, 2016). The CCN typically is used for acquiescing and studying the hospital's budget reports (The Joint Commission, 2010). The mandate requires health plans and hospitals to be Medicare-certified, be assigned a CCN, be accredited, and demonstrate meeting all the conditions of the governing bodies (The Joint Commission, 2010). The Joint Commission accredits over 20,000 HCOs and subsidiaries in the U.S. A preponderance of state governments identifies the Joint Commission accreditation as a form of licensure and the receipt of Medicaid compensation (Fremgmen, 2010).

Government Mandates

Government mandates have also changed requirements and pay structures of HCOs for quality of care (Public Law 111-5, n.d.). Mandates are succors necessary to protect the treatment of specific health conditions, certain types of healthcare providers, and some categories of dependents (Bihari, 2014). Quantities of health care succors are mandated by either state law, federal law, or both. Amongst the federal government and the states, there are approximately 2000 health insurance mandates (Oxley 101, 2014). The most critical mandate serving as a regulator to avoid fraud is the Sarbanes-Oxley Act 2002 (SOX) for health plans in health care and other businesses (Oxley 101, 2014). The SOX specifically explain, guide, and educate through the process. The SOX is mandatory for all health plans, and they must comply with SOX's rules and regulations, as far as accounting and compliance for the health care sector, and most importantly to regulate their claims and all finances involved in patient care (Oxley 101, 2014).

HEALTH CARE REFORMS

Regulations and technologies have given patients control over their care and the autonomy to choose innovative physicians able to deliver personal service. Continuous adherence to government requirements and insurance carrier demands requires software, hardware, and related components to ensure success. HCO need to safeguard patient information with secure storage of all compliance-related documentation. Ensuring the ability to control access, add, or modify records from patient information to billing and reconciliation of data. Regulators closely monitor health plans, such as the Department of Managed Health Care (DMHC), the Centers for Medicare & Medicaid Services (CMS), Independent Medical Reviewers (IMR), and the National Committee of Quality Assurance (NCQA), and other independent entities (Department of Managed Health Care [DMHC], 2015).

Regulators are continually looking at electronic data and regulating health plans' performance. Based on health care reports and audits results, the outcomes reflect quality assurance for members to assure overall compliance. Policies, health regulations, and government regulations affect various Health Care organizations and their members. The health care reforms discussed will be

1. Patient Protection and Affordable Care Act (PPACA);
2. Health Information Technology for Economic and Clinical Health Act of 2009 (HITECH);
3. The American Recovery and Reinvestment Act of 2009 (ARRA);
4. Health Insurance Portability and Accountability Act of 1996 (HIPPA);
5. Privacy Act of 1974; and the
6. Readmissions Reduction Program.

Patient Protection and Affordable Care Act (PPACA)

The PPACA, frequently summarized the Affordable Care Act (ACA) is related to overall quality for any HCO. A part of the overall quality is the ability to understand the care (Rosenbaum, 2011). For patients to obtain the quality of care and service, Senate Bill (SB) 853 management for threshold languages, mandates patients to have their care discussed in their languages for a clear understanding (Wu, 2015). SB853 mandates for health plans and providers to assist members in their threshold languages, such as

Chinese, and Spanish (main required languages). Health plans and physicians must hire and provide translators, leading to patient safety (Wu, 2015). However, most hire bilingual employees who translate when necessary.

The PPACA entails ten separate legislative titles with similar goals. PPACA relates to quality; the goal is to increase health-care value and efficiency while lessening lavish expenditures, allowing health-care system to be more accountable (Rosenbaum, 2011). The PPACA also invests in the development of a multi-payer National Quality Strategy and the creation of multi-payer quality and efficiency procedures to stimulate price procuring. The PPACA allows for better patient safety and all-embracing health information systems across both public and private insurers (Public Law 111-148, 2010). The long-term goal of the PPACA is to build on the Health Information Technology for Economic and Clinical Health (HITECH) Act of 2009.

Vital health assistance is a set of health care service required to be protected by individual plans. The PPACA safeguards health plans to bolster their position in the individual and small group markets (HealthCare.gov, n.d.). The Health Insurance Marketplace is compromising a comprehensive array of pieces and services, known as essential health benefits with Off Exchange Members (OEMs) (HealthCare.gov, n.d.). Vital health assistances requirements consist of 10 classifications. The classifications are as follows:

1. Ambulatory patient;
2. Emergency services;
3. Hospitalization; maternity and baby care;
4. Mental health and substance use malady services;
5. Behavioral health management;
6. Prescription drugs; rehabilitative and rehabilitative services and equipment;
7. Research laboratory services;
8. Preemptive and wellness services; and
9. Chronic disease management;
10. Pediatric services, containing oral and vision care (HealthCare.gov, n.d.).

Insurance policies have requirements including succors to be qualified and obtainable in the Health Insurance Marketplace (HealthCare.gov, n.d.). States expanding their Medicaid programs must provide the required benefits to people newly eligible for Medicaid, and who are in the low-income category (HealthCare.gov, n.d.).

The PPACA launched the Institute for Comparative Clinical Effectiveness Research (CCER). PPACA and CCER support the type of research essential to identifying the most appropriate and efficient health care for diverse patient populations (Rosenbaum, 2011). The initiatives of the PPACA and CCER are to improve quality and material, underlining efforts to accumulate statistics about health (Berenson, Paulus, & Kalman, 2012). Health care inequalities permit the U.S. HCOs opportunities to enhance measures of advancement with the prominent possibility for reduced health outcomes for both the population and subpopulations as well (Berenson, Paulus, & Kalman, 2012). For example, the sharing of standard databases has the possibility of assisting in the efficient conduct of business (Copeland, n.d).

The sharing could lead to an investigation in enterprise data warehousing, data mining, and data analytics capabilities for HCOs. Data mining combines techniques including statistical analysis, visualization, induction, and neural networks to explore large amounts of data and discover relationships and patterns that shed light on business problems (Rogers & Joyner, n.d.). HCOs can use the findings for more efficient, proactive decision making and obtaining a competitive advantage. Data mining is designed for exploiting massive amounts of data. The process can be more efficient initially if the organization problem is clearly identified followed by a explicit determination of the amount of data needed to solve the problem (Rogers & Joyner, n.d.).

A possible solution is intentionally recruiting upper level management during the infancy of the problem through the potential Return on Investment (ROI) or problem solving process. While applying a "bottom-up" method of data mining results in attainable goals and more widely accepted procedures (Rogers & Joyner, n.d.). Another initiative SOX protects the public and shareholders from accounting errors and fraud, and it provides accuracy for corporate organizations (Oxley 101, 2014). SOX audits all health plans to make sure health plans are up-to-date with their accounting ledgers and compliant. Some of the SOX requirements deal more with compliance than others, but mostly for-profit health plans (Oxley 101, 2014).

Health Information Technology for Economic and Clinical Health (HITECH) Act of 2009

The HITECH Act was ratified into law in 2009 as a measure of the American Recovery and Reinvestment Act of 2009 (ARRA) (Public Law 111-5, 2009). The Act attempted to increase the performance of health care systems from end to end through the use of technology, such as EHRs (Blumenthal, 2010). The HITECH Act focused on health organizations using certified EHRs. The Act expanded the federal government's ability to establish a national electronic patient records system by 2014 (APA Practice Organization, 2014). According to the requirements of the PPACA, the deadline has passed, and a national electronic patient records system has yet to be established. HCOs are trying to comply with the Act and are in a situation of influx, which needs addressing (Affordable Care Act [ACA], 2015).

The HITECH Act involves health consumers, hospitals in their care, and connects entire communities into more patient self-awareness. Leadership is critical for transforming challenges into opportunities. Some of the possibilities would promote preventive care at an affordable price, rather than paying higher premiums, depending on an individual's health care needs (Bentkover, 2012). The most critical task of leadership is establishing a mindset at the top of the organization and functioning to infuse a culture of excellence throughout the organization (Bentkover, 2012). HCOs progress when treating their members with integrity, value, and are single-mindedly committed to achieving a defined objective responsively for improved health care outcomes (Bentkover, 2012).

American Recovery and Reinvestment Act (ARRA) of 2009

Due to the economic crisis of 2008, the ARRA had three straightforward goals: creating new jobs while saving existing jobs, spurring economic activity, and investing in long-term growth fostering more accountability and transparency in government spending (Healthcare IT New, 2015). The law directed nearly $150 billion in new funds to the healthcare industry spending (Healthcare IT New, 2015). Commonly referred to as the Recovery Act, promoted performance reporting on a system-wide source allowing patients to readily access information about their health care and how their health-care providers perform (Public Law 111-5). The law also affirmed health care be consistent with quotas of the Health Care and Education Reconciliation Act (HCERA) of 2010 and the Student Aid and Fiscal

Responsibility Act along with the PPACA (Public Law 111-5). The Acts seeked to overhaul the current healthcare system. "ObamaCare" H.R. 3590, or Affordable Care Act (ACA) for short, turned out to be the most extensive renovation to health care reform since Medicare and Medicaid was signed into law in 1965 (Obamacare Facts, n.d.).

Health Insurance Portability and Accountability Act (HIPPA) of 1996

The introduction of HIPPA affected all health care providers, one-physician offices, health plans, employers, public health authorities, life insurers, clearinghouses, billing agencies, information systems vendors, service organizations and universities (Val Derde Regional Medical Center, 2015). For instance, physicians had to update their Business Associate Agreements (BAAs) and their Notices of Privacy Practices (NPPs) and ensure physicians understand the importance of encryption electronic protected health information (American Medical Association [AMA], 2015). Each health organization is not the same, and compliance responses are not standardized. For example, an organization with a computer network is required to implement one or more security authentication access mechanisms based on their network environment. The access mechanism may consist of user-based, role-based, and context-based access (Val Derde Regional Medical Center, 2015). Effective compliance requires organization-wide implementation.

Privacy Rule enforcement began on April 14, 2003, with implementation and enforcement controlled out of the Office of Civil Rights within the Department of Health and Human Services (DHHS). Civil and felonious consequences for non-compliance ranging from $100 to $250,000 per offense and up to 10 years incarceration. A presentation by Seymour (2010), posited the essential and relevant terms of the Privacy Rule are:

1. Covered entities: All health care providers, health plans and clearing houses which maintain patient data.
2. Protected Health Information (PHI): All individually identifiable health information and other information on treatment and care.
3. The patient retains protected Health Information: HIPAA gives patients' rights as to how PHI used. The Notice of Privacy Practices grants the right to view, inspect and copy one's PHI.
4. Individually Identifiable Health Information: A subset of PHI, including demographic information collected from an individual.
5. Consent: The communication process between caregiver and patient, referring to the use or disclosure of protected health information (PHI) to carry out treatment, payment or health care operations.
6. Authorization: The mechanism for obtaining consent from a patient for the use and disclosure of health information for nontreatment, payment or health care operations. For example, a written authorization required before a patient's health information included on a list for marketing purposes (para II HIPPA D Important and Relevant Terms).

The U.S. Department of Health and Human Services (HHS) adopted the rule, often referred to as the final "HIPAA Omnibus Rule." The rule began from changes made under the HITECH Act which is part of the same law creating EHR Incentive Programs under Medicare and Medicaid. The ACA expanded on provisions in HIPAA supporting administrative simplification. The requirements included operating rules for the HIPAA-named standards, a standard for electronic funds transfer, and a national health plan identifier.

Privacy Act of 1974

Since both the HIPPA and ARRA relate to privacy and record keeping, it is essential to understand the background of the Privacy Act of 1974. The Privacy Act of 1974 "protects records retrieved by personal recognizers such as a name, social security number, or other recognizing number or symbol" (U.S. Department of Health & Human Services{HHS}, n.d., para 2). The law prohibits the disclosure of records without the written consent of the individuals unless one of the twelve disclosure exceptions listed in the Act applies. The Privacy Act of 1974 created the System of Records Notices (SORNs) which necessitated health organizations to construct and retain SORNs. "A system of records consists of any item, collection, or grouping of information about an individual, where those records can be retrieved by the name of the individual or by some other type of identifier unique to the individual" (HHS, n.d., para 5). Shifting onto the Privacy Impact Assessments (PIAs), the "E-Government Act of 2002, requiring government agencies to assess the impact on privacy for systems that collect personally identifiable information in PIAs" (HHS, n.d., para 6).

Readmissions Reduction Program

Based on the PPACA, CMS computes the middle risk-adjusted, 30-day hospital-readmission amounts for patients with myocardial infarction, pneumonia, or heart failure via claims data (Berenson, Paulus, & Kalman, 2012). When a hospital's risk-adjusted readmission rate for such patients exceeds average risk, CMS and health plans discipline the hospital. The subsequent year for all Medicare admissions in part to its amount of excess readmissions of patients for the target conditions. A maximum punishment was set at 1% for 2013, ultimately reaching 3% of a hospital's Medicare payments. The CMS implementation reduces the potential penalties to 0.2% of federal Medicare payments in 2013 (Berenson, Paulus, & Kalman, 2012).

Except when they are at full capability, hospitals face two significant economic disincentives to dropping readmissions for the identified diagnoses: the direct costs of the program itself and decreased revenues resulting from effective interferences. Interferences to generate and withstand decreases in readmissions average $100 to $200 per discharge, typically (Berenson, Paulus, & Kalman, 2012). Overflowing can reduce hospitalizations for non-targeted diagnoses and drop readmissions from any cause even outside the 30-day window and across payers. Although the effects of reducing hospitalizations for non-targeted diagnoses and dropping readmissions are desirable outcomes for patients and payers, readmissions adversely mark hospitals' finances (Berenson, Paulus, & Kalman, 2012).

QUALITY HEALTH CARE DELIVERY, REPORTING AND INDICATORS

The health care reforms reflected the need to poise privacy protections with the public obligation to protect public health, conduct medical research, fight health care fraud and abuse, and improve the quality of care delivery (Val Derde Regional Medical Center, 2015). There has to be a focus on the quality of health care delivery and tools instrumental in the process (Department of Community and Family

Medicine, 2014). Before quality of health care delivery can be improved tools such as Involuntary Reporting, Patient Saefty Indicators (PSIs). Prevention Quality Indicators (PQIs); and Inpatient Quality Indicators(IQIs) need to be implemented by HCOs to provide better health care to patients (Val Derde Regional Medical Center, 2015).

Quality of Health Care Delivery

Quality of health care delivery is problematic because there is no clear and concise definition of quality and quality frequently depends on the patient (Department of Community and Family Medicine, 2014). The Health Services Research (HSR) evaluation of the quality of care established quality is an unspecified science and multidimensional. Even though the description is reasonably straightforward there is still no clear-cut definition (Steinwachs & Hughes, 2008). The intricacy in measuring quality derives from cracks in our understanding concerning diagnosis plans for patients. In turn the lack of understanding increases the probability of anticipated health outcomes changing (Steinwachs & Hughes, 2008).

Patients do not have to have the same anticipated health outcomes. Resulting in changes in the care for the same health problem for different patients, supplementary obscuring the measurement of quality of care patient (Department of Community and Family Medicine, 2014). In a succession of reports, the Institute of Medicine (IOM) termed ineffective care coordination as a cause of inadequate health care and introduced a series of reports recommended HIT to advance its quality process (National Research Council [NCR], 2013). Defined clinical benefits were:

1. Adequately maintained patient records.
2. No misplaced charts, notice of prescription medicine interactions.
3. Access to the most current educational information.
4. Printed prescriptions.
5. Improved patient communication options (NCR, 2013).

The IOM report requested changes in the delivery of health care or the medical model, focusing on the system rather than individual health care providers (Bleach, 2005).

After the recommendation, Congress created the Center for Patient Safety within the Agency for Healthcare Research and Quality (AHRQ) to augment the patient safety knowledge base (Bleach, 2005). The Center for Patient Safety led to the creation of specific research agendas; distributing grants for research on patient safety; and funding from the Centers of Excellence (Bleach, 2005). Having an understanding of policies and regulations, including the economics and financing of health care, facilitate the leadership process. Being a change agent and using continuous improvement to stay competitive in an ever-changing environment of health care leadership (Bleach, 2005). Three elements of using resources and assessments to help health care professionals identify their personality types, strengths, and other variables incorporated into a job or career fit:

1. The self-examination, which is the process of checking to make sure the person is going in the right direction.
2. The ability to rely on instinct and make decisions at times, coupled with the capacity to try to collect data to make the best decision possible.

3. Structure in an organization that will keep a leader focused and on track. When it comes to strengths, the race does not always go to the swiftest. The key is to stay persistent and never give up (Bleach, 2005).

Involuntary Reporting

The advantages of involuntary reporting include direct surveillance of providers or chart evaluation using initiate tools (AHRQ, 2014). Involuntary reporting remains a prominent foundation of information because the reporting is usually readily accessible. Frequently, involuntary reporting is used to attain an accurate account of what went wrong (Murff, Patel, Hripcsak, & Bateset, 2003). The limitations of voluntary reporting are there are no set procedures to review records. For example, in the studies, the data was provided by a two-step review process (Murff et al., 2003). If the health care provider's reviewers differ or if an adverse event occurred, the health care providers will try to come to an agreement or involve a third party (Murff et al., 2003). Typically, only a tiny portion of the charts are reviewed independently by two health care providers (Murff et al., 2003).

Notwithstanding the effectiveness of voluntary reporting systems in other industries, voluntary reporting in health care has been relatively ineffective (Murff et al., 2003). A framework accentuates analysis of the voluntary reporting and detailing progression improvements ascending from the analysis, rather than inspiring voluntary reporting for the sake of reporting (AHRQ, 2014). When there is no data and metrics, there is no reference point to know how the health care organization is doing. Without knowing how health care organizations compare to each other, there is no way to judge whether HCOs strategies are making a difference (Healthcare IT News, 2014).

Patient Safety Indicators (PSIs)

PSIs are a set of measures screening for contrary episodes patients experience as a consequence of contact with the U.S. health care system level (Agency for Research and Quality Indicators [AHRQ], 2006). The episodes are to be expected to range from amenable to prevention by changes at the system or provider level (AHRQ, 2006). PSIs make available a measure of possibly avoidable complication for patients receiving initial care and the difficulty of care within the same hospitalization (AHRQ, 2006). PSIs comprised of only episodes where a secondary diagnosis code flags a possibly avoidable difficulty. PSIs improve patient care by employing measures for the development and responsibility of patient care (AHRQ, 2006).

Prevention Quality Indicators (PQIs)

PQIs are utilized with hospital inpatient discharge information to recognize the quality of care for "ambulatory care delicate situations." Situations, where adequate outpatient care can theoretically avert the need for hospitalization or prompt interference, can avert difficulties or more severe diseases (AHRQ, n.d.a). Other preventive care services included are annual mammograms, preventive Ultrasounds, vision screenings, weight loss programs, and cholesterol screenings (AHRQ, n.d.a). The PQIs are populace based and adjusted for covariates. The gauges are grounded on hospital inpatient information, delivering understanding into the public health care system, or services external to the hospital setting (AHRQ, n.d.a).

Problem areas in health care need an auxiliary inquiry. Inquiries offer a fast check on primary care. Patient contact is common by using patient data established in hospital discharge abstract to aid public HCOs and other societies (AHRQ, n.d.a). An example of quality prevention indicator is a patient hospitalized for diabetes with diabetic difficulties. When the examination of the patient's circumstances is not practical or if a patient training requirement is needed for the proper self-management (AHRQ, n.d.a). PQIs are designed using voluntarily available hospital administrative information. The PQIs are a selection of instruments to aid finding a perspective on preventive care (AHRQ, n.d.a).

Inpatient Quality Indicators (IQIs)

IQIs are a method of delivering a viewpoint on hospital quality of care using hospital administrative information. IQIs reveal the quality of care esoteric to hospitals and comprise inpatient mortality for hospital quality and safety performance (Agency for Research and Quality Indicators, [AHRQ] n.d.b). Hospitals use of measures for which indication can advance the volume of procedures as it relates to lower mortality events (AHRQ, n.d.b). The IQIs are utilized to aid hospitals in recognizing impending difficult areas. Some areas require additional education by offering chances to evaluate the quality of care (AHRQ, n.d.b).

Esoteric to a hospital by authoritative information established in the general discharge record. The discharge records include mortality indicators for conditions. Indicators differ from hospital to hospital with varying processes; results connected to the bulk of the processes executed (AHRQ, n.d.b). Vendors have implemented standardized communication protocols such as the Health Level 7 (HL7). Interoperability has enhanced the exchange of information (Health Level 7 [HL7], 2009). The (HL7) criterion allowed information to be ascribed as a viewer for self-reporting, to provide a determination of contradictory information as standards were not universally accepted (HL7, 2009).

Some HIT modules can connect without alteration, while others need improvement to ensure data can be collected, stored, and shared. Despite the fact moving from legacy HIT systems to innovative systems is perplexing, particularly in general practitioner practices (Zandieh, Yoon-Flannery, & Kuperman, 2008). The American Recovery and Reinvestment Act of 2009 offer incentives for a national standard of HIT systems. Most hospitals can alter their HIT systems, patient intake observations, and internal usage. Clinics need organization headquarters to make modifications. The commitment and provision of a hospital's IT department are significant to the achievement of efforts (AHRQ, 2014).

DISCUSSION

The previous ten years have seen numerous industries enter an age of progressively sudden transformation. The most recent global decline, which began in December 2007, has contributed to an environment many believe is fundamentally different from ten years ago (Petrie, 2015). A starting point for organizations may come from aiding their people through redefining what is meant by the term leadership. There has been a significant trend among organizational theorists to shift the focus from leadership as an individual or as a role to leadership as a process (Petrie, 2015). To understand leadership as a shared process, rather than an individual skill set, senior executives must contemplate the best way to help leadership flourish in their respective organizations (Petrie, 2015).

The variances in career experiences are possible influences on the development of leadership skills (Russell & Kuhnert, 1992). The common trait of leadership theories is useful leadership performance. Having the right person in the leadership role who has intellectual depth and insight is paramount in solving issues arising in the HCO. Even though numerous HCO's have created and implemented training initiated to assist leaders with higher performance outcomes, regrettably, the training has not created higher performing leaders (Russell & Kuhnert, 1992). Policymakers realized the significant investment required in human resources as critical to the success of the organization to hasten the method of economic development (Hinami, Whelan, Konetzka, & Meltzer, 2012).

A possible solution is combining different leadership theories or career path development influenced by leaders in different roles to gain higher performance out of HCO leadership (Russell & Kuhnert, 1992). HCOs leadership understanding of the patient's definition of quality is problematic (Hinami, Whelan, Konetzka, & Meltzer, 2012). There is no precise definition of quality; frequently quality depends on the patient's health. Therefore, HCOs leaders are continually implementing new safety patient conduct. When viewing a patient's definition of quality from the standpoint of understanding systems and key processes, developing a concrete definition in a performance improvement project is a difficult task (Hinami, Whelan, Konetzka, & Meltzer, 2012).

From a mapping standpoint, critical for the health care professional to determine how proficiently they understand the mechanism of patient safety, quality, and quality improvement (Hinami, Whelan, Konetzka, & Meltzer, 2012). Additionally, preferences and understandings about provider roles are not uniform; different preferences exist around decision-making processes. Variations between providers and patients result in dissatisfaction and even malpractice. While constructive uniformities in studies have shown the potential to form continuing relationships (Hinami, Whelan, Konetzka, & Meltzer, 2012). HCO leadership can envision chances for improvement (HRSA, 2011). Giving the opportunity to improved procedures in comparison to currently practiced procedures (HRSA, 2011).

HCO leaders maneuver in an environment of ambiguity and overwhelming density. Problems are no longer straightforward; problems are involved, and at times, contain no clear-cut answers. The environment is creating a new thinking process for effective leaders to maintain success (HRSA, 2011). The problem should be viewed differently, due to the challenges mentioned above and patient safety as well as active communication. The use of a system's approach makes creating a new system more accessible than fixing or eliminating an old system, due to high expenses in health care (HRSA, 2011).

Sociologist Robert K. Merton devised the phrase "goal displacement" to define conforming to rigid procedures becoming the goal, rather than looking at the whole organization (Reed, 2006). The world was imagined by theorists such as Isaac Newton, as having the features of a clock. Mechanisms of the clock are possibly understandable by the progression of exploration and the systematic method (Reed, 2006). Reed (2006) implied the fundamental premise as follows:

1. Identify a system, not all things are systems. Some systems are straightforward and predictable, while other systems are complex and dynamic.
2. Explain the behavior or properties of the entire system. Focus on the whole systems is the process of synthesis. The exploration looks into things while synthesis looks out of things.
3. Explain the actions or properties of the thing to be explained regarding the role(s) or function(s) of the whole.

Transformational Leadership

The role of the health care organization and its leadership in implementing and sustaining continuous performance improvement is essential in enabling patient-centered care (Frampton, et al., 2008). Leadership and change-management strategies comprised of the patient and staff rounding, fireside or chair-side chats, and clinician, employee and board engagement, are effective ways to reinforce the foundation for patient-centered care (Frampton, et al., 2008). When describing and discussing leadership requirements essential to leading a productive organization. Leadership competencies are imperative. Leadership competencies are leadership talents and activities giving a higher performance for leaders (Society for Human Resource Management [SHRM], 2015).

To become an active HCO describing and discussing HCO leadership requirements is vital. Leadership competencies are leadership talents and activities yielding higher performance (SHRM, 2015). Constructing a distinctive leadership brand via leadership competencies yielding results to stakeholders, organizations gain a competitive advantage and a better image (SHRM, 2015). Leaders have grasped the need to address patient challenges and the realities of the branding processes. Agents at the Center for Creative Leadership recognized a couple of essential leadership competencies, constant among all organizations. The table separates the structure into competencies for leading the organization, leading the self, and leading others in the organization (SHRM, 2015). Shown in Table 1 are the constant competencies.

For a transformative change to be an active development, the change needs to meet each person where the "person is and open the door" (Center for Creative Leadership [CCL], 2015). Transformational leaders have reliability and high Emotional Intelligence (EI). Transformational leaders motivate individuals with a collective vision of the future, and they communicate well (CCL, 2015). Transformational leaders frequently are self-aware, genuine, and compassionate (CCL, 2015). Transformational leaders convince members to be responsible because they anticipate the best in individuals and hold themselves responsible for their actions, while simultaneously treating their members with respect and integrity (CCL, 2015). Using transformational leadership leads to high efficiency and commitment towards patient care and communication(CCL, 2015). Leadership is not a "one size fits all" concept; frequently, leaders must adapt leadership approach to fit the circumstances and must make rational decisions (CCL, 2015).

Table 1: Leadership Competencies Adapted from McCauley (2006).

Leading the Organization:	Leading the Self:	Leading Others:
Managing change	Demonstrating ethics and integrity	Communicating effectively with patient safety
Solving problems and making decisions	Displaying drive and purpose	Developing others
Managing politics and influencing others	Exhibiting leadership stature	Valuing diversity and difference
Taking risks and innovating	Increasing capacity to learn	Building and maintaining relationships
Setting vision and strategy	Managing oneself	Managing effective teams and workgroups
Managing the work	Increasing self-awareness	Delivering quality services
Enhancing business skills and knowledge	Developing adaptability	Educating others
Understanding and navigating the organization	Self-growth	Attaining membership

Strategies

Chathoth and Olsen (2002) emphasized the significance of organizational leadership, while other research focused on being central to the success of organizations. Organizational leadership is particularly for entities such as HCOs which are international and vibrant worldwide (Chathoth & Olsen, 2002). Direction and change management strategies, comprising of the patient and staff rounding, fireside or chair-side chats, clinician, employee and board engagement (Framptin et al., 2008). The strategies are effective ways to reinforce the foundation for patient-centered care Quality improvement in the U.S. health care industry is best defined by examining the driving forces affecting the industry (Framptin et al., 2008).

How can U.S. HCOs lower cost, raise quality, and remain competitive? In the past, businesses have amassed growing amounts of data in large databases (Rogers & Joyner, n.d.) The stockpiles mainly contain customer or patient data, the unique "gold" the competition lacks (Rogers & Joyner, n.d.). The data's hidden value, the potential to predict business trends and customer behavior, has mostly gone untapped. The opportunity to tap data's vast knowledge for better, faster and more accurate clinical diagnosis has mostly been unused (Rogers & Joyner, n.d.).

The model for use in health care analytics was developed by Dale Sanders, who during his work in the U.S. military, saw the same patterns in data engineering as those in software engineering before Object-Oriented Programming (OOP) (Ahier, 2014). While employed by TRW Inc., Mr. Sanders was sponsored in the late 1990s by the Pentagon to study advanced decision support in nuclear warfare operations, a project called the Strategic Execution Decision Aid (Ahier, 2014). For reinforcement, Mr. Sanders turned to the health care industry for role-model samples of computer-aided analytics to drive better decisions in time-critical, life-critical conditions (Ahier, 2014). Unfortunately, Mr. Sanders found nearly no examples, with the notable exception of a scattered few such as the Intermountain Healthcare in Salt Lake City (Ahier, 2014). Technology is a valuable tool for health plans to provide better care and quality assurance using analytics (DMHC, 2015).

Meaningful Use enticement payments seem to be stimulating implementation. EHRs may improve the ability for HCOs to collect useful data by increasing public and inhabitant's health (HealthCare.gov, n.d.). Consequently, gathering information in a form used across many HCOs, influenced quality improvement and deterrence undertakings (HealthCare.gov, n.d.). A notable example of quality improvement and deterrence undertakings is EHRs used to increase reporting capabilities through public health recording and scrutiny. Thus, allowing a more accessible path for HCOs to gather standardized, methodical data (HealthCare.gov, n.d.).

Health plans must be ready at any time to be audited by SOX to demonstrate best practices to avoid fraud (Oxley 101, 2014). In conjunction with the accessibility of newer and better EHR tools and the increasing focus on assimilating care in Accountable Care Organizations (ACO) (Oxley 101, 2014). Data collected from the EHR can improve quality through syndromic scrutiny data compliance, immunization registries, and electronic laboratory reporting. Providers can convey public and populace health statistics to public health officials (HealthCare.gov, n.d.). With the abundant availability of data accessible, public health organizations can enhance monitoring, preventing, and managing of diseases (HealthCare.gov, n.d.).

North Carolina initiated a planned program influencing EHRs to use public health alerts to providers on specific conditions in patients' records (Lurio, Morrison, Pichardo Berg, Buck, Wu, Kitson, Mostashari, & Calman, 2010). Electronic health information on the general population of patients allow for addressing the needs of patients indirectly and improving overall health care (Lurio, et al., 2010). An

HCOs ability to prevent disease enables providers the opportunity to send prompts to patients for preventive/follow-up care, and provide physicians' notes and updates on medical procedures (HealthCare.gov, n.d.). As a result, implementing continuous process improvements and quality management in health care can improve patient care (Lurio, et al., 2010). In conjunction with communication among health care providers and public health officials, including patient safety Quality measurement has progressed significantly, resting primarily in the early development stage (Lurio, et al., 2010).

The insurance industry has started using Electronic Data Interchange (EDI) for health care claims, procedure authorization, and payments. EDI "is defined as the direct computer-to-computer exchange of standard business forms" (References for Business, n.d. p. 1). The critical idea involved is the exchange of documents that allow a business application to take place without human intervention (References for Business, n.d.). Data communication is required for the exchange to take place. Universities are using EDI for sending grade transcripts, interlibrary material requests, and student loan information (References for Business, n.d.).

Retailers are sending EDI inventory data to suppliers and charging them with oversight of inventory levels and shipment initiation (References for Business, n.d.). The federal government and most states are now using EDI to collect tax filings. EDI is well established as a useful technology, reducing costs and increasing efficiency (References for Business, n.d.). EDI technologies are approximately the same age as Internet technologies (Copeland, n.d.). As the two technological communities begin to merge and as the business community sees the advantages of this merger, EDI and the Internet will eventually become ubiquitous (Copeland, n.d.).

The EDI working group at present has a charter for an interoperability standard for process-to-process EDI. Once that standard is in place, real-time EDI over the Internet will replace normal time-delayed, batch-style interactions (Copeland, n.d). An Enterprise Data Warehouse (EDW) forms the foundation for health care analytics. Most large HCOs have hundreds of different technology solutions from various vendors (Health Catalyst, 2014). There is a need to bring all data into a single foundation of organizational truth; it is difficult to provide reliable and repeatable reporting and analysis. From the foundation of the EDW, organizations can progress to registries and reports, population health, clinical and financial risk modeling (Health Catalyst, 2014).

CONCLUSION

Health care system must work to distinguish all relevant resources, real-time access information, and analyze what-if scenarios (Prior, 2006). In multifaceted HCOs, efficiency goals are not the ultimate level of success. HCOs need to realize efficiency goals to assist with meeting more difficult targets (Frampton, et al., 2008). The general atmosphere must utilize a remarkably designed method in the quest for quality management (James, n.d.). Health care reforms such as the Affordable Care Act, which represented two distinct pieces of legislation, the PPACA (P.L. 111-148) and the HCERA (P.L. 111-152) have changed the standards for improvement (Public Law 111-148, 2010).

Continuous improvement necessitates a transformation from the way HCOs have customarily provided care. HCOs leadership must improve patients' communication devise strategies and other strategies for connecting with patients (Department of Community and Family Medicine, 2014). A central degree of quality is defined as the extent to which patients' necessities and anticipations encountered to their liking (HRSA, 2011). Patients share involvement and or apprehension in the continuous improvement process

(Department of Community and Family Medicine, 2014). The vision for the CMS Quality Strategy is to optimize health outcomes by leading clinical quality improvement, and health system transformation (Centers for Medicare and Medicaid Services.gov, 2016).

The CMS Quality Strategy built from the foundation of the CMS Strategy, NCQA, and the Health Human Services (HHS) National Quality Strategy (NQS) (Centers for Medicare and Medicaid Services. gov, 2016). Like the NQS, the CMS Quality Strategy developed through a participatory, transparent, and collaborative process, including the contribution of a wide array of stakeholders (Prior, 2006). For more than a year, a group of leaders from across CMS met and developed the strategy. The group also sought out advice and input from other HHS agencies, the community, and CMS beneficiaries to inform their efforts (Prior, 2006). Driving quality improvement, and patient safety is a core function of CMS. Commitment is necessary for CMS to enhance partnerships with a delivery system. The goal is for providers to achieve maximum outcomes in health care and lower overall health care cost (NCR, 2013).

REFERENCES

Affordable Care Act (ACA). (2015). *Affordable Care Act and Title X Program*. Retrieved from: http://www.hhs.gov/opa/affordable-care-act/index.html

Agency for Healthcare Research and Quality (AHRQ). (2014). *Voluntary Patient Safety Event Reporting (Incident Reporting)*. Retrieved from: http://psnet.ahrq.gov/primer.aspx?primerID=13

Agency for Research and Quality Indicators. (2006). *Patient Safety Indicators*. Retrieved from: https://www.qualityindicators.ahrq.gov/Downloads/Modules/PSI/V30/2006-Feb-PatientSafetyIndicators.pdf

Agency for Research and Quality Indicators. (n.d.a). *Inpatient Quality Indicators Overview*. Retrieved from: www.ualityindicators.ahrq.gov/Modules/iqi_resources.aspx

Agency for Research and Quality Indicators. (n.d.b). *Prevention Quality Indicators Overview*. Retrieved from: www.qualityindicators. ahrq.gov/Modules/pqi_resources.aspx

Ahier, B. (2014). *Healthcare Analytics: Realizing the Value of Health IT*. Retrieved from: https://www.healthcatalyst.com/analytics-realizing-the-value-of-health-it

APA Practice Organization. (2014). *The Health Information Technology For Economic and Clinical Health Act (HITECH Act)*. Retrieved from:httptp://www.apapracticecentral.org/advocacy/technology/hitech-act.aspx

Ardey, R., & Ardey, R. (2015). Patient Perceptions and Expectations From Primary Health-care Providers in India. *Journal of Family Medicine and Primary Care*, *4*(1), 53–63. doi:10.4103/2249-4863.152254 PMID:25810990

Bentkover, J., & Ph, D. (2012). Executive Master of Healthcare Leadership, Brown University. *Leadership is Central to Healthcare System Reform*. Retrieved from: http://www.beckershospitalreview.com/hospital-management-administration/leadership-is-central-to-healthcare-system-reform.html

Berenson, R., Paulus, R., & Kalman, N. (2012). Medicare's Readmissions-Reduction Program - A Positive Alternative. *The New England Journal of Medicine*, *366*(15), 1364–1366. doi:10.1056/NEJMp1201268 PMID:22455754

Bihari, M. (2014). *Mandated Benefits - Understanding Mandated Health Insurance Benefits: Health Benefit Mandates Are Controversial*. Retrieved from: http://healthinsurance.about.com/od/reform/a/mandated_benefits_overview.htm

Bleach, S. (2005). *Medical Errors: Five Years After the IOM Report. Issue Brief*. Retrieved from: http://www.commonwealthfund.org/usr_doc/830_Bleich_errors.pdf

Blumenthal, D. (2010). Launching HITECH. *The New England Journal of Medicine*, 362–385. PMID:20042745

Cantrill, S. (2010). Computers in Patient Care: The Promise and the Challenge. *Communications of the ACM*, *53*(9), 42–47. doi:10.1145/1810891.1810907

Center for Creative Leadership (CCL). (2015). *Nearly 70% of all change efforts fail. We can do better*. Retrieved from: http://www.ccl.org/leadership/landing/leadingContinousChange.aspx

Centers for Medicare and Medicaid Services.gov. (2016). *CMS Quality Strategy Update*. Retrieved from: www.cms.gov/Medicare/Quality-Initiatives-Patient-Assessment-Instruments/QualityInitiativesGenInfo/Downloads/CMS-Quality-Strategy.pdf

Chathoth, P., & Olsen, M. (2002, April-September). Organizational Leadership and Strategy in the Hospitality Industry. *Journal of Services Research*, *2*(1).

Copeland, W. (n.d.). *Electronic Data Interchange: Concepts and Effects*. Retrieved from: https://www.isoc.org/inet97/proceedings/C5/C5_1.HTM

Department of Community and Family Medicine. (2014). *What is Quality Improvement? How Do You Define Quality?* Retrieved from: http://patientsafetyed.duhs.duke.edu/module_a/introduction/define_quality.html

Department of Managed Health Care (DMHC). (2015). *DMHC regulates Health Plans and Helps health plan members and providers*. Retrieved from: http://www.dmhc.ca.gov

E-Source. (n.d.). *Behavioral and Social Science Research. Evaluating the Quality of Health Care*. Retrieved from: www.esourceresearch.org/Portals/0/Uploads/Documents/Public/Cleary_FullChapter.pdf

Frampton, S., Guastello, S., Brady, C., Hale, M., Horowitz, S., Smith, S. B., & Stone, S. (2008). *The Patient-Centered Care Improvement Guide*. Derby, CT: The Planetree Association and The Picker Institute.

Fremgmen, B. (2010). *Medical Law and Ethics Prentice* (3rd ed.). Upper Saddle River, NJ: Prentice Hall.

Haj, H., Lamrini, M., & Rais, N. (2013). Quality of Care Between Donabedian Model and ISO9001V2008. *International Journal of Quality Research, 7*(1), 17–30.

Health Catalyst. (2014). *Late-Binding™ Data Warehouse Platform*. Retrieved from: https://www.healthcatalyst.com/late-binding-data-warehouse-platform

Health Industry Insights, an IDC Company. (2009). *The Future of Business and Clinical Intelligence in the U.S. Provider Market.* Retrieved from: http://www-07.ibm.com/solutions/au/healthcare/presentations/downloads/The_Future_of_Business_Clinical.pdf

Health Level 7. (2009). *What is HL7?* Retrieved from: www.hl7.org/about/hl7about.htm

Healthcare, I. T. New. (2014). *Deaths by medical mistakes hit records: The way IT is designed remains part of the problem.* Retrieved from: http://www.healthcareitnews.com/news/deaths-by-medical-mistakes-hit-records

Healthcare, I. T. New. (2015). *American Recovery and Reinvestment Act (ARRA).* Retrieved from: http://www.healthcareitnews.com/directory/american-recovery-and-reinvestment-act-arra

HealthCare.gov. (n.d.). *Essential Health Benefits.* Retrieved from: www.healthcare.gov/glossary/essential-health-benefits

Hinami, K., Whelan, C. T., Konetzka, R. T., & Meltzer, D. O. (2012). Provider expectations and experiences of comanagement. *Journal of Hospital Medicine, 6*(7), 401–404. doi:10.1002/jhm.914 PMID:21916002

Institute for Quality and Efficiency in Health Care. (2004). *The Institute.* Retrieved from: https://www.iqwig.de/en/home.2724.html

James, B. (n.d.). *Quality Management for Health Care Delivery. The Hospital Research and Educational Trust of the American Hospital Association.* Retrieved from: www.ghdonline.org/uploads/QMMP.pdf

Kumar, A., & Shim, S. J. (2005). Using computer simulation for surgical care process reengineering in hospitals. *Information Systems and Operational Research, 43*(4), 303–319. doi:10.1080/03155986.2005.11732732

Lesselroth, B., Felder, R., Adams, S., Cauthers, P., Dorr, D., Wong, G., & Douglas, D. (2009). Design and implementation of a medication reconciliation kiosk: The Automated Patient History Intake Device (APHID). *Journal of the American Medical Informatics Association, 16*(3), 300–304. doi:10.1197/jamia.M2642 PMID:19261949

Lurio, J., Morrison, F. P., Pichardo, M., Berg, R., Buck, M. D., Wu, W., ... Calman, N. (2010). Using electronic health record alerts to provide public health situational awareness to clinicians. *Journal of the American Medical Informatics Association, 17*(2), 217–219. doi:10.1136/jamia.2009.000539 PMID:20190067

McCauley, C. (2006). *Developmental Assignments: Creating Learning Experiences without Changing Jobs.* Retrieved from: www.worldcat.org/title/adaptability-responding-effectively-to-change/oclc

Murff, H. J., Patel, V. L., Hripcsak, G., & Bateset, D. W. (2003). Detecting adverse events for patient safety research: A review of current methodologies. *Journal of Biomedical Informatics, 36*(1), 131–143. doi:10.1016/j.jbi.2003.08.003 PMID:14552854

National Committee for Quality Assurance (NCQA). (2016). *Health Insurance Plan Rankings.* Retrieved from: http://www.ncqa.org/report-cards/health-plans/health-insurance-plan-rankings

National Research Council. (2013). *Core Measurement Needs for Better Care, Better Health, and Lower Costs: Counting What Counts: Workshop Summary*. Washington, DC: The National Academies Press.

O'Donnell, J., Pham, S., Pashos, C., Miller, D., Smith, M. (2009). *Health Technology Assessment: Lessons Learned from Around the World—An Overview. Value In Health*. Wiley-Blackwell. doi:10.1111/j.1524-4733.2009.00550.x

Obamacare Facts. (n.d.). *Obamacare Bill: Full PPACA & Related Laws*. Retrieved from: http://obamacarefacts.com/obamacarebill

Operations Research. (2007). *The Science of Better*. Retrieved from: The Science of Better website: www.scienceofbetter.org

Otani, K., Kurz, R. S., & Harris, L. E. (2005). Managing primary care using patient satisfaction measures. *Journal of Healthcare Management, 50*(5), 311–325. doi:10.1097/00115514-200509000-00007 PMID:16268410

Oxley 101. (2014). *Confused by SOX Compliance?* Retrieved from: www.sarbanes-oxley-101.com

Petrie, N. (2015). *Future Trends in Leadership Development*. Retrieved from: http://www.ccl.org/wp-content/uploads/2015/04/futureTrends.pdf

Prior, D. (2006). Efficiency and total quality management in health care organizations: A dynamic frontier approach. *Annals of Operations Research, 145*(1), 281–299. doi:10.100710479-006-0035-6

Public Law 111-148. (2010). *The American Recovery and Reinvestment Act (ARRA)*. Retrieved from: www.gpo.gov/fdsys/pkg/PLAW-111publ148/pdf/PLAW-111publ148.pdf

Public Law 111-5. Medicaid.gov. (n.d.). *Affordable Care Act*. Retrieved from: http://www.gpo.gov/fdsys/pkg/PLAW-111publ148/pdf/PLAW-111publ148.pdfPublic Law 111-5.

Reed, G. E. (2006). *Leadership and Systems Thinking*. Defense AT&L. Retrieved from: www.au.af.mil/au/awc/awcgate/dau/ree_mj06.pdf

References for Business. (n.d.). *Electronic Data Interchange (EDI) eCommerce Fulfillment*. Retrieved from: http://www.referenceforbusiness.com/encyclopedia/Eco-Ent/Electronic-Data-Interchange-EDI.html

Rogers, R., & Ellen, J. (n.d.). *Mining your Data for Health Care Quality Improvement*. Retrieved from: http://www2.sas.com/proceedings/sugi22/EMERGING/PAPER139.PDF

Rosenbaum, S. (2011). The Patient Protection and Affordable Care Act: Implications for Public Health Policy and Practice. *Public Health Reports, 126*(1), 130–135. doi:10.1177/003335491112600118 PMID:21337939

Ruffin, T. R. (2015). Health Information Technology and Business Process Reengineering. In M. Khosrow-Pour (Ed.), Encyclopedia of Information Science and Technology (3rd ed.; pp. 3355–3365). Hershey, PA: IGI Global. doi:10.4018/978-1-4666-5888-2.ch329

Russell, C., & Kuhnert, K. (1992). Integrating skill acquisition and perspective-taking capacity in the development of leaders. *The Leadership Quarterly, 3*, 109–135. doi:10.1016/1048-9843(92)90029-F

Seymour, M. (Presenter). (2002). *The Method and the Magic: Ethics and Information Management*. CASE District VII Conference, Anaheim, CA. Retrieved from: http://www.usc.edu/dept/source/HIPPA.html

Society for Human Resource Management (SHRM). (2015). *Leadership Competencies*. Retrieved from: http://www.shrm.org/research/articles/articles/pages/leadershipcompetencies.aspx

Steinwachs, D. M., & Hughes, R. G. (2008). Health Services Research: Scope and Significance. In *Patient Safety and Quality: An Evidence-Based Handbook for Nurses*. Rockville, MD: Agency for Healthcare Research and Quality (US). Retrieved from: http://www.ncbi.nlm.nih.gov/books/NBK2660

The Joint Commission. (2010). *Frequently Asked Questions about Accrediting Hospitals in Accordance with their CMS' Certification Number (CCN)*. Retrieved from: www.jointcommission.org/faqs_ccn/default.aspx

United States Congress House of Representatives. (1967). *Committee on Science and Astronautics. Technology assessment*. Statement of Emilio QDaddario, chair, Subcommittee on Science, Research, and Development. Washington: 90th Congress, 1st session; 1967. pp. 9–13.

United States Department of Health & Human Services (HHS). (n.d.). *Privacy*. Retrieved from: http://www.hhs.gov/foia/privacy

United States Department of Health and Human Services Health Resources and Service Administration (HRSA). (2011). *Quality Improvement. Part 1: Quality Improvement (QI) and the Importance of QI*. Retrieved from: www.hrsa.gov/quality/toolbox/methodology/qualityimprovement

Val Derde Regional Medical Center. (2015). *Health Insurance Portability and Accountability Act (HIPAA)*. Retrieved from: http://www.vvrmc.org/hipaa.html

Wu, E. (2015). *SB853 Bill Health Care language assistance*. Retrieved from http://cpehn.org/policy-center/cultural-and-linguistic-competency/sb-853-health-care-language-assistance-act

Zandieh, S. O., Yoon-Flannery, G. J., Kuperman, D., Langsam, D. J., Hyman, D., & Kaushal, R. (2008). Challenges to EHR implementation in electronic- versus paper-based office practices. *Journal of General Internal Medicine*, *23*(6), 755–761. doi:10.100711606-008-0573-5 PMID:18369679

KEY TERMS AND DEFINITIONS

Center for Creative Leadership: A website used by many for leadership development to assist with developing a framework for leaders in the healthcare industry.

Healthcare Organizations: Organized bodies of medical practitioners with a goal to deliver quality care to patients.

Healthcare Reform: Policies or regulation adopted to assist with the development and growth of quality in healthcare.

Leadership: The action of leading a group of people in a healthcare organization.

Organizational Development: A practice committed to increasing knowledge and efficiency of people in leadership positions to become more successful in healthcare organizations.

Quality Indicators: Created to measure the accessibility, success, and performance of healthcare.

Quality Management: The processes of ensuring healthcare services are consistent throughout healthcare organizations.

Society for Human Resource Management: A website used for by human resources for strategic management process in healthcare organizations.

Technology: The application of scientific knowledge to improve healthcare outcomes in the healthcare industry.

Transformational Leadership: Leadership approach implementing positive changes in followers and acts as a change agent in healthcare organizations.

Chapter 10
Health Literacy in School

S. M. Yasir Arafat
Bangabandhu Sheikh Mujib Medical University, Bangladesh

Md. Anwarul Azim Majumder
The University of the West Indies, Barbados

Russell Kabir
Anglia Ruskin University, UK

Konstantinos Papadopoulos
Middlesex University, UK

Md. Saleh Uddin
Chittagong Medical College Hospital, Bangladesh

ABSTRACT

Health literacy is a core element of patient-centered healthcare. Poor health literacy is a silent epidemic across the globe as it affects every aspect of health. Schools bear an important role in increasing health literacy. Improving health literacy in adolescence is supposed to improve the later life as adolescents are used to carry their modified behavior lifelong. Various school-based interventions covering physical and mental health have been studied and found to be effective. International bodies recommend incorporation of health-related tasks into school lessons and considered that teaching the young people will be a good investment for future. Multisectoral collaborations and locally proved effective strategies are the practical challenges. This chapter aims to focus on health literacy, global scenario of health literacy, measurement tools, role of school, interventions, limitations, and challenges of health literacy.

INTRODUCTION

In this contemporary and consumer driven world, education is considered as an important tool to increase income, reduce poverty, employ equality and justice, ensure sustainable growth and improve quality of health (United Nations General Assembly, 2015). Since 2000, preprimary education enrollment increased almost two third globally (UNESCO, 2015). According to UNESCO institute for statistics (2015), the

DOI: 10.4018/978-1-5225-4074-8.ch010

youth literacy is 91% and adult rate is 85% around the globe (UNESCO, 2014). Health literacy is a domain which is directly connected to education. As a term "Health literacy" was mentioned first in 1974 in an article titled "Health Education as Social Policy" (Mancuso, 2008; Peerson & Saunders, 2009). In past 30 years, more attention has been given to health literacy and it has gained popularity in most parts of the world (Berkman, Davis, & McCormack, 2010). But, still the definition of health literacy is yet to be unified and different authors, organizations, institutions, such as American Medical Association (AMA), WHO and Institute of Medicine (IOM) (Palumbo, 2015; Serper et al., 2014; Dickson-Swift, Kenny, Farmer, Gussy, & Larkins, 2014; Sørensen et al., 2012), defined it differently. Most widely used definition mentioned, health literacy as an "individual skills to obtain, process and understand health information and services necessary to make appropriate health decisions" (Dickson-Swift, Kenny, Farmer, Gussy, & Larkins, 2014; Sørensen et al., 2012). Dan Nutbeam preferred three typologies of health literacy mentioned as functional health literacy, interactive health literacy, and critical health literacy (Nutbeam, 2008; Nutbeam, 2000; Sørensen et al., 2012). For the better understanding about health literacy and school involvement in health issues, authors reviewed updated researches and documents. This chapter thoroughly described about global status of health literacy, measurement tools of health literacy, role of school in health literacy, interventions in school setting to improve health literacy, limitations & challenges of health literacy.

BACKGROUND

Health literacy (HL) is an important determinant of both public health as well as individual healthcare and is considered a core element of patient centered healthcare (Altin, Finke, Kautz-Freimuth, & Stock, 2014) where patients play a greater role in gaining and utilizing information about their health (Manganello, 2008). Although the concept prevailed before the term health literacy was coined first in 1974 in discussions regarding health education (Peerson & Saunders, 2009; Sørensen et al., 2012), since then its importance has increased as it is concerned with the individual's capacity to meet the complex health needs in this modern world (Sørensen et al., 2012). It covers the fields of health and education and builds an individual's ability to enjoy good health throughout the life span (Ghanbari, Ramezankhani, Montazeri, & Mehrabi, 2016).

Healthcare sector around the world rotates an ostensibly endless process of communicating health information clearly and tries to make sure that it is comprehended clearly. To provide safe and effective practice in the healthcare sector, the system is designed in such a way that structure, processes, tools and techniques should be in place for proper delivery of health information. Health care system should include and provide facilities related to health literacy (Osborne, 2012). It has been considered as a key determinant of health (Watson, 2011; Kickbusch, 2001) and its improvement is a practical approach to implement preventive strategies among the general population (Diemer et al, 2017). Recent evidence suggests that, health literacy has gained increased importance in public health, health promotion and clinical care (Liu, Liu, Li, & Chen, 2015). It is closely linked with knowledge, motivation, competency to access, understand, appraise and apply information to form and to make decisions related to healthcare (Sørenson, 2013). For adults with limited literacy or numeracy skills and with reduced functional skills, health literacy is viewed as a contemporary effort to foster adults' ability to manage their health (Marks, 2012).

HEALTH LITERACY

Global Scenario

Currently optimum health literacy is a prime concern globally and poor literacy in health is a silent epidemic that is threatening the health service across the globe (Palumbo, 2015; Sørensen et al., 2012; Parker & Ratzan, 2010). Inadequate health literacy is a concerning problem both in developed and developing countries and the portion with poor health literacy ranges from a quarter to a third of the population (How, 2011). In United States National Assessment of Adult Literacy (NAAL) in 2003 revealed only 12% of US adults were found to have proficient health literacy (Koh et al., 2012), 52% were found to have intermediate health literacy, 22% were found to have basic percent, 14% were found to have below basic health literacy (Vernon, Trujillo, Rosenbaum, & Debuono, 2007), & approximately 90 million (Safeer & Keenan, 2005) of adult American peoples have below basic or basic health literacy (Koh et al., 2012; Bailey et al., 2014; Cajita, Cajita, & Han, 2016; McCaffery et al., 2013; Vernon, Trujillo, Rosenbaum, & Debuono, 2007; How, 2011; Muscat et al., 2016). The proportion was found more in Australia, where it was about 60% (Muscat et al., 2016). A comparative report on health literacy in eight European Union state members revealed that 12% of all respondents have inadequate general health literacy and 35% have problematic health literacy. Therefore, limited health literacy in Europe is a significant burden which does not affect a minority of the population. However, there are marked differences between different countries as demonstrated by the European Health Literacy Survey (HLS-EU) which was conducted in 2011 in eight European countries (Fig 1) (HLS-EU Consortium, 2012). In Asia, research in health literacy is not a priority. In India, a study was conducted to see dental health literacy among patients and it revealed that, 60.4% having low health literacy score (D'Cruz, & Aradhya, 2013). In Bangladesh, the literacy rate and the enrollment in the schools are increasing day by day but the health literacy is still untapped (Arafat & Ahmed, 2017). Moreover, there prevails multiple misconceptions those direct the people to pursue abnormal health seeking behaviors such as attending the traditional healers instead of registered physicians even in the major illnesses (Arafat, 2017a). Inadequate health literacy is much worse in case of older persons. Previous studies in different cultures revealed majority of patients older than 60 years found to have the lowest levels of literacy, and 80 percent were found to have limited skills to fill out forms when they were asked even in the waiting rooms (Safeer & Keenan, 2005). One of the major effects to poor health literacy is failure to take medications results in approximately 125,000 deaths annually in US, that costs from $106 to $238 billion yearly (Bailey et al., 2014; How, 2011).

Importance in Relation to Health Outcome

People with poor health literacy often perceive poor self-efficiency in regards to deal with their health conditions (Palumbo, 2015; Serper et al., 2014; Andrus & Roth, 2002); usually are not willing to take part in the health care services appropriately; associated with inadequate in management of chronic health conditions and diseases, prone to greater risk of hospital admission and increased mortality (Palumbo, 2015; Serper et al., 2014; Koh et al., 2012; Cajita, Cajita, & Han, 2016; Andrus & Roth, 2002; Vernon, Trujillo, Rosenbaum, & Debuono, 2007; Berkman, Sheridan, Donahue, Halpern, & Crotty, 2011; Muscat et al., 2016). Limited health literacy is also likely to exhibit impairment in recalling the provided health information (Palumbo, 2015; Cajita, Cajita, & Han, 2016; DeWalt & Hink, 2009; Manganello, 2008). People with lower HL, are less efficacious in understanding the prescription as well as taking medications

Figure 1. European Health Literacy Survey (HLS-EU): Levels of general health literacy index in selected European countries (Source: Sorensen et al., 2015)

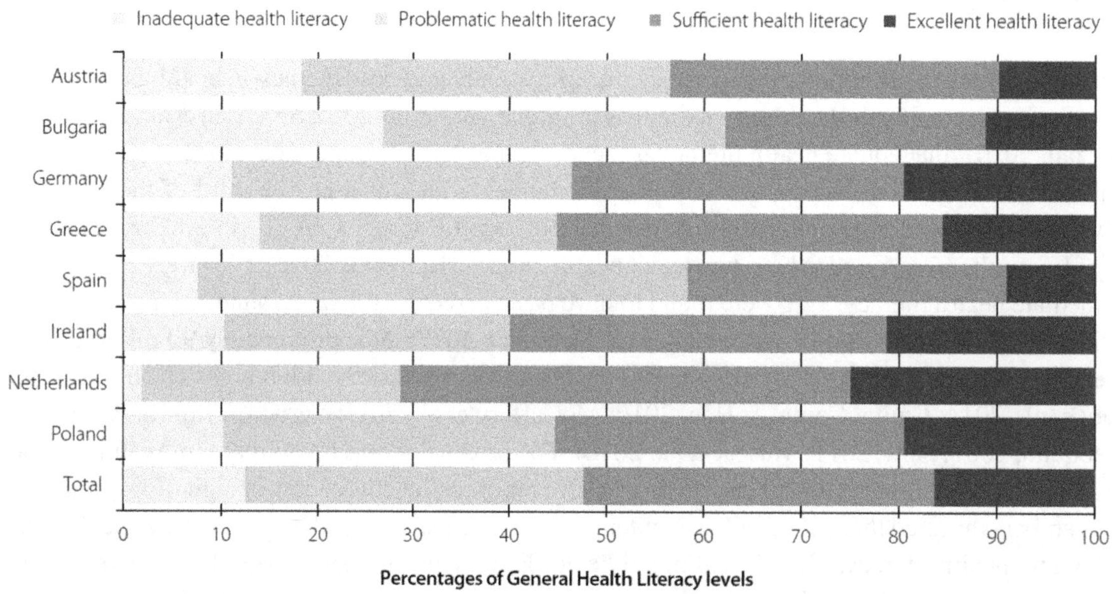

as per direction, unable to implement appropriate strategy to improve the compliance (DeWalt & Hink, 2009; Andrus & Roth, 2002; Cajita, Cajita, & Han, 2016; Palumbo, 2015; Koh et al., 2012); usually show serious medication errors repeatedly (Palumbo, 2015; Koh et al., 2012; Safeer & Keenan, 2005; Manganello, 2008; Vernon, Trujillo, Rosenbaum, & Debuono, 2007) that ultimately tolls high medical expenses (Palumbo, 2015; DeWalt & Hink, 2009; Manganello, 2008; Vernon, Trujillo, Rosenbaum, & Debuono, 2007; Muscat et al., 2016). Low health literacy is associated with poor knowledge in health, unhealthy behavioral pattern, lower preventive health services utilization (Vernon, Trujillo, Rosenbaum, & Debuono, 2007; Dickson-Swift, Kenny, Farmer, Gussy, & Larkins, 2014) ultimately acts as a strong barrier to access health care services (Palumbo, 2015; Kabir & Khan, 2013); as a catalyst of poor health and high hospitalization (Dickson-Swift, Kenny, Farmer, Gussy, & Larkins, 2014; Cajita, Cajita, & Han, 2016; Safeer & Keenan, 2005; Andrus & Roth, 2002; Vernon, Trujillo, Rosenbaum, & Debuono, 2007). Importantly poor health literacy affects three points as mentioned in access and utilization of health care, interaction with services provider and self-care (Osborn, Paasche-Orlow, Bailey, & Wolf, 2011; Sørensen et al., 2012) and negatively influence the motivation of the patient, problem solving ability, self-efficacy, appropriate self-care behavior (Osborn, Paasche-Orlow, Bailey, & Wolf, 2011). It is troublesome to process health information for the people with low health literacy those affects reading, understanding the medication labels, making appointments as well as understand the appointment slips, comprehending the verbal communications with health care services providers, understand and follow the educational and self-care materials to adapt the preventive services (Cajita, Cajita, & Han, 2016). Better or improved status of health literacy leads to improved health status, lowered health expense, shorter hospital stay, less frequent hospitalization, less utilization of the health resources (Sørensen et al., 2012; Safeer & Keenan, 2005). Adequate functional health literacy enables to understand the risks and related health services, improved compliance; adequate interactive health literacy enables to improve individual motivation, self-reliant capacities, as well as to be self-sufficient; adequately critical health literacy enables to be resilient to surrounding adversities such as social and economic (Sørensen et al., 2012). Along with the enormous personal benefits adequate health literacy ensures very impactful community and social benefits. Adequate functional health literacy increases the participation in community health programs; interactive health literacy accelerates influencing capacity of an individual to affect the social norms and more interactions between the surrounding societies; critical health literacy enhances community based empowerment and enables to act as social and economic determinants of health (Sørensen et al., 2012). Low, inadequate, poor health literacy substantially affects treatment compliance, self-control for chronic diseases and ultimately the treatment costs (Safeer & Keenan, 2005). Previous studies revealed a significant difference in health outcome between the highest and lowest health literacy groups and the finding recommended to improve the health literacy of lower group (How, 2011). Even poorly literate people are unable to pick up the benefits aimed from media campaigns, interventions, and educational programs (Manganello, 2008). With this increasing importance previous authors like to consider health literacy as the sixth vital sign along with other traditional vital signs mentioned as temperature, pulse, respirations, blood pressure, and pain and it should be assessed in the same way other vital signs are assessed (Heinrich, 2012).

Health Literacy and Economic Growth of a Nation

Key international declarations considered literacy as a right, both for children and adults. The Hamburg Declaration conceived literacy "as the basic knowledge and skills needed by all in a rapidly changing world, is a fundamental human right" (UNESCO, 1997). Everyone should have 'the same opportunities for access to programs of continuing education, including adult and functional literacy programs'. Literacy skills provide a number of benefits to individual e.g. informed decision-making, personal empowerment, participation in social activities etc.

Link Between General Literacy and Health

The impact of education or general literacy on population and public health, especially women's health, is a well-researched (Kickbusch, 2001) and it was demonstrated that literacy program also has a greater impact on health. Many studies reported the positive impact of education and literacy on population health, in particular women's' health and the health of children (Bledsoe, Casterline, Jonson-Kuhn, & Haaga, 1999; Sen, 1999; Nussbaum, 2000). Female literacy rate is considered to be one of the 10 key indicators to assess 'women's well-being' (Save the Children, 2000; Kabir, Rahman, Monte-Serrat, & Arafat, 2017). In a study in Nicaragua, lower infant mortality was recorded among mothers who had participated in an adult literacy campaign than those who had not (Sandiford et al., 1995). Other studies showed literacy and basic education programs (Burchfield et al., 2002a), and radio broadcasts and other health interventions (Burchfield et al., 2002b) improved health-related knowledge and health seeking behavior of the women.

Impact of Low Health Literacy on Health Development

Health literacy is increasingly becoming important area to support people to utilize the opportunities available in the healthcare to improve and manage their own health. The Center for Health Care Strategies

Inc. (Center for Health Care Strategies, 2013) used a simple definition of health literacy: "the degree to which individuals have the capacity to obtain, process, and understand basic health information and services needed to make appropriate health decisions." Health literacy helps people to "obtain, process, and understand basic health information and services needed to make appropriate health decisions" (U.S. Department of Health and Human Services, 2000). The relationship between literacy and health is complex and widely studied area. It represents a group of skills required for public and patients to understand and interpreted healthcare information and take necessary action in a health care environment when necessary. These skills include interpretation, print literacy, numeracy, and oral literacy (Agency for Health Care Research and Quality, 2011). So, health literacy is more than reading which also encompasses writing, numeracy, listening, speaking, and conceptual knowledge. Effective communication is critical to successful health care. Low health literacy is linked to poorer health status, higher morbidity, mortality, lack of medical care knowledge, more hospital visits and hospitalization, lack of knowledge about medical conditions, utilization of expensive services (e.g. emergency care and inpatient admissions), non-utilization of health promotion services, low self-reported health profile, poorer compliance rates with treatment modalities, and increased health care costs (Andrus & Roth, 2002; IOM, 2004; Agency for Health Care Research and Quality, 2011). Low health literacy can result in: medication errors; low rates of treatment compliance due to poor communication between providers and patients; reduced use of preventive services and unnecessary emergency room visits; ineffective management of chronic conditions, due to inadequate self-care skills; longer hospital stays and increased hospital re-admissions; poor responsiveness to public health emergencies; and higher mortality (Berkman, et al, 2004). Improving health literacy reduces health care costs and increases the quality of health care. It is now well-established that there is a relationship between educational attainment, literacy skills and economic growth (Coulombe, Tremblay, & Marchand, 2004).

Economic Implications of Health Illiteracy

Health care sectors in both developed and developing countries deal with limited resources. Healthcare activities, especially in developed countries, consume a large portion of economic resources. Healthcare spending has grown from 13.2% of GDP in 2000 to 17% in 2010. Low health literacy has a huge impact on a country and it is one of the important causes of economic inefficiency. The average annual health care costs of persons with very low literacy were found to be four times greater than for the general population (Weiss et al., 1994). It was found that adults with low health literacy experience 6% more hospital visits, 1.5 times more physician visit, 3 times more prescriptions and 2 day-longer hospital stays in comparison to those with proficient health literacy (The Ohio State University-Office of Outreach & Engagement, 2008). All these unintended activities as a result of low health literacy cost the U.S. economy up to $236 billion every year which represents between 7-17% of all personal health care expenditures (Vernon et al., 2007). As a whole, low functional literacy causes 3 to 6% greater health care expenditures (The Ohio State University-Office of Outreach & Engagement, 2008). This is a real blow for other sectors of the economy not only in the USA, the picture is the same for all developed and developing countries. This situation places health care system and the economy of a country at risk. The combination of low health literacy, demographic and epidemiological shifts, technological advances, and patients' high expectations places additional financial burden on the health care system and in a long run hinders economic growth of country.

Health literacy is also becoming increasingly important public health issue and found to contribute to social, economic and health development of a nation (Kickbusch, 2001). Health literacy enables individuals to protect themselves, their family and their community from various disasters and able them to take control of their health. It is evident that people with higher levels of health literacy are more likely to adopt healthier behaviors and decrease the undue utilization of healthcare. Moreover, they are far more able to understand available health-related information and would be empowered to make healthier choices. Benefits can be achieved across the life course and inter-generationally and the saved resources can be utilized to support priority health issues or can be channeled to other sectors for positive economic growth (WHO, 2016).

Access to reliable health information and usable health services are fundamental for the economic growth of a nation (Adams & Corrigan, 2003). The promises of medical research, health technology and healthcare delivery can only be implemented when a national action plan has been designed. The action plan needs to have specific steps connected to this direction. No single action will be sufficient. Actions should include partnerships among all levels of educators, health care providers, public and private healthcare institutions and government; should be based on feasibility, effectiveness and suitability; should evaluate the short and long-term effects of the efforts; and should involve continued public education, law and other policies to support health literacy (U.S. Department of Health and Human Services, Office of Disease Prevention and Health Promotion, 2010).

MEASUREMENTS OF HEALTH LITERACY

There are many measures globally which can qualify and quantify the status of health literacy. The tools aim to detect physical health literacy are: Rapid Estimate of Adult Literacy in Medicine (*REALM*) (Safeer & Keenan, 2005), Test of functional literacy in Adult (*TOFHLA*) (Baker, 2006), Wide Range Achievement Test-Revised (*WRAT-R*) (Bass, Wilson, & Griffith, 2003), Medical Achievement Reading Test (*MART*) (Hanson-Divers, 1997), Slosson Oral Reading Test (*SORT-R*), Peabody Individual Achievement Test Revised (*PIAT-R*) (Ojio, 2015), Instrument for Diagnosis of Reading (*IDL*) (Vernon, Trujillo, Rosenbaum, & Pfizer, 2007), Newest Vital Sign (*NVS*) (Peerson & Saunders, 2009), European health literacy questionnaire (*HLS-EU-Q47*) (Duong et al., 2017), High Blood Pressure-Health Literacy Scale (*HBP-HLS*) (Zhang et al., 2016), Health Literacy on Social Determinants of Health Questionnaire (*HL-SDHQ*) (Matsumoto & Nakayama, 2017), The Health Literacy Questionnaire (*HLQ*) (Nolte et al., 2017), The Eastern-Middle Eastern Adult Health Literacy (*EMAHL13*) (Nair, Satish, Sreedharan, & Ibrahim, 2016) etc.

Many reading cognition tools to assess patient's knowledge about health care terminologies are available and among them *REALM* is one of the most widely used instrument that can measure functional health literacy within 2 to 3 minutes by nurse or other staff (Safeer & Keenan, 2005). *TOFHLA* measures reading literacy, consists of 50 items assessing prose reading and 17 items assessing capacity to read and understand actual hospital documents and labeled prescription vials (Baker, 2006). The *WRAT-R* is a 57-item test that requires 3 to 5 minutes to respond and can measure reading, spelling and arithmetic (Bass et al., 2003). *MART* is designed to resemble a prescription label with its use of small print size, glossy cover, and medical terminology. This design allows practitioners and researchers to assess patients' inability to read the test (Hanson-Divers, 1997). *PIAT-R* is an individually administered tool measure six domain like: General information, Reading recognition, Reading comprehension, Mathematics, Spelling and Written expression (Ojio, 2015). Instrument for Diagnosis of Reading (*IDL*) is a reading comprehension bilingual (English-Spanish) tool for all ages. Subjects given time to read text of their own and then examiner asks series of questions of various difficulties (Andrus & Roth, 2002). Health literacy survey questionnaire (*HLS-EU Q47*) consists of 47 items that assess the capability to deal with health information like: access or obtain, understand, appraise, judge or evaluate, and apply or use health information) in three domains: health care, disease prevention, and health promotion (Duong et al., 2017). High Blood Pressure-Health Literacy Scale (*HBP-HLS*) is the only available hypertension specific HL instrument consists of 43 items assess knowledge about hypertension and its management (Zhang et al., 2016). *HLSDHQ* consists of 33 items clarifies 10 social determinants of health (Matsumoto & Nakayama, 2017). Health Literacy Questionnaire (*HLQ*) composed of 44 items which can assess nine distinct domains of health literacy like: support of health care providers, having adequate information for managing health, active management of health, social support for health, appraisal of health information, active engagement with health care providers, navigating health care system, ability to find good health information and understanding health information well enough to know what to do (Nolte et al., 2017). Eastern-Middle Eastern Adult Health Literacy (*EMAHL 13*) is brief screening tool can assess patient's ability to distinguish health and non-health related items (Nair et al., 2016).

In addition, regarding mental health literacy, a recent systemic review by Kutcher et al found 16 different tools in 17 studies mentioning mental health literacy tool (Wei, McGrath, Hayden, & Kutcher, 2016). The tools that measures knowledge about schizophrenia are: Knowledge About Schizophrenia Questionnaire (*KASQ*), Knowledge Questionnaire on Homecare of Schizophrenia (*KQHS*) and Knowledge about Schizophrenia Test (*KAST*). To detect literacy about overall mental health and illness there are few tools and these are: Multiple-Choice Knowledge of Mental Illnesses Test (*MC-KOMIT*), Mental Health Knowledge Schedule (*MAKS*), Mental Health Literacy Scale (*MHLS*), Journey of Hope (*JOH*) Outcome Survey, Knowledge of Mental Disorders (*KMD*), Mental Health Disorder Recognition questionnaire (*MDRQ*), Mental Health Knowledge Questionnaire (*MHKQ*). Others tools to detect knowledge about depression, anxiety and ADHD are: Depression Multiple Choice Question (*DMCQ*), Depression Literacy (*D-Lit*), Knowledge about Depression and Mania Inventory (*KDMI*), Adolescent Depression Knowledge Questionnaire (*ADKQ*), Anxiety Literacy Questionnaire (*A-Lit*), Test of Knowledge About ADHD (*KADD*). (Wei, McGrath, Hayden, & Kutcher, 2016).

KASQ consists of 25 multiple choice questions, *KQHS* contains 32 item multiple choice questionnaire on four aspects and *KAST* is 21 multiple choice questions on knowledge of schizophrenia. and *MC-KOMIT* is 33 multiple-choice items on knowledge of common mental illnesses, *MAKS* is 6-point Likert scale on 12 items of stigma knowledge of mental illness. *DMCQ* is 27 multiple-choice items, D-Lit is 22 true/false items, *ADKQ* is a tool consists of 13 dichotomous and 2 fill-in-the- blank questions and *KDM* is consists of 44 true false questions. *MC-KOMIT, MAKS, MHLS* tool containing multiple choice on 35 items regarding knowledge and attitudes about help-seeking, and ability to recognize disorders, *JOH* is a 4-point Likert scale on 15 items on mental health, *KMD* is tool having "Yes, "No", and "I don't know" responses to assess knowledge on the name and characteristics of mental disorders and ability to distinguish them from somatic illnesses, *MDRQ* is a 7-point Likert scale on 20 statements of mental illness descriptions in which 15 are real and 5 are false, *MHKQ* is tool having "yes", and "no" responses to 20 general mental health knowledge questions. *KDD* is tool containing 22 error-choice items to assess knowledge and attitudes toward students with ADHD. Among the measuring tools having good internal consistency are *DMCQ, KDD, JOH, KMD* and *ADKQ*. The tools having good to excellent content validity are: *KQHS, KAST, MC KOMIT, MAKS, KDM,* and *MHLS. KAST* and *KDM* are the two tools having fair criteria validity (Wei, McGrath, Hayden, & Kutcher, 2016).

ROLE OF SCHOOL IN HEALTH LITERACY

In 1986, WHO declared the Ottawa Charter and applauded the health promotion concept as health promotion is more than the disease prevention (Arafat, 2017b). Schools can have a very important role in health promotion and development of the future of the nation as well as the globe. Health literacy is a concept that can be extensively embraced by schools (St Leger, 2001). Schools across the world can play an important role in facilitating the achievements of health literacy as a public health goal along with the other educational commitments (Nutbeam, 2000). Nutbeam (2000) proposed a three-level hierarchy in health literacy. This would include: a) basic/functional literacy, b) through communication/interactive literacy and c) critical literacy. Critical literacy is generally defined as a set of skills that enable people to obtain, understand and use information to improve their health and is something that can be developed, thus; it should be an important goal of school education (Chinn, 2011). Although school may play an important role, in health literacy, it is important to be pointed that their core business is education, whilst the level of expertise in health issues is limited. Children are supposed to spend about 80% of their waking hours in school (Wang, Li, Siahpush, Chen, & Huberty, 2017) and they are also engaged in different school related tasks before and after school (Karczewski, Carter, & DeCator, 2016). Moreover, large numbers of adolescents work with childrenin schools to get them engaged (Demissie & Brener, 2017). In addition, schools are responsible for social and emotional knowledge along with the academic education (Weisman, Kia-Keating, Lippincott, Taylor, & Zheng, 2016). With the gradual physical and mental development adolescents are involved with their health care, interact with the health system and like to have access to health information (Manganello, 2008) as they pose both the responsibility and freedom. Addressing the health literacy positively at early age can have global improvement in aspects of interactions with the health system that ultimately drives to positive health outcome across life (Manganello, 2008). Schools can empower the youths by promoting health literacy (Hagell, Rigby, & Perrow, 2015). Schools can provide an excellent opportunity and critical facility in which many agencies can work together for the betterment of the youths as well as the economy. Schools play a facilitative role to bring the societal components together in which children act members of families, peers, schools, and communities (Valois & Hoyle, 2005). Like a silent epidemic, appropriate educational programs are necessary even before the assessment of health literacy in the clinical settings and schools can be most appropriate point to start (Heinrich, 2012). Moreover, adolescence is usually the starting point of different chronic diseases such as asthma, diabetes, cystic fibrosis and mental illness between the age ranging from 0–17 years (Manganello, 2008). Usually with the increase spread of internet, teenagers are more interested in seeking information regarding the management of their illness and health service providers consider the habit as an important one for the youths with chronic illness to have adequate health literacy skills to perceive the right meanings (Manganello, 2008). With physical, emotional, cognitive change, greater freedom and autonomy, improved reasoning and abstract thinking adolescence is to begin thinking about health literacy interventions (Gray, Klein, Noyce, Sesselberg, & Cantrill, 2005; Ghanbari, Ramezankhani, Montazeri, & Mehrabi, 2016; Manganello, 2008). Working on health literacy in adolescence would improve health literacy in later life and adolescents are used to carry their modified behavior across the life as they transition into adulthood (Manganello, 2008). IOM proposed to incorporate health-related tasks into lesson plans of schools and recommended that teaching the young people will be a good investment for future population health (Gray, Klein, Noyce, Sesselberg, & Cantrill, 2005; Manganello, 2008). Previous literature has shown that there is a strong relation between good health and educational achievement (World Bank, 1993; WHO, 1996). Therefore, a perception has been developed by schools and educators that if health and social issues will be addressed in schools, the learning outcomes will also be maximized (Cameron and McBride, 1995). St Leger and Nutbeam (2000) suggested that the health promoting school contributes to four main school-related outcomes: (i) lifelong learning skills; (ii) competencies and behaviors; (iii) specific cognate knowledge and skills; and (iv) self-attributes. Of course, these four school-related health/education outcomes are closely related to the three-level hierarchy in health literacy proposed by Nutbeam (2000) provided that they have been achieved by the students.

The effectiveness of school health and its outcomes has been reported by several reports and meta-analyses (Peters and Paulussen, 1994). Overall, the role of school in health literacy should include the following characteristics (adopted by St Leger, 2001):

1. Focusing on cognitive and social outcomes in conjunction with behavior change within an educational framework;
2. Occurring over several years and be relevant to young people's social and cognitive development;
3. Be adequately resourced;
4. Provision of significant professional development for teachers;
5. Be holistic in addressing strategic combinations of the curriculum, the school's physical environment, the school's social environment, health services, partnerships with parents and the local community and school policies;
6. Be based on effective learning theories; and recognize the limitations and opportunities of schools in bringing about substantial health improvements.

INTERVENTIONS IN SCHOOL TO IMPROVE THE HEALTH LITERACY

General Interventions

Some authors suggested a focus on the formal educational systems across the years such as elementary schools, high schools, junior schools, colleges and universities (Freedman et al., 2009). The approach should focus to prepare the students to address the public health concerns in from multiple perspectives rather to build them as public health specialist (Freedman et al., 2009). Educational materials distribution to the youths by health providers, schools and intervention programs can effective but further attention is needed regarding the readability of materials should be evaluated and sometimes it might be difficult for the youths to guide their choices about health behavior if they fail to understand the provided materials (Manganello, 2008). However, previous research revealed that school newsletters are being underutilized as a source of health promotion and health literacy in the school community (Merga & Hu, 2016).

Judicious use of media for the adolescents is a crucial part of health literacy as media is an important source of information nowadays. Past research revealed that youths aged 8–18 spend almost 6.5 hours per day with some type of media and their physical, social, mental, moral development is influenced by media. Educational television has been found to be linked with advances in literacy. Moreover, media is linked to development of health behavior and health literacy. So, justified use of media is an important area to improve health literacy in schools (Manganello, 2008) and limited abilities of using media should also be considered (Ghanbari, Ramezankhani, Montazeri, & Mehrabi, 2016). Educational programs implemented in schools or conducted via the mass media, can teach adolescents about health issues though the success of the interventions is dependent on their target group having the ability to understand the provided messages (Manganello, 2008). Creating a health promoting school environment is not just the focusing on the youths but also focusing the entire work force and a holistic approach involving every part is the best way to combat (Hagell, Rigby, & Perrow, 2015).

In this 21st century internet plays an important role in health, literacy, health literacy as well as internet has also a threatening role in regard to the novelty & validity of the available information (Ghanbari, Ramezankhani, Montazeri, & Mehrabi, 2016). Recent studies revealed respondents aged 15–24 years surfed internet for their expected information and they surfed several regular topics such sexual health, mental health, weight change, cancer, diabetes (Gray, Klein, Noyce, Sesselberg, & Cantrill, 2005). Limited internet facility, limited search abilities, low literacy skills affect the outcome and make difficult for adolescents to find, perceive the quality information. If there is nothing in the school health curriculum the adolescents would not achieve adequate health literacy (Ghanbari, Ramezankhani, Montazeri, & Mehrabi, 2016).

Specific Interventions

There are various school based interventions related to health literacy including physical and mental health. Specifically addressed areas are regarding: Obesity, Oral health, HIV, Fruit and vegetables intake, Nutrition, Bully behavior, Food literacy, Hand washing, Physical exercise, Adolescent dating violence, School based health centers (*SBHC*), Evidence based curriculum, Health Promotion School (*HPS*), School based health education, Physical education, Mental health teachers curriculum etc.

Interventions for Physical Health

High prevalence of childhood obesity predisposes children to various morbidities like insulin resistance, hypertension, dyslipidemia and liver disorders and risk of developing type 2 diabetes and cardiovascular diseases (Levy, Saenger, Steffes, & Delvin, 2017). In a study, school based health promotion program through scheduled extra school-day physical activities result increased habit of doing more aerobic activity among school children. "*KidMinutes*" is an easy measure that evaluates school activity program (Cluss et al., 2016). However, School-based intervention including counseling is not effective in reducing BMI or key obesogenic behaviors (Pbert et al., 2016). School based obesity prevention program is an effective approach to influence BMI among students (Karczewski, Carter, & DeCator, 2016). Academic lessons regarding physical activity has positive effect on BMI (de Greeff et al., 2016). The HealthCorps program is an effective health literacy program which significantly increases students' knowledge and behavior on issues like: nutrition, physical activity and mental health (Moonseong et al., 2016). It is evident that schools having Physical Exercise Lesson (*PEL*) program result more Physical Activity (PA) in both boys and girls (Frömel, Svozil, Chmelík, Jakubec, & Groffik, 2016). A Physical Activity program focusing school teachers is effective to increase PA and also improves early literacy (Kirk & Kirk, 2016). Go Wild with Fruits and Veggies (*GWWFV*) and fruit and vegetables snack program (FFVSP) is another curriculum based school program that increases the fruit and vegetables intake among students.

Building a Healthy Me (*BHM*) is an effective nutrition intervention for classroom and family (Larsen et al., 2017). Team Nutriathlon is another school based program that can raise vegetables, fruits and dairy product consumption (Loosier et al., 2016; Drapeau, V. Savard, BA. Gallant, A. Nadeau, L. Gagnon, 2016). Brighter Bites is a school based intervention that includes three components like: fresh produce deliveries, recipe demonstration and nutrition education. The intervention helps to learn some crucial lessons like: importance of leveraging existing infrastructure of food banks and engagement of parent, school and staff (Sharma et al., 2017). There is a discrepancy in the knowledge and comprehension about oral health differs from dental professional to students. In a study researcher used mouth drawing as tool of measuring health literacy among students prior and after health education. The study finds that 72.8% students answered better after the health education then they answered about the health education queries prior education (Ueno et al., 2014). Over the last 10 years, the Health Promoting School (*HPS*) concept developed and provided positive outcomes. HIV risk is not proportionate among sexual and gender minority (SGM) youth. School can play a valuable role for educating young students regarding primary prevention measures regarding such issue (Rose & Friedman, 2017).

Interventions for Mental Health

There are many specific interventions or programs focusing mainly on student's mental health. The Guide mental health literacy curriculum for school students is an effective way in raising mental health literacy. An MHL resource from Canada (*The Guide*) is the curriculum contains basic understanding of mental health, mental disorders and treatment in brief, about stigma, about help seeking behavior (Mcluckie, Kutcher, Wei, & Weaver, 2014). Teen Mental Health First Aid (*teen MHFA*) is training program for students effective to raise mental health literacy (Hart, Mason, Kelly, Cvetkovski, & Jorm, 2016). "Mental health education program", "Mental health for everyone" are the similar approaches to raise mental health literacy among students (Ojio, 2015; Mcluckie, Kutcher, Wei, & Weaver, 2014). To assess the status of knowledge and attitude about mental health and improving that issue can be solved by Focus Group Discussion (*FGD*) (Okello, Abbo, Muhwezi, Akello, & Ovuga, 2014). Other than these intervention, school based interventions were tried previously in different ways. Among them intervention for bully prevention reduces bully behavior among students (Educational Intervention Using the Integrated Model for Behavior Change, 2016), community based dating violence prevention program reduces dating violence behavior in adolescent school students (Joppa, Rizzo, Nieves, & Brown, 2016). In a review, it was found that sexual abuse among children age group occurs frequently in family setting and abuse victims are often bullied and isolated in school. In order to prevent serious mental health problems, teachers and school counsellors play an important role in identifying and offering help (Sawyerr & Bagley, 2017). A good portion of adult mental health and substance use (MH& SU) disorders starts in adolescent age. In another review it was found that, along with other intervention school can take part a significant role in prevention program (Dunne et al., 2016). Continuing innovation, adaptation and evaluation of programs is now required, especially in low-income countries, to integrate mental health promotion in the public health agenda of countries worldwide (Herrman & Jané-llopis, n.d.). Suicide is the second leading cause of death for adolescents. Whereas school-based prevention programs are effective, obtaining active consent for youth participation in public health programming concerning sensitive topics is challenging. The current authors explored several active consent procedures for improving participation rates. Although passive consent produces the highest student participation, these methods are not always appropriate for programs addressing sensitive topics in schools. In-person active consent procedures may be the best option when prioritizing balance between parental awareness and successful student recruitment ("Procedures for School Programming: Addressing the Sensitive Topic of Suicide," 2017). Differences in the use of school-based behavioral health services (autism, attention deficit hyperactivity disorder [ADHD], conduct/oppositional defiant disorder, and ''other'') by racial and ethnic groups suggest the need for culturally appropriate outreach and tailoring of services to improve service utilization (Locke et al., 2017). Findings suggest that school engagement is a potentially modifiable target for interventions aiming to ameliorate the negative influence of mental health problems on school functioning for adolescent girls with histories of abuse or neglect (Threlfall, Auslander, Gerke, Mcginnis, & Myers, 2017).This study tested the influence of a training intervention to improve teachers' ability to accurately identify preschool children's emotional and behavioral problems in 24 schools in Addis Ababa, Ethiopia. Sensitivity and specificity of teacher identification, and overall agreement with an established measurement criterion (*Strengths and Difficulties Questionnaire*) were examined 2 years following training compared to pre- intervention baseline, and a non-intervention control group of 12 schools. Results indicate that the teacher training was significantly associated with more accurate identification of children's problem (Desta et al., 2017). Depression and anxiety often emerge for the first time during youth. The school environment provides an ideal context to deliver prevention programs, with potential to offset the trajectory towards disorder. These results suggest that the refinement of school-based prevention programs have the potential to reduce mental health burden and advance public health outcomes (Newby & Christensen, 2016).

CONTROVERSIES IN HEALTH LITERACY

In recent years, the volume of research on health literacy has grown. However, the definition of health literacy is yet to be universal. Moreover, few authors compare the concept as a repackaged form of health promotion (Sørensen et al., 2012; Nutbeam, 2000; Tones, 2002; Chinn, 2011). Some authors, clinicians and scholars like to consider health literacy as an individual responsibility and consider that itis the personal fault of the patient to have low health literacy (Koh et al., 2012; Serper et al., 2014). On the other hand, others consider health literacy as a dynamic & complex issue this reflects the available health information and service availability (Koh et al., 2012). IOM recommended it as a shared function of the society and the individual (Sørensen et al., 2012). IOM explains the source of relationship is the interaction of individual's skills and the sociomiety system demands. Health literacy is generated in the society as a whole but it can also be originated in an individual context based on different programs such as educational learning in the family setting, health promotion in the school, patient education programs, different patient self-management programs (Eichler, Wieser, & Brügger, 2009). WHO, IOM as well as different other professional societies mentioned repeatedly that poor health literacy is the result of low education, poor opportunity and limited healthcare access (Bailey et al., 2015). In addition, as mentioned in previous chapters, although schools may play an important role, in health literacy, it is important to be pointed that their expertise includes general education, whilst the level of expertise in health issues is limited (Chinn, 2011). Literature shows that educational programs particularly in schools, can promote the increase of the literacy levels of health care through a health curriculum however; at the moment there is no agreement on what a healthcare school curriculum design should include, probably because of the long-term nature of these educational programs (Parker and Kreps, 2004). Another limitation of school but also of other health literacy educational programs is that they focus solely on reading, writing, speaking, and listening skills and not on the larger set of communication strategies that consumers need to get the most out of the modern health care system (Cegala, 2003; Jones, Kreps & Cresskill, 1995).

RECOMMENDATIONS

Educators, school administrators and policy makers need to be well informed about the strengths and limitations of the current database on the effectiveness of currently available health literacy programs in schools (Schachter et al., 2008). Effectiveness of school-based health literacy programs will help establish strong foundation for addressing health promotion, prevention and intervention among adolescents in school establishments. Provider (teacher) health literacy is as important as student health literacy and taking full advantage of provider-student relationship in child and adolescent health promotion helps the preparation of the teacher (Peterson et al, 2001) and to achieve them teachers needed to adopt, learn and practice about new concepts such as critical health literacy and successive changes required in school structure to achieve beneficial outcomes which heavily depends on funding (St. Leger, 2001).

However, applications of interventions not know to be effective could be a waste of the limited public funds (Wei et al., 2013). According to AMA four areas should be further explored for research such as screening of the health literacy, communication improvement focusing the low literacy patients, expenses and outcome of inadequate health literacy, and causal relationship of low health literacy and health (Sørensen et al., 2012). Authors recommended that schools can act as a vehicle for promoting health literacy as well as overall health though there is limited evidence to support any specific level of school such as primary or secondary (Hagell, Rigby, & Perrow, 2015). Health promoting school concept is recommended to be embraced to initiate and sustain the positive changes (Valois & Hoyle, 2005). As schools influence directly both the education and development of the youths, IOM highlighted the need for playing important role in improving the health literacy (Manganello, 2008). WHO recommends few things after reassessment of the effectiveness of Health Promoting Schools such as curriculum modification with inputting the issues, changing the school ethos and further engagement of the families and communities (Hagell, Rigby, & Perrow, 2015).Parents play an important role in the lives of students and teachers should engage parents during the process delivery of health education which is a great part of family life (Begoray et al, 2009).

CONCLUSION

Health literacy is a global concern of this century. Although healthcare is moving towards the patient-centered approach poor health literacy is still a silent epidemic that affects health outcomes holistically. School is a potential area to improve the health literacy nationally and globally. Different measures are available to assess literacy. As schools influence directly both the education and development of the youths,

IOM highlighted the need for playing important role in improving the health literacy. After reassessment of the effectiveness of Health Promoting Schools, the WHO recommends curriculum modification with inputting the issues, changing the school ethos and further engagement of the families and communities. Multiple interventions are implemented across the globe. Educational programs particularly in schools, can promote the increase of the literacy levels of healthcare through a health curriculum however; at the moment there is no agreement on what a healthcare school curriculum design should include, probably because of the long-term nature of these educational programs. Moreover, health literacy educational programs focus solely on reading, writing, speaking, and listening skills and not on the larger set of communication strategies that consumers need to get the most out of the modern healthcare system. Multisectoral collaboration such as health, education, finance, media, communication; and locally proved effective strategies should be considered as a priority.

REFERENCES

Adams, K., & Corrigan, J. M. (2003). *Priority areas for national action: Transforming health care quality*. Washington, DC: National Academies Press.

Agency for Health Care Research and Quality (AHRQ). (2011). *Health Literacy Interventions and Outcomes: an Update of the Literacy and Health Outcomes Systematic Review of Literature*. Author.

Altin, S. V., Finke, I., Kautz-Freimuth, S., & Stock, S. (2014). The evolution of health literacy assessment tools: A systematic review. *BMC Public Health*, *14*(1), 1207. doi:10.1186/1471-2458-14-1207 PMID:25418011

Andrus, M. R., & Roth, M. T. (2002). Health Literacy: A Review. *Pharmacotherapy*, *22*(3), 282–302. doi:10.1592/phco.22.5.282.33191 PMID:11898888

Arafat, S. M. Y. (2017a). Abnormal Health Believes with Frequent Presentations: Ethnographic Observation from Primary Care of Bangladesh. *International Journal of Perceptions in Public Health*, *1*(2), 85–86.

Arafat, S. M. Y. (2017b). Mental Health Promotion or Public Mental Health: The Time Demanded Area. *Journal of Behavioral Health*, *6*(1), 1–3. doi:10.5455/jbh.20161121095655

Arafat, S. M. Y., & Ahmed, S. (2017). Burden of Misconception in Sexual Health Care Setting: A Cross-Sectional Investigation among the Patients Attending a Psychiatric Sex Clinic of Bangladesh. *Psychiatry Journal*, *2017*, 4. doi:10.1155/2017/9827083 PMID:28740851

Bailey, S. C., Brega, A. G., Crutchfield, T. M., Elasy, T., Herr, H., Kaphingst, K., ... Schillinger, D. (2014). Update on health literacy and diabetes. *The Diabetes Educator*, *40*(5), 581–604. doi:10.1177/0145721714540220 PMID:24947871

Bailey, S. C., Fang, G., Annis, I. E., O'Conor, R., Paasche-Orlow, M. K., & Wolf, M. S. (2015). Health literacy and 30-day hospital readmission after acute myocardial infarction. *BMJ Open*, *5*(6), e006975. doi:10.1136/bmjopen-2014-006975 PMID:26068508

Baker, D. W. (2006). The meaning and the measure of health literacy. *Journal of General Internal Medicine, 21*(8), 878–883. doi:10.1111/j.1525-1497.2006.00540.x PMID:16881951

Bass, P. F., Wilson, J. F., & Griffith, C. H. (2003). A Shortened Instrument for Literacy Screening. *Journal of General Internal Medicine, 18*(12), 1036–1038. doi:10.1111/j.1525-1497.2003.10651.x PMID:14687263

Begoray, D. L., Wharf-Higgins, J., & MacDonald, M. (2009). High school health curriculum and health literacy: Canadian student voices. *Global Health Promotion, 16*(4), 35–42. doi:10.1177/1757975909348101 PMID:20028667

Berkman, N. D., Davis, T. C., & McCormack, L. (2010). Health literacy: What is it? *Journal of Health Communication, 15*(Suppl 2), 9–19.

Berkman, N. D., Dewalt, D. A., Pignone, M. P., Sheridan, S. L., Lohr, K. N., Lux, L., ... Bonito, A. J. (2004). *Literacy and Health Outcomes: AHRQ Evidence Report Summaries.* Agency for Healthcare Research and Quality.

Berkman, N. D., Sheridan, S. L., Donahue, K. E., Halpern, D. J., & Crotty, K. (2011). Low health literacy and health outcomes: An updated systematic review. *Annals of Internal Medicine, 155*(2), 97–107. doi:10.7326/0003-4819-155-2-201107190-00005 PMID:21768583

Bledsoe, C. H., Casterline, J. B., Jonson-Kuhn, J. A., & Haaga, J. G. (1999). *Critical Perspectives on Schooling and Fertility in the Developing World.* Washington, DC: National Academy Press.

Burchfield, S., Hua, H., Baral, D., & Rocha, V. (2002b). *A Longitudinal Study of the Effect of Integrated Literacy and Basic Education Programs on the Participation of Women in Social and Economic Development in Nepal.* Washington, DC: United States Agency for International Development Office of Women in Development.

Burchfield, S., Hua, H., Iturry, T. S., & Rocha, V. (2002a). *A Longitudinal Study of the Effect of Integrated Literacy and Basic Education Programs on the Participation of Women in Social and Economic Development in Bolivia.* Washington, DC: United States Agency for International Development Office of Women in Development.

Cajita, M. I., Cajita, T. R., & Han, H.-R. (2016). Health Literacy and Heart Failure: A Systematic Review. *The Journal of Cardiovascular Nursing, 31*(2), 121–130. doi:10.1097/JCN.0000000000000229 PMID:25569150

Cameron, I., & McBride, N. (1995). Creating health promoting schools: Lessons from the west Australian school health project. *Health Promotion Journal of Australia, 5*, 4–10.

Cegala, D. J. (2003). Patient communication skills training: A review with implications for cancer patients. *Patient Education and Counseling, 50*(1), 91–94. doi:10.1016/S0738-3991(03)00087-9 PMID:12767592

Center for Health Care Strategies Inc. (2013). *What is Health Literacy?* Retrieved from https://www.chcs.org/media/CHCS_Health_Literacy_Fact_Sheets_2013.pdf

Chinn, D. (2011). Critical health literacy: A review and critical analysis. *Social Science & Medicine, 73*(1), 60–67. doi:10.1016/j.socscimed.2011.04.004 PMID:21640456

Cluss, P., Lorigan, D., Kinsky, S., Nikolajski, C., McDermott, A., & Bhat, K. B. (2016). School-Based Health Promotion Initiative Increases Children's Physical Activity. *American Journal of Health Education, 47*(6), 343–354. doi:10.1080/19325037.2016.1219287

Coulombe, S. Tremblay, J., & Marchand, S. (2004). *Literacy scores, human capital and growth across fourteen OECD countries.* Statistics Canada Catalogue number 89-552-MIE200411.

D'Cruz, A. M., & Aradhya, M. R. S. (2013). Health literacy among Indian adults seeking dental care. *Dental Research Journal, 10*(1), 20–24. PMID:23878559

de Greeff, J. W., Hartman, E., Mullender-Wijnsma, M. J., Bosker, R. J., Doolaard, S., & Visscher, C. (2016). Effect of Physically Active Academic Lessons on Body Mass Index and Physical Fitness in Primary School Children. *The Journal of School Health, 86*(5), 346–352. doi:10.1111/josh.12384 PMID:27040472

Demissie, Z., & Brener, N. (2017). Demographic Differences in District-Level Policies Related to School Mental Health and Social Services-United States, 2012. *The Journal of School Health, 87*(4), 227–235. doi:10.1111/josh.12489 PMID:28260247

Desta, M., Deyessa, N., Fish, I., Maxwell, B., Zerihun, T., Levine, S., … Garland, A. F. (2017). *Teachers to Identify Mental Health Problems : A Task-Sharing Intervention in Ethiopia.* Academic Press.

DeWalt, D. A., & Hink, A. (2009). Health Literacy and Child Health Outcomes: A Systematic Review of the Literature. *Pediatrics, 124*(Supplement), S265–S274. doi:10.1542/peds.2009-1162B PMID:19861480

Dickson-Swift, V., Kenny, A., Farmer, J., Gussy, M., & Larkins, S. (2014). Measuring oral health literacy: A scoping review of existing tools. *BMC Oral Health, 14*(148), 13. PMID:25472659

Diemer, F. S., Haan, Y. C., Nannan Panday, R. V., van Montfrans, G. A., Oehlers, G. P., & Brewster, L. M. (2017). Health literacy in Suriname. *Social Work in Health Care, 56*(4), 283–293. doi:10.1080/00981389.2016.1277823 PMID:28271964

Drapeau, V., Savard, B. A., Gallant, A., Nadeau, L., & Gagnon, J. (2016). The Effectiveness of A School-Based Nutrition Intervention on Children's Fruit, Vegetables, and Dairy Product Intake. *The Journal of School Health, 86*(5), 353–362. doi:10.1111/josh.12385 PMID:27040473

Dunne, T., Bishop, L., Avery, S., & Darcy, S. (2016). A Review of Effective Youth Engagement Strategies for Mental Health and Substance Use Interventions. *The Journal of Adolescent Health, 60*(5), 487–512. doi:10.1016/j.jadohealth.2016.11.019 PMID:28087268

Duong, T. V., Aringazina, A., Baisunova, G., Nurjanah, Pham, T. V., Pham, K. M., … Chang, P. W. (2017). Measuring health literacy in Asia: Validation of the HLS-EU-Q47 survey tool in six Asian countries. *Journal of Epidemiology, 27*(2), 80–86. doi:10.1016/j.je.2016.09.005 PMID:28142016

Eichler, K., Wieser, S., & Brügger, U. (2009). The costs of limited health literacy: A systematic review. *International Journal of Public Health, 54*(5), 313–324. doi:10.100700038-009-0058-2 PMID:19644651

(2016).. . *Following an Educational Intervention Using the Integrated Model for Behavior Change., 86*(11), 813–822.

Freedman, D. A., Bess, K. D., Tucker, H. A., Boyd, D. L., Tuchman, A. M., & Wallston, K. A. (2009). Public Health Literacy Defined. *American Journal of Preventive Medicine*, *36*(5), 446–451. doi:10.1016/j.amepre.2009.02.001 PMID:19362698

Frömel, K., Svozil, Z., Chmelík, F., Jakubec, L., & Groffik, D. (2016). The Role of Physical Education Lessons and Recesses in School Lifestyle of Adolescents. *The Journal of School Health*, *86*(2), 143–151. doi:10.1111/josh.12362 PMID:26762826

Ghanbari, S., Ramezankhani, A., Montazeri, A., & Mehrabi, Y. (2016). Health Literacy Measure for Adolescents (HELMA): Development and Psychometric Properties. *PLoS One*, *11*(2), e0149202. doi:10.1371/journal.pone.0149202 PMID:26881933

Gray, N. J., Klein, J. D., Noyce, P. R., Sesselberg, T. S., & Cantrill, J. A. (2005). The Internet: A window on adolescent health literacy. *The Journal of Adolescent Health*, *37*(3), 243.e1–243.e7. doi:10.1016/j.jadohealth.2004.08.023 PMID:16109345

Hagell, A., Rigby, E., & Perrow, F. (2015). Promoting health literacy in secondary schools: A review. *British Journal of School Nursing*, *10*(2), 82–87. doi:10.12968/bjsn.2015.10.2.82

Hanson-Divers, E. C. (1997). Developing a medical achievement reading test to evaluate patient literacy skills: A preliminary study. *Journal of Health Care for the Poor and Underserved*, *8*(1), 56–69. doi:10.1353/hpu.2010.0304 PMID:9019026

Hart, L. M., Mason, R. J., Kelly, C. M., Cvetkovski, S., & Jorm, A. F. (2016). "teen Mental Health First Aid": A description of the program and an initial evaluation. *International Journal of Mental Health Systems*, *10*(1), 3. doi:10.118613033-016-0034-1 PMID:26788123

Heinrich, C. (2012). Health literacy: The sixth vital sign. *Journal of the American Academy of Nurse Practitioners*, *24*(4), 218–223. doi:10.1111/j.1745-7599.2012.00698.x PMID:22486837

Herrman, H., & Jané-llopis, E. (n.d.). The Status of Mental Health Promotion. *Public Health Reviews*, *34*(2), 1–21.

HLS-EU consortium. (2012). *Comparative report of health literacy in eight EU member states*. The European health literacy survey HLS-EU. Retrieved from http://www.health-literacy.eu

How, C. H. (2011). A review of health literacy: Problem, tools and interventions. *Proceedings of Singapore Healthcare*, *20*(2), 119–125. doi:10.1177/201010581102000209

Jones, J. A., Kreps, G. L., & Phillips, G. M. (1995). *Communicating with your doctor: getting the most out of health care*. Cresskill, NJ: Hampton Press.

Joppa, M. C., Rizzo, C. J., Nieves, A. V., & Brown, L. K. (2016). Pilot Investigation of the Katie Brown Educational Program: A School-Community Partnership. *The Journal of School Health*, *86*(4), 288–297. doi:10.1111/josh.12378 PMID:26930241

Kabir, R., & Khan, H. T. A. (2013). Utilization of antenatal care among pregnant women of urban slums of Dhaka City, Bangladesh. *IOSR Journal of Nursing and Health Science*, *2*(2), 55–59. doi:10.9790/1959-0221519

Kabir, R., Rahman, S., Monte-Serrat, D. M., & Arafat, S. M. Y. (2017). Exploring the decision-making power of Bangladeshi women of reproductive age: Results from a national survey. *South East Asia Journal of Medical Sciences*, *1*(1), 4–8.

Karczewski, S. A., Carter, J. S., & DeCator, D. D. (2016). The Role of Ethnicity in School-Based Obesity Intervention for School-Aged Children: A Pilot Evaluation. *The Journal of School Health*, *86*(11), 778–786. doi:10.1111/josh.12433 PMID:27714874

Kickbusch, I. S. (2001). Health literacy: Addressing the health and education divide. *Health Promotion International*, *16*(3), 259–267. doi:10.1093/heapro/16.3.289 PMID:11509466

Kirk, S. M., & Kirk, E. P. (2016). Sixty Minutes of Physical Activity per Day Included Within Preschool Academic Lessons Improves Early Literacy. *The Journal of School Health*, *86*(3), 155–163. doi:10.1111/josh.12363 PMID:26830501

Koh, H. K., Berwick, D. M., Clancy, C. M., Baur, C., Brach, C., Harris, L. M., & Zerhusen, E. G. (2012). New federal policy initiatives to Boost health literacy can help the nation move beyond the cycle of costly "crisis care.". *Health Affairs*, *31*(2), 434–443. doi:10.1377/hlthaff.2011.1169 PMID:22262723

Larsen, A. L., Liao, Y., Alberts, J., Huh, J., Robertson, T., & Dunton, G. F. (2017). RE-AIM Analysis of a School-Based Nutrition Education Intervention in Kindergarteners. *The Journal of School Health*, *87*(1), 36–46. doi:10.1111/josh.12466 PMID:27917488

Levy, E., Saenger, A. K., Steffes, M. W., & Delvin, E. (2017). Pediatric Obesity and Cardiometabolic Disorders: Risk Factors and Biomarkers. *EJIFCC*, *28*(1), 6–24. PMID:28439216

Liu, Y. B., Liu, L., Li, Y. F., & Chen, Y. L. (2015). Relationship between Health Literacy, Health-Related Behaviors and Health Status: A Survey of Elderly Chinese. *International Journal of Environmental Research and Public Health*, *12*(8), 9714–9725. doi:10.3390/ijerph120809714 PMID:26295246

Locke, J., Kang-Yi, C. D., Pellecchia, M., Marcus, S., Hadley, T., & Mandell, D. S. (2017). Ethnic disparities in school-based behavioral health service use for children with psychiatric disorders. *The Journal of School Health*, *87*(1), 47–54. doi:10.1111/josh.12469 PMID:27917490

Loosier, P. S., Doll, S., Lepar, D., Ward, K., Gamble, G., & Dittus, P. J. (2016). Effectiveness of an Adaptation of the Project Connect Health Systems Intervention: Youth and Clinic-Level Findings. *The Journal of School Health*, *86*(8), 595–603. doi:10.1111/josh.12414 PMID:27374349

Mancuso, J. M. (2008). Health literacy: A concept/dimensional analysis. *Nursing & Health Sciences*, *10*(3), 248–255. doi:10.1111/j.1442-2018.2008.00394.x PMID:18786068

Manganello, J. A. (2008). Health literacy and adolescents: A framework and agenda for future research. *Health Education Research*, *23*(5), 840–847. doi:10.1093/her/cym069 PMID:18024979

Marks, R. (2012). *Health literacy and school-based health education*. Emerald Group Publishing.

Matsumoto, M., & Nakayama, K. (2017). Development of the health literacy on social determinants of health questionnaire in Japanese adults. *BMC Public Health*, *17*(1), 30. doi:10.118612889-016-3971-3 PMID:28056903

McCaffery, K. J., Holmes-Rovner, M., Smith, S. K., Rovner, D., Nutbeam, D., Clayman, M. L., ... Sheridan, S. L. (2013). Addressing health literacy in patient decision aids. *BMC Medical Informatics and Decision Making*, *13*(Suppl 2), S10. doi:10.1186/1472-6947-13-S2-S10 PMID:24624970

Mcluckie, A., Kutcher, S., Wei, Y., & Weaver, C. (2014). Sustained improvements in students¿ mental health literacy with use of a mental health curriculum in Canadian schools. *BMC Psychiatry*, *14*(1), 1694. doi:10.118612888-014-0379-4 PMID:25551789

Merga, M. K., & Hu, Q. M. (2016). Health education beyond the school gates: Use of school newsletters to communicate health messages to parents and their families. *Australian Journal of Education*, *60*(1), 73–85. doi:10.1177/0004944115627567

Moonseong, H., Erica, I., Natania, O., Carmen, I., Shawn, H., & Judith, W.-R. (2016). Behaviors and Knowledge of HealthCorps New York City High School Students: Nutrition, Mental Health and Physical Activity. *The Journal of School Health*, *86*(2), 84–95. doi:10.1111/josh.12355 PMID:26762819

Muscat, D. M., Smith, S., Dhillon, H. M., Morony, S., Davis, E. L., Luxford, K., ... Buchbinder, R. (2016). Incorporating health literacy in education for socially disadvantaged adults: An Australian feasibility study. *International Journal for Equity in Health*, *15*(1), 84. doi:10.118612939-016-0373-1 PMID:27259476

Nair, S. C., Satish, K. P., Sreedharan, J., & Ibrahim, H. (2016). Assessing health literacy in the eastern and middle-eastern cultures. *BMC Public Health*, *16*(1), 831. doi:10.118612889-016-3488-9 PMID:27538529

Newby, M., & Christensen, H. (2016). NU SC. *Clinical Psychology Review*.

Nielsen-Bohlman, L., Panzer, A. M., & Kindig, D. A. (2004). Health Literacy: A Prescription to End Confusion. Washington, DC: The National Academy of Sciences.

Nolte, S., Osborne, R. H., Dwinger, S., Elsworth, G. R., Conrad, M. L., Rose, M., ... Zill, J. M. (2017). German translation, cultural adaptation, and validation of the Health Literacy Questionnaire (HLQ). *PLoS One*, *12*(2), 12. doi:10.1371/journal.pone.0172340 PMID:28234987

Nussbaum, M. C. (2000). *Women and Human Development. The Capabilities Approach*. Cambridge, UK: Press Syndicate of the University of Cambridge. doi:10.1017/CBO9780511841286

Nutbeam, D. (2000). Health literacy as a public health goal: A challenge for contemporary health education and communication strategies into the 21st century. *Health Promotion International*, *15*(3), 259–267. doi:10.1093/heapro/15.3.259

Nutbeam, D. (2008). The evolving concept of health literacy. *Social Science & Medicine*, *67*(12), 2072–2078. doi:10.1016/j.socscimed.2008.09.050 PMID:18952344

Ojio, Y. (2015). Development of a mental health literacy program for secondary school students and its effects: In-school mental health literacy education. *School Mental Health: Global Challenges and Opportunities*, (3).

Okello, E. S., Abbo, C., Muhwezi, W. W., Akello, G., & Ovuga, E. (2014). Mental health literacy among secondary school students in North and Central Uganda: A qualitative study. *World Cultural Psychiatry Research Review*, *9*(3), 70–80. PMID:26113883

Osborn, C. Y., Paasche-Orlow, M. K., Bailey, S. C., & Wolf, M. S. (2011). The mechanisms linking health literacy to behavior and health status. *American Journal of Health Behavior, 35*(1), 118–128. doi:10.5993/AJHB.35.1.11 PMID:20950164

Osborne, H. (2012). *Health Literacy from A to Z: Practical Ways to Communicate Your Health Message*. Jones & Bartlett Publishers.

Palumbo, R. (2015). Discussing the Effects of Poor Health Literacy on Patients Facing HIV: A Narrative Literature Review. *International Journal of Health Policy and Management, 4*(7), 417–430. doi:10.15171/ijhpm.2015.95 PMID:26188806

Parker, R., & Kreps, G. L. (2005). Library outreach: Overcoming health literacy challenges. *Journal of the Medical Library Association: JMLA, 93*(4), S81–S85. PMID:16239962

Parker, R., & Ratzan, S. C. (2010). Health Literacy: A Second Decade of Distinction for Americans. *Journal of Health Communication, 15*(sup2), 20–33.

Pbert, L., Druker, S., Barton, B., Schneider, K. L., Olendzki, B., Gapinski, M. A., ... Osganian, S. (2016). A School-Based Program for Overweight and Obese Adolescents: A Randomized Controlled Trial. *The Journal of School Health, 86*(10), 699–708. doi:10.1111/josh.12428 PMID:27619760

Peerson, A., & Saunders, M. (2009). Health literacy revisited: What do we mean and why does it matter? *Health Promotion International, 24*(3), 285–296. doi:10.1093/heapro/dap014 PMID:19372101

Peters, L., & Paulussen, T. (1994). *School Health: A Review of the Effectiveness of Health Education and Health Promotion*. Utrecht: Dutch Centre for Health Promotion.

Peterson, F. L., Cooper, R. J., & Laird, J. A. (2001). Enhancing Teacher Health Literacy in School Health Promotion A Vision for the New Millennium. *The Journal of School Health, 71*(4), 138–144. doi:10.1111/j.1746-1561.2001.tb01311.x PMID:11354982

Rose, I. D., & Friedman, D. B. (2017). Schools. *The Journal of School Nursing, 33*(2), 109–115. doi:10.1177/1059840516678910 PMID:28288553

Safeer, R. S., & Keenan, J. (2005). Health literacy: The gap between physicians and patients. *American Family Physician, 72*(3), 463–468. PMID:16100861

Sandiford, P. J., Cassel, M., & Sanchez, G. (1995). The impact of women's literacy on child health and its interaction with access to health services. *Population Studies, 49*(1), 5–17. doi:10.1080/0032472031000148216

Save the Children. (2000). *State of the World's Mothers*. Westport, CT: Save the Children.

Sawyerr, A., & Bagley, C. (2017). Child Sexual Abuse and Adolescent and Adult Adjustment : A Review of British and World Evidence, with Implications for Social Work, and Mental Health and School Counselling. *Advances in Applied Sociology, 7*(01), 15. doi:10.4236/aasoci.2017.71001

Schachter, H. M., Girardi, A., Ly, M., Lacroix, D., Lumb, A. B., van Berkom, J., & Gill, R. (2008). Effects of school-based interventions on mental health stigmatization: A systematic review. *Child and Adolescent Psychiatry and Mental Health, 2*(1), 18. doi:10.1186/1753-2000-2-18 PMID:18644150

Sen, A. (1999). *Development as Freedom*. Oxford, UK: Oxford University Press.

Serper, M., Patzer, R. E., Curtis, L. M., Smith, S. G., O'Conor, R., Baker, D. W., & Wolf, M. S. (2014). Health literacy, cognitive ability, and functional health status among older adults. *Health Services Research, 49*(4), 1249–1267. doi:10.1111/1475-6773.12154 PMID:24476068

Sharma, S. V., Chow, J., Pomeroy, M., Raber, M., Salako, D., & Markham, C. (2017). Lessons Learned From the Implementation of Brighter Bites: A Food Co-op to Increase Access to Fruits and Vegetables and Nutrition Education Among Low-Income Children and Their Families. *The Journal of School Health, 87*(4), 286–295. doi:10.1111/josh.12497 PMID:28260244

Sorensen, K. (2013). *Health literacy: a neglected European public health disparity*. Maastricht: Universitaire Pers Maastricht.

Sørensen, K., Pelikan, J. M., Röthlin, F., Ganahl, K., Slonska, Z., Doyle, G., ... Brand, H. (2015). Health literacy in Europe: Comparative results of the European health literacy survey (HLS-EU). *European Journal of Public Health, 25*(6), 1053–1058. doi:10.1093/eurpub/ckv043 PMID:25843827

Sørensen, K., Van den Broucke, S., Fullam, J., Doyle, G., Pelikan, J., Slonska, Z., & Brand, H. (2012). Health literacy and public health: A systematic review and integration of definitions and models. *BMC Public Health, 12*(1), 80. doi:10.1186/1471-2458-12-80 PMID:22276600

St. Leger, L. (2001). Schools, health literacy and public health: Possibilities and challenges. *Health Promotion International, 16*(2), 197–205. doi:10.1093/heapro/16.2.197 PMID:11356758

St. Leger, L., & Nutbeam, D. (2000). A model for mapping linkages between health and education agencies to improve school health. *The Journal of School Health, 70*(2), 45–50. doi:10.1111/j.1746-1561.2000.tb07239.x PMID:10715824

The Ohio State University-Office of Outreach & Engagement. (2008). *Health Literacy: It's Time To Take It Seriously!* AHEC Clear Health Communication Program.

Threlfall, J. M., Auslander, W., Gerke, D., Mcginnis, H., & Myers, S. (2017). Mental Health and School Functioning for Girls in the Child Welfare System : The Mediating Role of Future Orientation and School Engagement. *School Mental Health, 9*(2), 194–204. doi:10.100712310-017-9207-6 PMID:28572859

Tones, K. (2002). Health literacy: New wine in old bottles? *Health Education Research, 17*(3), 287–290. doi:10.1093/her/17.3.287 PMID:12120844

Ueno, M., Takayama, A., Adiatman, M., Ohnuki, M., Zaitsu, T., & Kawaguchi, Y. (2014). Application of visual oral health literacy instrument in health education for senior high school students. *International Journal of Health Promotion and Education, 52*(1), 38–46. doi:10.1080/14635240.2013.845412

United Nations Educational Scientific and Cultural Organization. (1997). *The Hamburg Declaration on Adult Learning (CONFINTEA V)*. Author.

United Nations Educational Scientific and Cultural Organization. (2014). Adult and Youth Literacy. Institute for Statistics, (32), 1–4.

United Nations Educational Scientific and Cultural Organization. (2015). *Education For All 2000-2015: Achievements and Challenges. EFA Global Monitoring Report*. Author.

United Nations General Assembly. (2015). *Transforming our world: The 2030 agenda for sustainable development*. Author.

U.S. Department of Health and Human Services. (2000). *Healthy People 2010*. Washington, DC: U.S. Government Printing Office.

U.S. Department of Health and Human Services, Office of Disease Prevention and Health Promotion. (2010). *National Action Plan to Improve Health Literacy*. Washington, DC: Author.

Valois, R. F., & Hoyle, T. B. (2005). Health in Education: The Challenge Continues. *American Journal of Health Education*, *36*(1), 43–47. doi:10.1080/19325037.2005.10608156

Vernon, J. A., Trujillo, A., Rosenbaum, S. J., & Pfizer, B. D. (2007). *Low Health Literacy: Implications for National Health Policy*. Academic Press.

Wang, H., Li, T., Siahpush, M., Chen, L.-W., & Huberty, J. (2017). Cost-Effectiveness of Ready for Recess to Promote Physical Activity in Children. *The Journal of School Health*, *87*(4), 278–285. doi:10.1111/josh.12495 PMID:28260240

Watson, R. (2011). Europeans with poor" health literacy" are heavy users of health services. *British Medical Journal*, 343. PMID:22127773

Wei, Y., Hayden, J. A., Kutcher, S., Zygmunt, A., & McGrath, P. (2013). The effectiveness of school mental health literacy programs to address knowledge, attitudes and help seeking among youth. *Early Intervention in Psychiatry*, *7*(2), 109–121. doi:10.1111/eip.12010 PMID:23343220

Wei, Y., McGrath, P. J., Hayden, J., & Kutcher, S. (2016). Measurement properties of tools measuring mental health knowledge: A systematic review. *BMC Psychiatry*, *16*(1), 297. doi:10.118612888-016-1012-5 PMID:27553955

Weisman, H. L., Kia-Keating, M., Lippincott, A., Taylor, Z., & Zheng, J. (2016). Mental Health Stigma Prevention: Pilot Testing a Novel, Language Arts Curriculum-Based Approach for Youth. *The Journal of School Health*, *86*(10), 709–716. doi:10.1111/josh.12427 PMID:27619761

Weiss, B. D., Blanchard, J. S., McGee, D. L., Hart, G., Warren, B., Burgoon, M., & Smith, K. J. (1994). Illiteracy among Medicaid recipients and its relationship to health care costs. *Journal of Health Care for the Poor and Underserved*, *5*(2), 99–111. doi:10.1353/hpu.2010.0272 PMID:8043732

World Bank. (1993). *World Development Report 1993. Investing in Health*. Oxford, UK: Oxford University Press.

World Health Organization. (1996). *The Status of School Health*. Geneva: WHO.

World Health Organization. (2016). *Policy brief 4: Health literacy*. Retrieved from http://www.who.int/healthpromotion/conferences/9gchp/policy-brief4-health-literacy.pdf?ua=1

Zhang, Q., Huang, F., Liu, Z., Zhang, N., Mahapatra, T., Tang, W., ... Zhang, J. (2016). Cross-Cultural Validation of the High Blood Pressure Health Literacy Scale in a Chinese Community. *PLoS One*, *11*(4), 12. doi:10.1371/journal.pone.0152182 PMID:27116336

Chapter 11
An Overview of Global Health Initiatives and Practices

Kijpokin Kasemsap
Suan Sunandha Rajabhat University, Thailand

ABSTRACT

This chapter presents the overview of global health literacy, the advances issues of global health literacy, global health literacy and the internet utilization, global health literacy and disease management, and global health literacy and diabetes. Global health literacy is the important subject that is related to the individual's ability to understand and manage any healthcare issue. Global health literacy should be enhanced through healthcare providers and healthcare organizations. Global health literacy can help people prevent their health problems, protect their health, and manage their healthcare problems in a timely and effective manner. People who understand health instructions usually make fewer mistakes when taking medicine or preparing for the medical procedures toward the reduction of medical errors in global healthcare.

INTRODUCTION

Effective health care delivery is an essential issue for citizens and communities across the globe (Wickramasinghe, 2017). The growing complexity associated with using the health care system creates serious barriers to health care quality and access (Knight, 2017). One such barrier is the limited health literacy (Knight, 2017). Health literacy is about how patients understand health information about health and health care, and how they apply that health information to their daily lives, utilize it to make health-related decisions, and act on it (Kasemsap, 2017a). Health literacy deals with health behavior and the utilization of health services toward affecting health outcomes and health costs in health care settings (Kasemsap, 2018a).

Limited health literacy may lead to poor health outcomes and inappropriate health care utilization, particularly in patients with chronic diseases (Zuercher, Diatta, Burnand, & Peytremann-Bridevaux, 2017). Health-related issues have considerable impact on the lives of senior citizens and their well-being (Reychav & Azuri, 2016). To successfully assist patients in understanding complex health information

DOI: 10.4018/978-1-5225-4074-8.ch011

and in navigating the health system, professionals must make the distinction between low literacy and low health literacy (Barnett & Kaske, 2012). Health care providers and nurses must have the ability to adapt care for patients with low health literacy, making health literacy education of medical and nursing students essential (Mosley & Taylor, 2017).

Health professionals can utilize a broad range of health communication strategies to ensure patients understand their options and share their health care decisions (Kasemsap, 2017b) with the utilization of mobile health systems (Kasemsap, 2018b) and health informatics (Kasemsap, 2018c). Health care workers need resources that focus on health literacy, and patients require the understanding of health care-related information in a user-friendly format (Faddoul, 2017). Incorporation of an educational program into clinical visits for patients with chronic disease improved disease-specific knowledge and prompted patients to become activated and involved in their care, improving health behaviors and outcomes (Eckman et al., 2012).

This chapter is based on a literature review of global health literacy. The extensive literature of global health literacy provides a contribution to practitioners and researchers by indicating the initiatives and practices of global health literacy in global health care.

BACKGROUND

Health literacy is a growing concern as its relationship with health outcomes becomes clearer (Mackert, Ball, & Lopez, 2011). Health literacy is defined as a person's ability to act upon information about health (Nielsen-Bohlman, Panzer, & Kindig, 2004) and to effectively utilize such information to improve their health (Kaas, Stasková, & Šulistová, 2016). People with lower levels of health literacy create the higher emergency and health care costs (Mantwill & Schulz, 2015). Between one-third and one-half of all adults struggle with health information, and at-risk groups, such as the elderly, ethnic minorities, and those of lower socioeconomic status are more likely to have low health literacy (Nielsen-Bohlman et al., 2004).

Health literacy is recognized as a crucial element of patient safety (McCune, Lee, & Pohl, 2016). Along with increased awareness of health literacy, creation of strategies and initiatives, such as shared decision, plain language, and decision aides, have improved patient-centered approaches to facilitating the patients' ability to obtain and understand health information to the extent that they are able to affect a level of health autonomy (McNeil & Arena, 2017). By offering effective health information materials, older adults can play a more active role in their health care (Andrade, Silva, & Martins, 2017).

Functional health literacy focuses on both reading and writing skills that enable individuals to effectively function in everyday situations (Nutbeam, 2008). Inadequate functional health literacy is associated with poor recall of correct medication name, dosage, and administering frequency (Backes & Kuo, 2012). Interactive health literacy includes advanced skills that allow a person to extract information, derive meaning from different forms of communication and apply new information to the changing circumstances (Nutbeam, 2008). Interactive health literacy is associated with patients' perceived ability to organize care, interact with health care providers, and perform self-care (van der Heide, Heijmans, Schuit, Uiters, & Rademakers, 2015). Critical health literacy encompasses more advanced skills for analyzing information and for using information to exert greater control over life events and situations (Nutbeam, 2008).

IMPORTANT ASPECTS OF GLOBAL HEALTH LITERACY

This section indicates the overview of global health literacy; the advances issues of global health literacy; global health literacy and the Internet utilization; global health literacy and disease management; and global health literacy and diabetes.

Overview of Global Health Literacy

Inadequate health literacy, namely the problematic individual's ability to navigate the health care system, has been recognized as a silent approach affecting a large part of the world population (Palumbo, Annarumma, Adinolfi, Musella, & Piscopo, 2016). There is still need for deeper understanding on the determinants of health literacy in relation to adolescents to guide the development of health literacy instruments and interventions (Parisod, Axelin, Smed, & Salanterä, 2016). Regular self-monitoring and high health literacy are positively related in global health care (Carels, Selensky, Rossi, Solar, & Hlavka, 2017).

Populations most likely to experience low-literacy levels are among those being asked to manage chronic conditions; these include older adults, ethnic minorities for whom English is a second language, people with low levels of income and education, and people with an already compromised health status (Wolf, Gazmararian, & Baker, 2005). Individuals often read several grade levels lower than the highest grade achieved in school, and their health literacy may be lower than their general literacy skills because of unfamiliar medical vocabulary and concepts (Sayah & Williams, 2012). Health literacy measurement can help improve health care service delivery (Stonbraker, Schnall, & Larson, 2015).

Health literacy has the impact on the effective use of health care-related knowledge (Castro-Sánchez, Chang, Vila-Candel, Escobedo, & Holmes, 2016). The implications of adopting a broader social ecological perspective to address low health literacy shifts the field from thinking about the individual educational interventions to how individual interventions can be effectively enhanced by the interventions at additional levels of influence (McCormack, Thomas, Lewis, & Rudd, 2017). Low health literate individuals face a range of problems, including longer and more frequent hospitalizations and more trouble managing chronic conditions (Weiss & Palmer, 2004).

Patients receive health information from a wide variety of medical and administrative staffs, so it is important all health care workers be sensitive to the needs of those with low health literacy to improve all aspects of providing health care, including interpersonal communication, the readability of patient forms and handouts, and flow of patients through a health care organization (Mackert et al., 2011). Patients with limited health literacy are often less prepared for diagnostic examinations, and as a result, tend to have the examinations of poorer diagnostic quality (Goguen, 2016).

Patients' comprehension of their injury, health care treatment, and health care provider's instructions plays an important role in health management and recovery from trauma (Roh et al., 2016). Low health literate patients must understand the physicians' explanations of their conditions with the support of health care recommendation, and this health literacy-related breakdown in communication contributes to poorer outcomes (Schillinger, Bindman, Wang, Stewart, & John, 2004).

Health literacy initiatives can be promoted by focusing on health care-related clients to develop domain-specific skills that increase the likelihood of using health information sources and accrue benefits (Suri, Majid, Chang, & Foo, 2016). Poor health literacy is a stronger predictor of a person's health than age, income, employment status, education level and race (Schillinger et al., 2002), and is associated with a wide range of adverse direct and indirect effects on care processes and health outcomes (Howard, Gazmararian, & Parker, 2005).

Advanced Issues of Global Health Literacy

Low health literacy is found to be associated with various issues, such as the lack of preventive-service utilization (Scott, Gazmararian, Williams, & Baker, 2002); delayed diagnoses (Wolf et al., 2006); alterations in physical and mental health (Wolf et al., 2005); decreased self-management skills (Williams, Baker, Parker, & Nurss, 1998); misunderstandings about medical conditions (Gazmararian, Williams, Peel, & Baker, 2002); poor self-rated health; increased mortality risk (Baker, Wolf, Feinglass, & Thompson, 2007); and higher utilization of services.

Limited health literacy is associated with restricted health-related knowledge (Ishikawa, Takeuchi, & Yano, 2008), and is linked to suboptimal health practices, such as limited utilization of preventive care (Howard, Sentell, & Gazmararian, 2006) and medication nonadherence (Osborn, Paasche-Orlow, Davis, & Wolf, 2007). Low-literate individuals are more likely to gain the poor health status (Wolf et al., 2005), functional limitations (Kim & Kim, 2009), and poor glycemic control (Powell, Hill, & Clancy, 2007). Thus, health care professionals should explore the patients' application of complementary and alternative approaches, and health literacy should be improved so that patients can be informed regarding the possible benefits and disadvantages of complementary and alternative therapies (Dişsiz & Yilmaz, 2016).

The development, implementation, and evaluation of health literacy interventions for older people with chronic conditions are important to increase medication adherence and improve patient outcomes (Lee, Yu, You, & Son, 2017). Decreased medication knowledge and medication adherence are linked to patients with low health literacy (Barnett & Kaske, 2012). Compared with individuals with adequate health literacy, the presence of limited or inadequate health literacy has been associated with poorer health status, decreased utilization of preventative care, increased application of medical resources through increased hospitalizations, and increased risk of premature death (Mullins, Blatt, Gbarayor, Yang, & Baquet, 2005).

Motivational determinants include traditional social cognition constructs (e.g., beliefs and attitudes), which are associated with access to health information and knowledge (Fransen, von Wagner, & Essink-Bot, 2012). Volitional determinants refer to both objective and subjective (e.g., self-efficacy) action controls, and include task-specific skills, such as information processing and navigational skills to acquire the specific knowledge about medication adherence regimens and cognitive skills (Fransen et al., 2012). Patients are called upon to be increasingly responsible for self-care at the same time that medical care becomes more complex and technical (Matsuyama et al., 2011). To improve self-care behaviors, health care providers should target improving self-efficacy, and enhancing health literacy can be considered as a potential strategy for improving self-efficacy (Lee et al., 2016).

Global Health Literacy and the Internet Utilization

The Internet represents an essential tool for knowledge translation to consumers of health information (Arocha & Hoffman-Goetz, 2008). For consumers, the Internet offers virtually limitless information on health, multiple health perspectives, and the ability to communicate with others concerning health issues (Willis, Wang, & Rodgers, 2013). Those with advanced electronic health (e-health) literacy skills can apply more efficient online search strategies and can identify higher-quality health information resources (Quinn, Bond, & Nugent, 2017). The effects of motivation for health-related Internet use on health literacy are mediated by both health-related Internet application and perceived health information overload (Jiang & Beaudoin, 2016).

The percentages of seeking health-related information on the Internet of those who live in the cities are higher than those who live in the rural areas (Yildirim & Çakir, 2017). Technological efforts should be made to make e-health services easily accessible to low-literacy individuals and to enhance individual health literacy through educational programs (Kim & Xie, 2017). E-health make it possible for health care providers to better manage patient care through the secure use and sharing of health information (Kasemsap, 2017c). Communication and patient education efforts should aim to raise awareness on online health information quality and to promote the application of established evaluation criteria, especially among low health literate citizens (Diviani, van den Putte, Meppelink, & van Weert, 2016).

Global Health Literacy and Disease Management

The World Health Organization (WHO) has supported the concept of therapeutic patient education as an essential strategy to increase the patients' active participation in the process of disease management (Maisano, 2006). However, low health literacy can describe a barrier to patient understanding and involvement in self-management programs (Ebright, Urden, Patterson, & Chalko, 2004). Regarding disease management, video images can enhance health care-related communication with patients (Frosch, Kaplan, & Felitti, 2003).

The addition of a video component to educational materials has promoted patients' knowledge about diseases and treatments, and has increased the involvement in treatment decisions (Wood & Duffy, 2004). There is the study involving patients with congestive heart failure describing the relationship between decreased medication knowledge and adherence with increased cardiovascular-related emergency-department visits (Backes & Kuo, 2012).

Global Health Literacy and Diabetes

Health literacy has been associated with many health care components and outcomes in individuals with chronic illnesses, including those with diabetes (Sayah & Williams, 2012). In individuals with diabetes, research studies present an association between low health literacy and worse glycemic control (Powell et al., 2007); higher risk of significant hypoglycemia (Sarkar et al., 2010); higher rates of retinopathy (Schillinger et al., 2002); less comprehension of medication instructions, dosing, timing and warnings (Wolf et al., 2007); poorer disease knowledge (Gazmararian et al., 2002), and poorer patient-physician communication (Castro, Wilson, Wang, & Schillinger, 2007).

FUTURE RESEARCH DIRECTIONS

The classification of the extensive literature in the domains of global health literacy will provide the potential opportunities for future research. Digital literacy is the ability to find, evaluate, utilize, share, and create the digital content (Kasemsap, 2017d) regarding ICT competency (Kasemsap, 2018d). Medical errors are caused by mistakes in drug prescription, dosing, and medical administration in inpatient and outpatient settings (Kasemsap, 2017e). Knowledge management (KM) is the functional application of knowledge and organizational resources (Kasemsap, 2018e). Knowledge transfer emphasizes the source of the knowledge and its receiver in order to distribute the determined knowledge among people (Kasemsap, 2018f). Investigating the relationships among global health literacy, digital literacy, health outcomes, KM, and knowledge transfer toward the reduction of medical errors in global health care should be further studied.

CONCLUSION

This chapter explained the overview of global health literacy; the advances issues of global health literacy; global health literacy and the Internet utilization; global health literacy and disease management; and global health literacy and diabetes. Global health literacy is the important subject that is related to the individual's ability to understand and manage any health care issue. Global health literacy should be enhanced through health care providers and health care organizations. Global health literacy can help people prevent their health problems, protect their health, and manage their health care problems in a timely and effective manner. People who understand health instructions usually make fewer mistakes when taking medicine or preparing for the medical procedures toward the reduction of medical errors in global health care.

REFERENCES

Andrade, I., Silva, C., & Martins, A. C. (2017). Application of the Health Literacy INDEX on the development of a manual for prevention of falls for older adults. *Patient Education and Counseling*, *100*(1), 154–159. doi:10.1016/j.pec.2016.07.036 PMID:27516436

Arocha, J. F., & Hoffman-Goetz, L. (2008). Improving Internet-based health knowledge through attention to literacy. In A. Kushniruk & E. Borycki (Eds.), *Human, social, and organizational aspects of health information systems* (pp. 331–346). Hershey, PA: IGI Global. doi:10.4018/978-1-59904-792-8.ch020

Backes, A. C., & Kuo, G. M. (2012). The association between functional health literacy and patient-reported recall of medications at outpatient pharmacies. *Research in Social & Administrative Pharmacy*, *8*(4), 349–354. doi:10.1016/j.sapharm.2011.08.001 PMID:22133649

Baker, D. W., Wolf, M. S., Feinglass, J., & Thompson, J. A. (2007). Health literacy and mortality among elderly persons. *Archives of Internal Medicine*, *167*(14), 1503–1509. doi:10.1001/archinte.167.14.1503 PMID:17646604

Barnett, S. G., & Kaske, B. (2012). Impact of a health literacy presentation during an introductory pharmacy practice experience. *Currents in Pharmacy Teaching and Learning*, *4*(1), 39–45. doi:10.1016/j.cptl.2011.10.001

Carels, R. A., Selensky, J. C., Rossi, J., Solar, C., & Hlavka, R. (2017). A novel stepped-care approach to weight loss: The role of self-monitoring and health literacy in treatment outcomes. *Eating Behaviors*, *26*, 76–82. doi:10.1016/j.eatbeh.2017.01.009 PMID:28189945

Castro, C. M., Wilson, C., Wang, F., & Schillinger, D. (2007). Babel babble: Physicians' use of unclarified medical jargon with patients. *American Journal of Health Behavior*, *31*(Suppl. 1), S85–S95. doi:10.5993/AJHB.31.s1.11 PMID:17931142

Castro-Sánchez, E., Chang, P. W. S., Vila-Candel, R., Escobedo, A. A., & Holmes, A. H. (2016). Health literacy and infectious diseases: Why does it matter? *International Journal of Infectious Diseases*, *43*, 103–110. doi:10.1016/j.ijid.2015.12.019 PMID:26751238

Dişsiz, G., & Yilmaz, M. (2016). Complementary and alternative therapies and health literacy in cancer patients. *Complementary Therapies in Clinical Practice*, *23*, 34–39. doi:10.1016/j.ctcp.2016.02.004 PMID:27157956

Diviani, N., van den Putte, B., Meppelink, C. S., & van Weert, J. C. M. (2016). Exploring the role of health literacy in the evaluation of online health information: Insights from a mixed-methods study. *Patient Education and Counseling*, *99*(6), 1017–1025. doi:10.1016/j.pec.2016.01.007 PMID:26817407

Ebright, P. R., Urden, L., Patterson, E., & Chalko, B. (2004). Themes surrounding novice nurse near-miss and adverse-event situations. *The Journal of Nursing Administration*, *34*(11), 531–538. doi:10.1097/00005110-200411000-00010 PMID:15586075

Eckman, M. H., Wise, R., Leonard, A. C., Dixon, E., Burrows, C., Khan, F., & Warm, E. (2012). Impact of health literacy on outcomes and effectiveness of an educational intervention in patients with chronic diseases. *Patient Education and Counseling*, *87*(2), 143–151. doi:10.1016/j.pec.2011.07.020 PMID:21925823

Faddoul, B. (2017). Gamification and health literacy. In I. Management Association (Ed.), Medical education and ethics: Concepts, methodologies, tools, and applications (pp. 51–62). Hershey, PA: IGI Global. doi:10.4018/978-1-5225-0978-3.ch003

Fransen, M. P., von Wagner, C., & Essink-Bot, M. L. (2012). Diabetes self-management in patients with low health literacy: Ordering findings from literature in a health literacy framework. *Patient Education and Counseling*, *88*(1), 44–53. doi:10.1016/j.pec.2011.11.015 PMID:22196986

Frosch, D. L., Kaplan, R. M., & Felitti, V. J. (2003). A randomized controlled trial comparing Internet and video to facilitate patient education for men considering the prostate-specific antigen test. *Journal of General Internal Medicine*, *18*(10), 781–787. doi:10.1046/j.1525-1497.2003.20911.x PMID:14521639

Gazmararian, J. A., Williams, M. V., Peel, J., & Baker, D. W. (2002). Health literacy and knowledge of chronic disease. *Patient Education and Counseling*, *51*(3), 267–275. doi:10.1016/S0738-3991(02)00239-2 PMID:14630383

Goguen, J. (2016). Health literacy and patient preparation in radiology. *Journal of Medical Imaging and Radiation Sciences*, *47*(3), 283–286. doi:10.1016/j.jmir.2016.06.002

Howard, D. H., Gazmararian, J. A., & Parker, R. M. (2005). The impact of low health literacy on the medical costs of Medicare managed care enrollees. *The American Journal of Medicine*, *118*(4), 371–377. doi:10.1016/j.amjmed.2005.01.010 PMID:15808134

Howard, D. H., Sentell, T., & Gazmararian, J. A. (2006). Impact of health literacy on socioeconomic and racial differences in health in an elderly population. *Journal of General Internal Medicine*, *21*(8), 857–861. doi:10.1111/j.1525-1497.2006.00530.x PMID:16881947

Ishikawa, H., Takeuchi, T., & Yano, E. (2008). Measuring functional, communicative, and critical health literacy among diabetic patients. *Diabetes Care*, *31*(5), 874–879. doi:10.2337/dc07-1932 PMID:18299446

Jiang, S., & Beaudoin, C. E. (2016). Health literacy and the Internet: An exploratory study on the 2013 HINTS survey. *Computers in Human Behavior*, *58*, 240–248. doi:10.1016/j.chb.2016.01.007

Kaas, J., Stasková, V., & Šulistová, R. (2016). The concept of health literacy in contemporary nursing. *Kontakt*, *18*(4), e219–e223. doi:10.1016/j.kontakt.2016.10.001

Kasemsap, K. (2017a). The fundamentals of health literacy. In N. Wickramasinghe (Ed.), *Handbook of research on healthcare administration and management* (pp. 507–527). Hershey, PA: IGI Global. doi:10.4018/978-1-5225-0920-2.ch030

Kasemsap, K. (2017b). Promoting health literacy in global health care. In N. Wickramasinghe (Ed.), *Handbook of research on healthcare administration and management* (pp. 485–506). Hershey, PA: IGI Global. doi:10.4018/978-1-5225-0920-2.ch029

Kasemsap, K. (2017c). Telemedicine and electronic health: Issues and implications in developing countries. In K. Moahi, K. Bwalya, & P. Sebina (Eds.), *Health information systems and the advancement of medical practice in developing countries* (pp. 149–167). Hershey, PA: IGI Global. doi:10.4018/978-1-5225-2262-1.ch009

Kasemsap, K. (2017d). Digital storytelling and digital literacy: Advanced issues and prospects. In D. Loveless, P. Sullivan, K. Dredger, & J. Burns (Eds.), *Deconstructing the education-industrial complex in the digital age* (pp. 151–171). Hershey, PA: IGI Global. doi:10.4018/978-1-5225-2101-3.ch009

Kasemsap, K. (2017e). The perspectives of medical errors in the health care industry. In M. Riga (Ed.), *Impact of medical errors and malpractice on health economics, quality, and patient safety* (pp. 113–143). Hershey, PA: IGI Global. doi:10.4018/978-1-5225-2337-6.ch005

Kasemsap, K. (2018a). Challenges and implications of health literacy in global health care. In M. Khosrow-Pour (Ed.), *Encyclopedia of information science and technology* (4th ed.; pp. 3734–3744). Hershey, PA: IGI Global. doi:10.4018/978-1-5225-2255-3.ch324

Kasemsap, K. (2018b). Mobile health systems and electronic health record: Applications and implications. In J. Machado, A. Abelha, M. Santos, & F. Portela (Eds.), *Next-generation mobile and pervasive healthcare solutions* (pp. 67–85). Hershey, PA: IGI Global. doi:10.4018/978-1-5225-2851-7.ch005

Kasemsap, K. (2018c). Advanced issues of health informatics and clinical decision support system in global health care. In J. Machado, A. Abelha, M. Santos, & F. Portela (Eds.), *Next-generation mobile and pervasive healthcare solutions* (pp. 153–170). Hershey, PA: IGI Global. doi:10.4018/978-1-5225-2851-7.ch010

Kasemsap, K. (2018d). Encouraging digital literacy and ICT competency in the information age. In M. Khosrow-Pour (Ed.), *Encyclopedia of information science and technology* (4th ed.; pp. 2253–2263). Hershey, PA: IGI Global. doi:10.4018/978-1-5225-2255-3.ch196

Kasemsap, K. (2018e). Knowledge management: Applications and implications. In A. Gyamfi & I. Williams (Eds.), *Evaluating media richness in organizational learning* (pp. 232–261). Hershey, PA: IGI Global. doi:10.4018/978-1-5225-2956-9.ch012

Kasemsap, K. (2018f). The role of knowledge transfer in modern organizations. In F. Di Virgilio (Ed.), *Social media for knowledge management applications in modern organizations* (pp. 190–217). Hershey, PA: IGI Global. doi:10.4018/978-1-5225-2897-5.ch009

Kim, H., & Xie, B. (2017). Health literacy in the eHealth era: A systematic review of the literature. *Patient Education and Counseling*, *100*(6), 1073–1082. doi:10.1016/j.pec.2017.01.015 PMID:28174067

Kim, S. H., & Kim, S. H. (2009). Health literacy and functional health status in Korean older adults. *Journal of Clinical Nursing*, *18*(16), 2337–2343. doi:10.1111/j.1365-2702.2008.02739.x PMID:19583664

Knight, G. D. (2017). Health literacy: An essential ingredient for better health outcomes –Overview of health literacy theoretical concepts. In I. Management Association (Ed.), Medical education and ethics: Concepts, methodologies, tools, and applications (pp. 22–50). Hershey, PA: IGI Global. doi:10.4018/978-1-5225-0978-3.ch002

Lee, Y. J., Shin, S. J., Wang, R. H., Lin, K. D., Lee, Y. L., & Wang, Y. H. (2016). Pathways of empowerment perceptions, health literacy, self-efficacy, and self-care behaviors to glycemic control in patients with type 2 diabetes mellitus. *Patient Education and Counseling*, *99*(2), 287–294. doi:10.1016/j.pec.2015.08.021 PMID:26341940

Lee, Y. M., Yu, H. Y., You, M. E., & Son, Y. J. (2017). Impact of health literacy on medication adherence in older people with chronic diseases. *Collegian (Royal College of Nursing, Australia)*, *24*(1), 11–18. doi:10.1016/j.colegn.2015.08.003 PMID:29218957

Mackert, M., Ball, J., & Lopez, N. (2011). Health literacy awareness training for healthcare workers: Improving knowledge and intentions to use clear communication techniques. *Patient Education and Counseling*, *85*(3), e225–e228. doi:10.1016/j.pec.2011.02.022 PMID:21474264

Maisano, G. (2006). *Therapeutic education of patients with coronary heart disease: Training guide for general practitioners*. Udine, Italy: World Health Organization.

Mantwill, S., & Schulz, P. J. (2015). Low health literacy associated with higher medication costs in patients with type 2 diabetes mellitus: Evidence from matched survey and health insurance data. *Patient Education and Counseling*, *98*(12), 1625–1630. doi:10.1016/j.pec.2015.07.006 PMID:26198546

Matsuyama, R. K., Wilson-Genderson, M., Kuhn, L., Moghanaki, D., Vachhani, H., & Paasche-Orlow, M. (2011). Education level, not health literacy, associated with information needs for patients with cancer. *Patient Education and Counseling*, *85*(3), e229–e236. doi:10.1016/j.pec.2011.03.022 PMID:21543182

McCormack, L., Thomas, V., Lewis, M. A., & Rudd, R. (2017). Improving low health literacy and patient engagement: A social ecological approach. *Patient Education and Counseling*, *100*(1), 8–13. doi:10.1016/j.pec.2016.07.007 PMID:27475265

McCune, R. L., Lee, H., & Pohl, J. M. (2016). Assessing health literacy in safety net primary care practices. *Applied Nursing Research*, *29*, 188–194. doi:10.1016/j.apnr.2015.04.004 PMID:26856512

McNeil, A., & Arena, R. (2017). The evolution of health literacy and communication: Introducing health harmonics. *Progress in Cardiovascular Diseases*, *59*(5), 463–470. doi:10.1016/j.pcad.2017.02.003 PMID:28216109

Mosley, C. M., & Taylor, B. J. (2017). Integration of health literacy content into nursing curriculum utilizing the health literacy expanded model. *Teaching and Learning in Nursing*, *12*(2), 109–116. doi:10.1016/j.teln.2016.12.005

Mullins, C. D., Blatt, L., Gbarayor, C. M., Yang, H. W., & Baquet, C. (2005). Health disparities: A barrier to high-quality care. *American Journal of Health-System Pharmacy*, *62*(18), 1873–1882. doi:10.2146/ajhp050064 PMID:16141106

Nielsen-Bohlman, L., Panzer, A., & Kindig, D. (2004). *Health literacy: A prescription to end confusion.* Washington, DC: National Academy of Sciences.

Nutbeam, D. (2008). The evolving concept of health literacy. *Social Science & Medicine*, *67*(12), 2072–2078. doi:10.1016/j.socscimed.2008.09.050 PMID:18952344

Osborn, C. Y., Paasche-Orlow, M. K., Davis, T. C., & Wolf, M. S. (2007). Health literacy: An overlooked factor in understanding HIV health disparities. *American Journal of Preventive Medicine*, *33*(5), 374–378. doi:10.1016/j.amepre.2007.07.022 PMID:17950402

Palumbo, R., Annarumma, C., Adinolfi, P., Musella, M., & Piscopo, G. (2016). The Italian health literacy project: Insights from the assessment of health literacy skills in Italy. *Health Policy (Amsterdam)*, *120*(9), 1087–1094. doi:10.1016/j.healthpol.2016.08.007 PMID:27593949

Parisod, H., Axelin, A., Smed, J., & Salanterä, S. (2016). Determinants of tobacco-related health literacy: A qualitative study with early adolescents. *International Journal of Nursing Studies*, *62*, 71–80. doi:10.1016/j.ijnurstu.2016.07.012 PMID:27459318

Powell, C. K., Hill, E. G., & Clancy, D. E. (2007). The relationship between health literacy and diabetes knowledge and readiness to take health actions. *The Diabetes Educator*, *33*(1), 144–151. doi:10.1177/0145721706297452 PMID:17272800

Quinn, S., Bond, R., & Nugent, C. (2017). Quantifying health literacy and eHealth literacy using existing instruments and browser-based software for tracking online health information seeking behavior. *Computers in Human Behavior*, *69*, 256–267. doi:10.1016/j.chb.2016.12.032

Reychav, I., & Azuri, J. (2016). Including elderly patients in decision making via electronic health literacy. In M. Cruz-Cunha, I. Miranda, R. Martinho, & R. Rijo (Eds.), *Encyclopedia of e-health and telemedicine* (pp. 241–249). Hershey, PA: IGI Global. doi:10.4018/978-1-4666-9978-6.ch020

Roh, Y. H., Lee, B. K., Park, M. H., Noh, J. H., Gong, H. S., & Baek, G. H. (2016). Effects of health literacy on treatment outcome and satisfaction in patients with mallet finger injury. *Journal of Hand Therapy*, *29*(4), 459–464. doi:10.1016/j.jht.2016.06.004 PMID:27765527

Sarkar, U., Karter, A. J., Liu, J. Y., Moffet, H. H., Adler, N. E., & Schillinger, D. (2010). Hypoglycemia is more common among type 2 diabetes patients with limited health literacy: The Diabetes Study of Northern California (DISTANCE). *Journal of General Internal Medicine*, *25*(9), 962–967. doi:10.100711606-010-1389-7 PMID:20480249

Sayah, F. A., & Williams, B. (2012). An integrated model of health literacy using diabetes as an exemplar. *Canadian Journal of Diabetes*, *36*(1), 27–31. doi:10.1016/j.jcjd.2011.08.001

Schillinger, D., Bindman, A. B., Wang, F., Stewart, A., & John, P. (2004). Functional health literacy and the quality of physician–patient communication among diabetes patients. *Patient Education and Counseling*, *52*(3), 315–323. doi:10.1016/S0738-3991(03)00107-1 PMID:14998602

Schillinger, D., Grumbach, K., Piette, J., Wang, F., Osmond, D., Daher, C., ... Bindman, A. B. (2002). Association of health literacy with diabetes outcomes. *Journal of the American Medical Association*, *288*(4), 475–482. doi:10.1001/jama.288.4.475 PMID:12132978

Scott, T. L., Gazmararian, J. A., Williams, M. V., & Baker, D. W. (2002). Health literacy and preventive health care use among Medicare enrollees in a managed care organization. *Medical Care*, *40*(5), 395–404. doi:10.1097/00005650-200205000-00005 PMID:11961474

Stonbraker, S., Schnall, R., & Larson, E. (2015). Tools to measure health literacy among Spanish speakers: An integrative review of the literature. *Patient Education and Counseling*, *98*(12), 1513–1523. doi:10.1016/j.pec.2015.07.012 PMID:26227578

Suri, V. R., Majid, S., Chang, Y. K., & Foo, S. (2016). Assessing the influence of health literacy on health information behaviors: A multi-domain skills-based approach. *Patient Education and Counseling*, *99*(6), 1038–1045. doi:10.1016/j.pec.2015.12.017 PMID:26794667

van der Heide, I., Heijmans, M., Schuit, A. J., Uiters, E., & Rademakers, J. (2015). Functional, interactive and critical health literacy: Varying relationships with control over care and number of GP visits. *Patient Education and Counseling*, *98*(8), 998–1004. doi:10.1016/j.pec.2015.04.006 PMID:25956070

Weiss, B. D., & Palmer, R. (2004). Relationship between health care costs and very low literacy skills in a medically needy and indigent Medicaid population. *The Journal of the American Board of Family Practice*, *17*(1), 44–47. doi:10.3122/jabfm.17.1.44 PMID:15014052

Wickramasinghe, N. (2017). *Handbook of research on healthcare administration and management*. Hershey, PA: IGI Global. doi:10.4018/978-1-5225-0920-2

Williams, M. V., Baker, D. W., Parker, R. M., & Nurss, J. R. (1998). Relationship of functional health literacy to patients' knowledge of their chronic disease. *Archives of Internal Medicine*, *158*(2), 166–172. doi:10.1001/archinte.158.2.166 PMID:9448555

Willis, E., Wang, Y., & Rodgers, S. (2013). Online health communities and health literacy: Applying a framework for understanding domains of health literacy. In I. Management Association (Ed.), User-driven healthcare: Concepts, methodologies, tools, and applications (pp. 180–196). Hershey, PA: IGI Global. doi:10.4018/978-1-4666-2770-3.ch010

Wolf, M. S., Gazmararian, J. A., & Baker, D. W. (2005). Health literacy and functional health status among older adults. *Archives of Internal Medicine*, *165*(17), 1946–1952. doi:10.1001/archinte.165.17.1946 PMID:16186463

Wolf, M. S., Knight, S. J., Lyons, E. A., Durazo-Arvizu, R., Pickard, S. A., Arseven, A., ... Bennett, C. L. (2006). Literacy, race, and PSA level among low-income men newly diagnosed with prostate cancer. *Urology*, *68*(1), 89–93. doi:10.1016/j.urology.2006.01.064 PMID:16844451

Wolf, M. S., Williams, M. V., Parker, R. M., Parikh, N. S., Nowlan, A. W., & Baker, D. W. (2007). Patients' shame and attitudes toward discussing the results of literacy screening. *Journal of Health Communication*, *12*(8), 721–732. doi:10.1080/10810730701672173 PMID:18030638

Wood, R. Y., & Duffy, M. E. (2004). Video breast health kits: Testing a cancer education innovation in older high-risk populations. *Journal of Cancer Education*, *19*(2), 98–104. doi:10.120715430154jce1902_10 PMID:15456666

Yildirim, F., & Çakir, M. (2017). Are adult women or men who use the Internet as a health information resource more health literate? In I. Management Association (Ed.), Medical education and ethics: Concepts, methodologies, tools, and applications (pp. 1208–1234). Hershey, PA: IGI Global. doi:10.4018/978-1-5225-0978-3.ch055

Zuercher, E., Diatta, I. D., Burnand, B., & Peytremann-Bridevaux, I. (2017). Health literacy and quality of care of patients with diabetes: A cross-sectional analysis. *Primary Care Diabetes*, *11*(3), 233–240. doi:10.1016/j.pcd.2017.02.003 PMID:28292571

KEY TERMS AND DEFINITIONS

Communication: The process of sending and receiving messages.

Healthcare: The practical execution of body health and mental health.

Information: The knowledge that can be gained and shared through several methods.

Knowledge: The information that can help individuals solve the problems.

Literacy: The state of being educated in the specific matter.

Patient: The person who requires the medical care.

Skill: The ability to manage the significant tasks.

Understanding: The condition of an individual who understands any subject.

Chapter 12
Health Literacy and Ethnic Minority Populations

Dela Idowu
Gift of Living Donation, UK

Gillian King
University of London, UK

ABSTRACT

This chapter will show how optimizing health literacy can benefit the delivery of healthcare to the population in a way that materially addresses the inequalities in the National Health Service (NHS). These inequalities adversely impact different population groups in different ways, for various reasons. However, ethnic minority populations are especially vulnerable to inequalities having an adverse effect on the delivery of healthcare to the population, thereby adversely affecting their access, engagement, and healthcare benefits and consequently their general health, wellbeing, and life expectancy. Optimizing health literacy in these populations will enable increased engagement and participation, thereby delivering healthcare more effectively to the population by tailoring it to their needs and addressing current inequalities.

INTRODUCTION

The delivery of healthcare to the UK population since 1948, has been achieved through a universal system of healthcare, the National Health Service (NHS). In post-war Britain, it was the aim of the government of the day to provide the entire population with a service which was universal and free at the point of need. The service remains free, although patients who are able, in certain circumstances contribute through paying for prescriptions, dental, and optical services. The service has remained the same in principle for almost 70 years, and has resisted attempts to introduce direct contributions despite a rapidly changing and aging population, and advances in medical science that drive up the cost of healthcare and the expectations of patients. The NHS is still the largest single pay system in the world, employing some 1.4 million people.

DOI: 10.4018/978-1-5225-4074-8.ch012

It could be argued, however, that the comprehensive nature of the delivery to the entire population produced a weakness which was not accounted for from the its inception (Asaria, 2017). Thus, inequalities developed, which according to Asaria (2017), have resisted various attempts over the years to mitigate.

The UK being a diverse[1] country made up of four nation, England, Wales, Scotland, and Northern Ireland, needed a service which would cater to the unique needs of the population. Early on, the system was unable to meet those needs, and inequalities appeared which can affect different populations in various ways.

It is well established that inequalities can arise from ethnicity (Szczepura, 2005), geographical location (Hacking et al., 2011), age (Raine et al., 2009), gender (Rein et al., 2010), type of illness (Emerson & Baines, 2011), and other aspects of disadvantage or vulnerability (Parry et al., 2007; Dixon-Woods et al., 2006) (as cited by Cookson, Propper, Asaria & Raine, 2016 p.1). As well as the aforementioned inequalities, there is also ample evidence that there are socio-economic inequalities in the NHS. Cookson et al (2016) concluded that despite "poorer individuals receiving a greater quantity of publicly funded NHS healthcare in terms of overall expenditure… richer patients tend to achieve better outcomes" (p.19).

Ethnic minority populations often bear the brunt of some of these inequalities as ethnicity has an impact on health inequalities (Matthews, 2015). It was established by Karlson & Nazroo (2000) that ethnicity has an impact on the health of the population and has been recognised as a crucial factor since the 1970s. (as cited by Matthews, 2015 p.18). Socio-economic inequalities affect ethnic minority populations disproportionately, as a greater proportion of them are in a lower socio-economic group and experience social deprivation in the form of unemployment, poverty, and poor housing more acutely than the rest of the population. This adversely affects their engagement with healthcare delivery, which invariably results in poorer health outcomes. Bécares (2013) has found that generally, people from black and minority ethnic backgrounds in Britain have poorer health than the rest of the population. (as cited by Matthews, 2015 p.19).

Further, Bécares (2013) found that geographical inequalities also affect ethnic minority populations more adversely, with London residents experiencing greater inequality than the rest of the population in Britain (as cited by Matthews, 2015 p.19). So, an individual of ethnic minority origin, who lives in London, can be up to three times more likely to have a long-term illness than their white counterpart. It is possible that the picture is much more complex, and indeed, Williams (2015) argues as much, but repeated research has found that these inequalities persist, despite many attempts through research and government policy to address them. (Asaria, 2017).

It has been argued that the inequalities persist due to a lack of consensus among academics and policy makers alike, as to their cause and origin. The concept of biological differences among the races has historically been used to interpret different epidemiology of the diseases of different races. However, Williams (2015) argues against this and contends that there is no evidence that biological differences exist between ethnicities as "different population groups have more biological commonalities than differences; variations that do exist are no greater than those in a single population group (White, 2013)". (Williams, 2015 p.18).

Therefore, it is logical to conclude that the inequalities persist due to the social and economic structures that contribute to the inequalities in our society, which is a conclusion Williams (2015) comes to, after he analyses the impact racism has on inequalities. Institutional racism is no doubt a factor in the way the NHS operates and relates to the ethnic minority population. A British social attitudes survey conducted in 2013 showed that, though consistently dropping since 1983, 30% of the British population still described themselves as racially prejudiced. (National Centre of Social Research, 2014). There is, therefore, ample support for the conclusion that racially prejudiced attitudes persist in British institutions of which the NHS is one.

The persistence of these inequalities for the ethnic minority population within the NHS has been previously identified and acknowledged. Following the McPherson Inquiry (1999),[2] Race Equality Action plan was launched to address the lack of diversity in the leadership of the NHS. It was necessary to launch subsequent plans in 2004 and 2015 as little progress was made in the previous strategies. As research now shows a link between patient experience and treatment of ethnic minority staff, it has become imperative to address the inequalities that are evident in the NHS as an institution (Kline, 2015). The author further asserts that "such research provides a powerful business case for tackling discrimination to improve patient care, especially when further strengthened by evidence that diversity in leadership benefits innovation and the likelihood that NHS organisations whose leadership more closely resembles that of the communities being served will be more sensitive to their needs" (Kline, 2015, para.3).

Health literacy is well placed to address these inequalities, as the main advantage of health literacy is patient engagement, which would enable the ethnic minority population to engage with their own health needs as well as with the healthcare professionals in delivering those needs to the population. An engaged population increases participation and empowerment of the patients which would improve health outcomes and decrease mortality rates. Berkman et al. (2011) showed that people who lack health literacy have poorer health outcomes and higher mortality rates (as cited by Batterham, Hawkins, Collins, Buchbinder & Osborne, 2016).

According to Berkman et al. (2011) health literacy is a relatively new concept and was first established in the 1970s to increase patients' ability to engage with their healthcare by being able to read and understand written health information (as cited by Batterham et al.2016 p. 3). The concept has recently become more prominent as a result of the European health policy framework, Health 2020. The policy builds on two European Health charters[3] which promote health in terms of human rights and has at its heart patient participation, improvements in leadership, and health governance that is participatory. This approach has been adopted by European countries including the UK since the WHO regional office Europe launched a strategic document, "Priorities for health systems strengthening in the WHO European Region 2015 – 2020: walking the talk on people centeredness" (Jakab et al., 2016). As the title suggests, the emphasis is people centred and is therefore an opportunity to optimize health literacy beyond just improving the ability of patients to understand written health information. There is potential for the health literacy of individuals to be harnessed for the benefit of the community and populations and to further enhance it in organisations to benefit the health system and population groups alike (Batterham et al., 2016).

This will enable health systems and population groups to work together to improve health literacy in vulnerable population groups and thereby improve the health outcomes and mortality of population groups where inequalities persist. It is also an opportunity in the UK to strengthen the leadership in the NHS in order that it may better serve the healthcare needs of the population groups.

The current structure of the NHS does not match the needs of the ethnic minority population. The reasons for this are complex, but it is at least in part due to the unrepresentative leadership. Senior management and decision-makers in the NHS, do not match the population they serve. It can therefore be a challenge for the voice of patients and patient groups to be heard, but if the healthcare system includes health literacy as part of its organisational structure this will produce organically, a more diverse leadership which could better serve the community. Kline (2014) concluded that, "it is surely time to urgently and decisively address the widespread, deep-rooted, systemic and largely unchanging discrimination that black and minority ethnic staff within the NHS face. The evidence is now clear that their treatment is a good predictor of the quality of patient care." (p.66).

This chapter will outline how health literacy can specifically address the inequalities already identified.

BACKGROUND

Health literacy was first introduced as a concept by Simonds (1974) as a means of improving healthcare delivery, by providing basic health education (as cited by Palumbo, 2016). It was thought that patients would be able to participate better in their health care if they were provided with written and numerical health information that they could understand, and this would aid in the delivery of their care.

However, there is not as yet a universal standard method of measuring individual health literacy, but different methods have been used which attempt to quantify the extent to which individuals are able to understand health information, which require both numerical and written skills. It has been suggested that the current measurement tools do not consider the way the modern broader definition of health literacy has evolved, and therefore constitutes a limitation on how health literacy may be used to improve inequalities (Batterham et al., 2016).

Nevertheless, in England, a recent study discovered that 43% of adults (16-65) found health information provided by the health system, such as medicine labels, health history, consent forms, education booklets, and brochures, difficult to understand. This rose to 61% when the information required numerical skills (Rowlands et al., 2016). It is worth noting that before this study, the level of health literacy in England was unknown. Further, as had been previously suggested by Batterham et al., (2016) and observed by Rowlands et al. (2016) there is still more work to be done on measuring health literacy before it can be useful in determining how to harness it and optimize it. However, it is evident from the literature review that individuals, health systems, and health professionals have a part to play in optimizing health literacy in order to improve health outcomes. Rowlands et al. (2016) found that "[General Practitioners] have a key literacy role through patient care and through their roles as health service commissioners. *Rigour* should be applied to the development of health materials" (Rowlands et al., 2016, emphasis added).

Even though the measurement of health literacy is still evolving, the concept has been further expanded from its basic form. It was described by Raynor (2012) as having three aspects; the ability to read and understand health information, a critical ability to engage with the health care process, and the removal of unnecessary barriers and complexities by the health care system which could prevent the patient from understanding the system and becoming involved.

HEALTH LITERACY IN THE COMMUNITY

The Scope of Health Literacy

The purpose of this chapter is to apply health literacy as a tool to improve health inequalities. To apply it as a tool however, it is necessary to acknowledge that health literacy includes multiple components and can be found in multiple settings (Batterham et al., 2016). In its report, The World Health Organisation Regional office for Europe (2013) suggested that "health literacy assessment can be used to improve clinical service delivery, community participation in health service planning, public health education, and policy development" (as cited by Batterham et al., 2016, p.4). Several definitions of health literacy have emerged over the years, as the concept is still evolving. However, the authors of this paper will mainly rely on the definition provided by the World Health Organisation (2013), which indicates that health literacy is the personal characteristics and social resources needed for individuals and communities to access, understand, appraise, and use information and services to make decisions about health.

This definition acknowledges that responsibility for tackling this lies with the community and health services and not just with individuals. Implicit within the definition is the idea that it is a critical empowerment strategy to increase people's control over their health, their ability to seek out information, and their ability to take responsibility.

Health literacy includes elements such as reading, verbal communication, numeracy skills, comprehension, and the ability to use information in key health care decision-making. Many people struggle regularly to understand these elements of health information, but the struggle is even harder for people from an ethnic minority background because of their unique cultural challenges and barriers. For example, illnesses such as sickle cell disease, high blood pressure, diabetes, and chronic kidney disease, are prevalent in the black population. However, as many are unaware of the link between their illnesses and their diet, it is often difficult for them to manage their condition as effectively as they are expected to by the health care professionals. There is also a barrier of poor language competence which is an issue for many first-generation immigrant adults who are aging and require specific health information. It therefore follows that by improving health literacy in these groups, together with increasing system and healthcare professional awareness of the challenges they face, there would be an opportunity to achieve optimum healthcare outcomes.

Health Literacy and the NHS

It is very important for the NHS to address health literacy in a country where people come from diverse backgrounds. This is especially relevant for NHS England, as people from ethnic minority backgrounds principally reside in England. Taking the black population as an example, at the time of the last census in 2011, around 3.1 million people identified themselves as Black or Black British and11% of the minority black population live in the Greater London area, a further 2% reside in the West Midlands. However, 78% of the African population and (61%) Caribbean population live in London. (Office for National Statistics, 2012).

NHS England has set up a National Health Literacy Collaborative with membership drawn from other arm's length bodies, government departments, representative and delivery organisations, and the voluntary sector. A national strategy for health literacy is being developed which includes a health literacy resource hub, which is a place for practitioners looking for resources and information.

Also being developed, is some health literacy demonstrator activity which aims to test out whether improving people's heath literacy can also enhance their ability to self-manage their long term condition. Further, NHS England's Supported Self Care programme (Berry, 2016) has been working hard to ensure that the language it uses is relevant, appropriate, and expressive for people with lived experience to ensure that people can relate to the use of the language. This is helpful for people with lower levels of health literacy. There is still much more to be done with health literacy in the NHS, but it is clear that there is an awareness of how health literacy can be optimized in the system, giving patients independence and some autonomy, as has been seen with self-care.

Health Literacy and the Patient

Health literacy is vital for routine patient care. It is vital for disease prevention, early screening, and self-care health management. Health literacy skills are needed for most aspects of people's lives in one form or another: dialogue and discussion, reading health information, making health care choices, and for the use of medical devices for personal or family health care. Insulin injections, blood pressure monitoring machines, home dialysis machines, inhalers, and calculating timing or dosage of medicines are just some of the ways health literacy is part of routine health care.

For most of the general population, their first engagement with health literacy is through their General practitioner (GP) Surgery and GP, as a result, both have a pivotal role in improving communication skills, and tailoring information not only to clinical needs but also to patient health literacy. This need was acknowledged by Rowlands et al. (2016) discussed earlier.

Practice Managers have a role to develop health systems and create environments that support patients' health literacy skills, both in understanding and using health information. This can be done by ensuring information and resources are easily accessible and meet the diverse needs of their cohort of patients. They can also make provisions for certain services required specifically for ethnic minority groups. In the UK, this might include specialist services for illnesses prevalent among black people such as sickle cell disease, because access to such services could help to improve health literacy.

Training for healthcare professionals is necessary in order for them to better support patients from ethnic minority backgrounds; it will also help to recognise key symptoms e.g. sickle cell crisis, high blood pressure in black patients, and improve levels of cultural awareness. In addition, health care organisations could improve health literacy in the ethnic minority population by recruiting more staff from ethnic minority backgrounds who can help to improve access to services for the ethnic minority population.

The Patient in the Community

Edwards, Wood, Davies & Edwards (2013) found that it is possible, that having accessed the health literacy of individuals in the health system, individuals with high literacy are able to *distribute* health literacy throughout the community to improve access, participation, and compliance (as cited by Batterham et al., 2016).

Ali, Ferguson, Mitha & Hanlon (2014) found that health care professionals find it challenging to communicate effectively with people with low literacy (as cited by Batterham, 2016). The fact that there is limited research in organizational health literacy led to the suggestion that this is because of lack of confidence and the inability to find helpful resources (Batterham, 2016). Chaudhry et al., (2011) established that there is inequality in health literacy among ethnic minority groups, therefore it is particularly useful to distribute health literacy among these populations, as it is more likely that results will be achieved by members of the community with high literacy communicating within their own community. Parashar (2005) found that the average literacy level for women in villages was a stronger indicator for childhood immunization than was the literacy levels of individuals. (as cited by Batterham, 2016). According to him, "this suggests that the sharing of information and experiences among mothers increased the likelihood that they would immunize their children." (Batterham, 2016 p.8)

This type of intervention would be particularly useful in ethnic minority populations as the experiences will be shared within the community group. This is the best place to understand the ways in which discussions about health occur within families and social networks and understand the cultural and religious norms that influence the way the people in the population think and act about their health. This type of intervention is needs based and will therefore develop the capacity for ethnic minority populations to make decisions that will promote health and better manage chronic health conditions.

This strategy is already being trialed in the UK, based on previous success in the Netherlands (Ismail, 2015) and the US (Waterman et al., 2015).

It was observed in the UK that patients with end stage renal failure (ESRF) who are of ethnic minority origin, spend up to twice as long on the waiting list (despite adjustments made for ethnicity and other factors) and are less likely to be recipients of living donors. In collaboration with NHS Blood and Transplant, Kidney Research UK and Gift of Living Donation (GOLD), a proposal was funded to train peer educators to share their experiences of kidney donation with potential donors and recipients. As a result, patients and their families become more knowledgeable about ESRF and are better equipped to make informed decisions about kidney donation. The expected outcome (the project is still at the pioneering stage) is that not only will live donors be increased in the black community, there will be increased awareness through education (distributed health literacy), which will lead to better health literacy across all transplant needs and better health outcomes and better mortality rates in the black community when it comes to kidney disease. This model could be used throughout the population for any vulnerable group facing inequalities.

For this type of intervention to be optimized however, it is necessary for the NHS to be health literate. The literature to date on health literacy, does establish that from the genesis of the development of health literacy as a concept, emphasis has been placed on individual health literacy, which the authors of this paper have sought to expand to communities through distributed health literacy. However, organizational health literacy is still in its infancy in term of research but is necessary for the intervention previously described to be effective (Palumbo, 2016).

Even where individuals have high literacy, it has been found through a recent literature review (Palumbo, 2016), that it is not merely sufficient for individuals to be health literate, but health organizations must also cultivate a health literate environment, through policy and culture, in which the patient with adequate health literacy skills can engage and participate. Though this is not yet the prevailing trend, it is possible to achieve if health organisations make health literacy a main organisational priority by involving the populations they serve in the "design, implementation and evaluation of health care services" (Palumbo, 2016 p.83). It could also be achieved by implementing health literacy strategies at any stage of the patient's experience, making health information accessible, and providing appropriate guidance for the patient through the system (Palumbo, 2016).

SOLUTIONS AND RECOMMENDATIONS

Community Engagement

The ethnic minority population in Britain is struggling with its identity[4], as evidenced by social problems such as racial discrimination, poverty, housing, employment, immigration, social status, and mistrust of the establishment which all have a profound effect on people achieving good health. This will always represent a major challenge for healthcare professionals, health service providers and policy makers, all of whom form part of the establishment. As Mathews (2015) concluded, we must not "...avoid analyzing the social and economic causes of inequality and consequently, fail to challenge the social and economic structures that create an inequitable society" (p.20).

It is possible to challenge these inequalities by paying attention to what is required by the community and implementing policies and processes at an institutional level that will enable the community to participate and thereby be empowered. Eliminating the impact of these inequalities and improving the social environment is a goal we must strive for as a central component of achieving optimal health by optimizing health literacy through community groups.

Ethnic minority community groups can also play a role by promoting greater empowerment among patients in their community. Achievable results are possible by helping individuals develop confidence to process, and understand basic health information and services needed to make appropriate health decisions. This may best be achieved through the peer support model of communication, and through targeted community-based educational outreach.

Culturally sensitive community based patient education can also provide a solution and improve health literacy. This type of health literacy is already helping patients to live with long term illnesses with the aim of achieving improved health outcomes in the UK.

Community Engagement in the US and the Netherlands

Community outreach patient educational programmes are widely used in the US as an effective intervention to increase health literacy in the African American population. One such successful community outreach programme evaluated the effectiveness of educational interventions in removing barriers to living donor kidney transplantation for Black patients, as they are less likely to receive a live donor kidney transplant (LDKT) than patients of all other races (Rodrigue et al., 2014). The study found that patients that had received intervention in their home for themselves and their guests were more likely to have donor inquiry and evaluation. They were also more likely to have higher knowledge, fewer concerns, and higher willingness to talk to others about donation six weeks after intervention. Rodrigue et al. (2014) concluded that the study highlighted the importance of including the patient's social network in LDKT education and the potential of the intervention to reduce racial inequality in LDKT rates.

Findings in the Netherlands also show proven success that community education can play a key role in helping to improve health literacy in ethnic communities; especially in the case of informing patients and their families about living kidney donation (Ismail et al., 2014). They found that home-based family intervention increased knowledge, communication, and living donation rates in a randomized controlled trial. The authors developed and tested an educational program to support well-informed decision making among patients and their social network regarding living donor kidney transplantation (LDKT). One hundred sixty-three patients who were unable to find a living donor were randomized to standard care or standard care plus home-based education. In the plus group, patients and members of their social network participated in home-based educational meetings and discussed renal replacement therapy options. Patients and invitees completed pre and post self-report questionnaires measuring knowledge, risk perception, communication, self-efficacy, and subjective norm. LDKT activities were observed for six months' post intervention. Patients in the experimental group showed significantly more improvements in knowledge and communication compared with the control group. The invitees showed pre and post increases in knowledge and attitude toward discussing renal replacement therapies, attitude toward donating a kidney, willingness to donate a kidney, and a decrease in risk perception.

Finally, there were significantly more inquiries, evaluations, and actual LDKTs in the experimental group compared with the control group. The conclusion was that home-based family education supports well-informed decision making and promotes access to LDKT.

Community Engagement in the UK

Another community education outreach effort that has proven highly successful and valuable is the role peer educators play in increasing health literacy. Kidney Research UK developed a peer educator outreach initiative to increase the number of ethnic minorities on the organ donor register (Buffin, Little, Jain & Warrens, 2015).

Peer Educators are lay people, usually from the local community, with a passion for promoting health and giving back to their communities. They have an empathy born out of experience, in terms of language, culture & religion; moreover, they have similar experiences with healthcare.

In the UK, this form of community outreach has benefited ethnic minority patients living with End Stage Renal Disease (ESRD). Ethnic minority patients with ESRD make up 30% of people on the UK's transplant waiting list, but they spend longer on dialysis than the rest of the general population due to the lack of matching donor kidneys. Culturally, people from ethnic minority populations are more amenable to living kidney donation than cadaveric donation. However, the numbers accessing living kidney donation are still disproportionate compared to white patients.

The UK Pilot

NHS Blood and Transplant (NHSBT), in partnership with The Living Donor Kidney Transplantation 2020 UK Strategy Implementation Group (LDKT 2020), Kidney Research UK, and Gift of Living Donation, a Black & Minority Ethnic (BME) community organisation, funded the first UK pilot peer educator LDKT home-based education programme.

The aim of the one-year pilot was to help identify the barriers affecting ethnic minority patients' access to living transplantation and improve engagement within the community. The pilot was the combination of the American model previously described and the Peer Educator Model developed by Kidney Research UK. The implementation of this unique programme offered patients a more culturally relevant educational approach to living kidney donation. It was also more accessible to a wider group of ethnic minorities who would never have considered living donation.

The culturally tailored model empowered patients to broach the difficult conversation of their need for a kidney with loved ones, it also engaged and educated family members on living kidney donation. The model uses culturally relatable DVDs, books, and printed materials to deliver its educational sessions.

The home education pilot was established to complement patient education provided in the hospital setting. By engaging with patients and their families in the home environment, the primary aim was to improve awareness and access to LDKT. The 'at home' element of the intervention offered: a more relaxed environment; easier access to family and friends; an opportunity to discuss barriers to LDKT; provide information, and build trust.

Background of UK Pilot

The pilot was established in two large UK transplant centres: Queen Elizabeth Hospital, University Hospitals of Birmingham (UHB) for South Asian communities, and Guy's and St. Thomas' NHS Foundation Trust (GSTT), London for Black communities. Key roles were recruited/identified locally for each site and included:

- 1 Peer Educator Coordinator (PEC).
- 1 Lead Nurse (Band 7/8).
- Up to 10 Peer Educator Volunteers – transplant donors & recipients.
- 3-4 Link Nurses representing each key clinical area.
    - Living donor coordination
    - Recipient coordination
    - Advanced kidney care/low clearance

Governance

- ACE Advisory and Dissemination Board (ADB) appointments.
- Donor and recipient volunteers recruited and inducted via Trust Voluntary Services.
- Link nurses identified for each clinical area to identify suitable patients and communicate directly with PEC.
- Policies, guidance, and procedures developed in line with Trust Governance requirements.
- Bespoke, documentation developed to underpin all aspects of the programme.
    - Job profiles
    - Risk assessments
    - Participant consent forms
    - Volunteer training programmes
- Agreed upon standards and guidelines for record-keeping.
- All documentation transferable to other Trusts with minor adaptations.

Education and Training

- All Peer Educator volunteers received Trust specific induction and accredited, bespoke training equivalent to an A level standard delivered by ADB members.
- On-going education and support from PECs, lead and link nurses, and core project team.

Patient Recruitment

Link nurses in each of the key clinical areas were identified patients from the relevant communities (Black or Asian) who were:

- Referred to advanced kidney care from nephrology or a failing transplant.
- Scheduled to attend group education meetings in preparation for renal replacement therapy (RRT).
- Poor attendees who may have disengaged with the healthcare team.

- On dialysis with no documented transplant plan.
- On the transplant waiting list without LDKT options identified/followed-up.

Deliverable Outcomes

To accommodate the short duration of the project, the deliverable outcomes were modified to achieve realistic targets:

Quantitative Measures

- Expressions of interest from enrolled patients and their families about LDKT.
- Uptake of and attendance at patient education sessions/events including prospective patients and lapsed attendees.
- Uptake of and attendance at home visits.

Qualitative Measures (Reflections and Opinions): Assessed by Questionnaire +/- Focus Groups

- Individual patients, family members, and friends.
- Multi-disciplinary team members.
- Peer Educator Volunteers.

Other Outputs

Retrospective participant (patients, potential donors, peer educator volunteers, and multi-disciplinary team) analysis to explore the identified barriers to LDKT; how they could best be overcome, and feedback on the pilot project itself

- Identify socio-economic determinant for future measurement or indicator.
- PEC involvement and role profile/experience and impact.

Toolkit template for dissemination to other Trusts e.g. applied learning, governance processes, volunteer recruitment and training and leadership (Peer Educator Coordinator, Peer Educator Volunteer and professional)

Outcomes and Shared Learning

Quantitative data collection was limited by the short timeframe of the project, delayed due to Trust volunteer recruitment and induction processes (on GSTT site) and recruitment of PEC (UHB site). Data collection commenced on the GSTT site from January 2017 and in April 2017 at UHB, where the project has been extended within the remaining budget until the 30 June 2017.

The uptake of attendance at the education sessions or engagement of lapsed attendees as a direct result of the project could not be analysed accurately in this short period. A direct referral from the GSTT advanced kidney care clinic in February, resulting in a home visit in March 2017.

Qualitative analysis was performed using a short Survey Monkey questionnaire to healthcare professionals and a paper questionnaire for all PEC, volunteer, and patient participants, tailored accordingly. Response rates as follows:

- Professionals: 89% (8/9).
- Peer Volunteers: 78% (7/9) GSTT (includes volunteers who withdrew) 66% (4/6) UHB (includes trained volunteers who had not received referrals).
- Patient and donor participants were surveyed separately after the home visit and all participants (2 potential donors, 1 patient) responded.

Essentials for Success

- Effective collaborations- strategic (within the core team); operational (between colleagues and key departments within individual Trusts) and good team dynamics at all levels.
- Strong leadership - core project team, early appointment of a PEC, and lead nurse to establish and sustain the project.
- Strong belief and commitment to success within the core project team and volunteers.
- Willing volunteers with insight into the donor or recipient experience.
- Recognise the challenge- a volunteer home intervention model is a 'first' for most Trusts; few existing policies and guidelines in place.
- Time- to embed the concept, establish acceptance, manage logistics, and provide practical solutions to local issues.

Participant Perspectives

- Healthcare professionals
  - Initially more skeptical about the likelihood of success in comparison with PECs and volunteers
  - Initially more concerned about volunteer recruitment, additional workload, and Trust engagement than volunteers
- Healthcare professionals and volunteers
  - Some volunteers withdrew due to local Trust volunteer recruitment and induction processes
  - All positive about success by the end of the pilot
  - Expressed concerns about future funding to sustain the project
- All participants (patients, donors, volunteers, and professionals)
  - Evaluated the pilot positively overall
  - Evaluated the home visit experience positively
  - Generated 2 live donor inquiries

Summary of UK Pilot

This pilot demonstrates to date 'proof of concept' - that it is feasible to set up a cost effective, sustainable home-based education programme using Peer Volunteers to complement hospital-based education. Further quantitative analysis is required to assess the impact of home-based intervention using this model. The qualitative analysis shows that the initiative was welcomed by patients and volunteers and healthcare professionals became more positive about success as the project progressed. A key output from this pilot will be the development of a comprehensive toolkit to provide a template for other UK Trusts who wish to adopt this approach (Burnapp, 2017)

SOLUTIONS AND RECOMMENDATIONS

To greatly improve health outcomes among its ethnic minority population, especially in the South East of England and the Midlands, the UK needs to move towards an inclusive model of health literacy. This model must seek to engage organisations, health care professionals, communities, and individuals, in a linked, multi sector collaboration.

Individual Level

The authors have shown that even when patients are health literate, interacting with healthcare professionals and navigating the complex nature of the healthcare system can be very intimidating, and stressful for the patient; especially if coupled with the fear of a new diagnosis or the fear associated with receiving instructions that require reading or form filling. Individuals who are unsure, lack the confidence to ask questions or need help completing health information paperwork or communicating their health needs, should be encouraged to seek the support of a family member, friend, or some other person from their social network, for medical appointments or consultations. This is a simple way of improving the health literacy of individuals. This helps to provide patients with an extra pair of ears to reinforce the information provided by GPs or healthcare professionals, seek clarification and understanding when needed or act as an interpreter. This support also benefits 1st generation ethnic minorities for who English may not be their 1st language or who find it difficult to understand some of the medical terminology and their diagnosis. This kind of support is common in ethnic minority communities where health decisions are made not just by individuals, but are strongly supported by family members. This form of engagement and family support will certainly improve access to health information and services for patients and should be encouraged.

Patient centred care would also improve healthcare literacy in ethnic minority individuals (Epstein, Fiscella, Lesser & Strange, 2010).

The phrase "patient-centred care" has become relevant since the launch of Health 2020, but its meaning is poorly understood. Epstein et al., (2010) describes patient-centred care, why it matters, and how policy makers can advance it in practice. Ultimately, patient-centred care is determined by the quality of interactions between patients and clinicians. The evidence shows that patient-centred care improves disease outcomes and quality of life, and that it is critical to addressing racial, ethnic, and socioeconomic disparities in health care and health outcomes. Policy makers need to look beyond such areas as health information technology to shape a coordinated and focused national policy in support of patient-centred care. The policies should help health professionals acquire and maintain skills related to patient-centred care, and it should encourage organizations to cultivate a culture of patient-centeredness.

Health Care Services and Health Care Professionals

A coordinated and focused approach is needed to make health literacy an integral aspect of healthcare services at all levels. For example, at the primary care level, a GP's ability to respond to ethnic minority patients with different health literacy needs requires them to develop strategies and skills to engage more effectively with their patients to enhance the quality of their health. These skills and strategies can be shared with other GPs as good practice standards and incorporated in the clinic, making it an integral and coordinated effort to routinely deliver on health literacy.

Many factors in the current UK health care system are organisational barriers which prevent even health literate individuals from engaging with the system. In the UK, the health care system is a large, sometimes bureaucratic, public institution which can be mildly annoying in other government bodies, but when a chronically ill patient relies on these institutional systems for their well-being, when they break down or don't work because they are too generalised, it can feel life threatening. It is incumbent on the institution to work to remove barriers that frustrate the efforts of patients who are health literate, from engaging with the processes and ensure they are designed for patients. This can be achieved by patients being a part of the decision making process, as patients, but also as part of the institutional leadership.

This may need to involve a major cultural shift in the UK, because the institutions tend to be top-heavy and centred around professionals, which is understandable, considering no one wants to be treated in hospital by an amateur, but what the studies in the US and the Netherlands, as well as the pilot in the UK has shown is that there is a gap between what the medical professionals can provide by way of information and diagnoses and treatment and what the patient needs in terms of emotional support. This is especially true when it comes to serious chronic illnesses, such as cancer and kidney disease. These are life threatening and life-changing diseases and can be frightening for even the most health literate (that is probably why doctors make the worst patients)! It has been proven that emotional and other forms of support through an illness can have a positive impact on compliance and outcomes for patients, so much more needs to be done to bridge this gap, and health care organisations have a role to play in optimizing health literacy to achieve these aims.

Community

Language, diverse backgrounds, and cultural barriers often keep the ethnic minority population from accessing optimum health care. However, healthcare systems will benefit from building networks with community and faith-based organisations and charities, as they are a good and powerful channel to promote and deliver targeted health information to diverse groups. This role can also be reversed, and community members can be involved where key decisions about the community's health are being discussed at a strategic and policy making level. Community leaders should attend health seminars and health promotion events to better educate themselves on health matters that affect their community. The different ethnic minority communities can play a vital role in maximising health outcomes for their population, they can include health information on radio shows, feature health articles in ethnic minority publications, use art, drama, and entertainment to deliver underlying health messages, and the community can involve people of the same ethnicity in the public eye to influence health behaviour changes in the ethnic minority community and raise awareness on health issues that mainly affect that population.

There are ethnic minority recognised events such as the Notting Hill Gate Carnival and the Black Hair and Beauty Show that can be utilized by both health care providers and community groups to promote health literacy on a larger scale. Faith groups also provide a platform to deliver health information to very large audiences. Information about illnesses prevalent in ethnic minority communities can be delivered and endorsed by faith leaders to encourage and spur community members to be more active and engaged when it comes to health information that could enhance the quality of life for members. Community participation is a major player in supporting health care systems to deliver an excellent standard of health literacy to ethnic minority populations but is currently undervalued and underutilised. Community leaders have a powerful voice and should use it loudly to orchestrate and advocate for better health outcomes for their people.

FUTURE RESEARCH DIRECTIONS

Health literacy has evolved a great deal in the last 30 years and has developed into a concept that can be employed in health systems to benefit patients individually, in the community, and in the health organisation. There is ample evidence through research and practice that optimizing health literacy can deliver the goals of Health 2020, to provide a health system focused on the needs of the people it serves.

As research has shown, there is still much to do to increase health literacy for individuals and the community and remove barriers inadvertently or advertently placed in the way of individuals trying to navigate the healthcare system, by the organisations with which they are trying to engage. (Palumbo,2016).

Therefore, more needs to be done to increase the health literacy levels in the population, because as evidenced by the studies in the US, the Netherlands, and the pilot in the UK, health literacy can be distributed through the community. More research needs to be done into the efficacy of existing methods and exploring new and more efficient ways to measure and thereby harness health literacy of individuals.

Further, there needs to be more research into how health originations can be more health literate by implementing methods and procedures already identified as necessary. (Palumbo, 2016)

It is conceivable that the organisations' structures can be adjusted to accommodate being more health literate because optimizing health literacy needs organisations and individuals to all be health literate in order to work together to tailor the healthcare delivery to the health needs of the community. It is entirely possible that once the individuals and community become more health literate, they will become more knowledgeable about what the community wants and needs.

For ethnic minority groups specifically, there is a lack of research on diseases prevalent in these populations and research about how and why it progresses in the community. There should be more collaborations with higher institutions in countries in Africa and Asia regarding diseases prevalent in those regions. Even something as fundamental as the Body Mass Index (BMI), which is calibrated for the Caucasian body, is not adjusted for differences in the ethnic minority body which are significant when calculating eGFR (Glomerular Filteration Rate) in kidney patients, for example, because it depends on body size, age, and gender. These are relevant to the patient, especially if they are health literate and want to engage in their care. More research around the diseases that affect ethnic minority populations and how and why they progress will help the health professionals and health systems better serve this community and impact the health inequalities that plague this population group.

It is an exciting prospect that optimizing health literacy might achieve what has previously eluded governments, policy makers, and social researchers alike.

CONCLUSION

There is health inequality in ethnic minority populations in the UK that adversely affects their access to healthcare, and thereby adversely affects their health outcomes. Optimizing health literacy is a proven way to address these health inequalities, as health literacy is wide in scope and form and can be applied to fit the community. However, there is still much to be done, as organizational health literacy is still in its infancy, and is needed, together with a development of individual and community health literacy to optimize health literacy and decrease inequalities.

There is an opportunity for health literacy in the community to overcome many of the difficulties of enhancing individual health literacy within health systems, but this can only be optimized when health organizations become more health literate by removing barriers that prevent individual patients (and by extension the community) from optimizing their health literacy.

ACKNOWLEDGMENT

This research was supported by the Community Interest Organisation, Gift of Living Donation (GOLD) and NHS Blood and Transplant (NHSBT).

REFERENCES

Asaria, M. (2017) *The economics of health inequality in the English NHS – the long view* (Centre for Health Economics Research Paper 142). University of York.

Batterham, R., Hawkins, M., Collins, P., Buchbinder, R., & Osborne, R. (2016). Health literacy: Applying current concepts to improve health services and reduce health inequalities. *Public Health Journal*, *132*, 3–12. doi:10.1016/j.puhe.2016.01.001 PMID:26872738

Berry, J. (2016). *Does Health Literacy Matter?* Retrieved on 24 May 2017 from https://www.england.nhs.uk/blog/jonathan-berry/

Buffin, J., Jain, N., Little, R., & Warrens, A. N. (2015). A peer outreach initiative to increase the registration of minorities as organ donors. *Clinical Kidney Journal*. Retrieved on 11 June 2017 from https://www.ncbi.nlm.nih.gov/pmc/articles/PMC4581384/

Burnapp, L. (2017). *Organ donation transplantation acceptance, empowerment and choice in living donor kidney transplantation* (Unpublished internal report). NHS Blood & Transplant Advisory and Dissemination Board.

Cookson, R., Propper, C., Asaria, M., & Raine, R. (2016). *Socioeconomic inequalities in health care in England* (Centre for Health Economics Research Paper 129). University of York.

Epstein, R. M., Fiscella, K., Lesser, C., & Stange, K. C. (2010). *Why the nation needs a policy push on patient-centered health care.* Retrieved on 11 June 2017 from http://content.healthaffairs.org/content/29/8/1489.short

Ismail, S. Y., Luchtenburg, A. E., Timman, R., Zuidema, W. C., Boonstra, C., Weimar, W., . . . Massey, E. K. (2014). *Home-based family intervention increases knowledge, communication and living donation rates: a randomized controlled trial.* Retrieved on 11 June 2017 from http://onlinelibrary.wiley.com/doi/10.1111/ajt.12751/

Jakab, Z., Celarc, M., & Ossinovski, J. (2016). Introducing the 20th Ljubljana Charter Anniversary issue. *Eurohealth (London), 22*(2), 2.

Kline, R. (2014) *The snowy peaks of the NHS: a survey of discrimination in governance and leadership and the potential impact on patient care in London and England.* Retrieved on 15 June 2017 from https://www.england.nhs.uk/wp-content/uploads/2014/08/edc7-0514.pdf

Kline R., (2015). *Beyond the snowy white peaks of the NHS?* Better Health. Retrieved on 31 May 2017 from Betterhealth.org.uk

Matthews, D. (2015). The impact of ethnicity on health inequalities. *Nursing Times, 111*(44), 18–20. PMID:26665383

McPherson, W. (1999). *The Stephen Lawrence inquiry – report of an inquiry* retrieved on 14 June 2017 from https://www.gov.uk/government/uploads/system/uploads/attachment_data/file/277111/4262.pdf

National Centre for Social Research. (2014). *30 years of British social attitudes self-reported racial prejudice data.* Retrieved on 15 June 2017 from https://diversityuk.org/wp-content/uploads/2014/06/selfreported-racial-prejudice-datafinal.pdf

Office for National Statistics. (2012). *Ethnicity and national identity in England and Wales: 2011.* Retrieved on 13 June 2017 from /www.ons.gov.uk/peoplepopulationandcommunity/culturalidentity/ethnicity/articles/ethnicityandnationalidentityinenglandandwales/2012-12-11

Palombo, R. (2016). Designing health-literate health care organization: A literature review. *Health Services Management Research, 29*(3), 79–87. doi:10.1177/0951484816639741

Raynor, D. K., (2012). Health literacy – Is it time to shift our focus from patient to provider? *British Medical Journal.* doi:102236/bmj.e2188

Rodrigue, J. R., Paek, M. J., Egbuna, O., Waterman, A. D., Schold, J. D., Pavlakis, M., & Mandelbrot, D. A. (n.d.). *Making house calls increases living donor inquiries and evaluations for blacks on the kidney transplant waiting list.* Retrieved on 24 May 2017 from https://www.ncbi.nlm.nih.gov/pmc/articles/PMC4218873/

Rowlands, G., Protheroe, J., Winkley, J., Richardson, M., Seed, P., & Rudd, R. (2015). A mismatch between population health literacy and the complexity of health information: An observational study. *The British Journal of General Practice, 65*(635), 296–297. doi:10.3399/bjgp15X685285 PMID:26009533

The European Network Against Racism. (2014). *Invisible visible minority – confronting Afrophobia and advancing equality for people of African descent and black Europeans in Europe*. Brussels: European Network Against Racism.

Waterman, A. D., Morgievich, M., Cohen, D. J., Butt, Z., Chakkera, H. A., Lindower, C., … LaPoint Rudow, D. (2015). Living donor kidney transplantation: improving education outside of transplant centers about live donor transplantation – recommendations from a concensus conference. *Clinical Journal of the American Society of Nephrology*. Retrieved 17 May 2017, from https://www.ncbi.nlm.nih.gov/pmc/articles/PMC4559502/

World Health Organisation. (2013). *Health literacy the solid facts*. Retrieved on 14 May 2017 from http://www.euro.who.int/__data/assets/pdf_file/0008/190655/e96854.pdf

ENDNOTES

1. The authors in this context do not merely refer to ethnic diversity, as the English, Scottish and Northern Irish population have distinct culture, habits, life style and characteristics which have an impact on their health and therefore healthcare delivery. There is also a political distinction, due to devolution, which means the delivery can be materially different in the different countries.
2. This was an inquiry into the conduct of the police following the death of a black teenager, Stephen Lawrence, which found that the police were institutionally racist.
3. The Ljubljana Charter on Reforming Health Care in Europe and The Tallinn Charter: Health Systems for Health and Wealth.
4. There is ample evidence that the disadvantages ethnic minority populations face results in discrimination throughout life and has an impact on identity. The European Network Against Racism (2014) published a book, Invisible Visible Minority, in which it asserted that European people of African descent (black Europeans) were so discriminated against in Europe that there should be a formal definition of racism against black people called Afrophobia.

Chapter 13
Health Literacy in the Development of Kidney Transplantation Programs in Low- and Middle-Income Countries

Jennie A. L. Jewitt-Harris
Transplant Links, UK

Andrew R. Ready
University Hospital Birmingham, UK

ABSTRACT

The need to introduce complex medical technologies in low- and middle-income countries (LMIC) is increasing, to improve quality of life and life expectancy. Despite improvements in medical infrastructure, many countries do not have the skills required to implement such technologies and need support from overseas organizations. Transplant Links (TLC) is a UK charity supporting the development of sustainable kidney transplant programs in LMIC countries. TLC's experience demonstrates health literacy challenges encountered in introducing a complex medical technology, of which transplantation is a good example. Such challenges were found to be wide-ranging, in a specialty already associated with low levels of health literacy. Nevertheless, such challenges need to be addressed and measures undertaken to improve the level of understanding of renal failure and transplantation by patients, families, healthcare workers, and other stakeholders including politicians, healthcare managers, and the media. These measures may be transferable to the development of other complex medical technologies.

DOI: 10.4018/978-1-5225-4074-8.ch013

INTRODUCTION

There is an increasing need to introduce complex medical technologies in low and middle-income countries (LMIC). New technologies often bring significant improvements in survival and quality of life, but their introduction can create major challenges. Many countries who have previously been unable to develop such healthcare measures are now able to put in place the required infrastructure but do not necessarily have the accompanying specialist skills to implement them. Such development often relies on the support of volunteer specialist health professionals from other countries through partnerships and charitable organisations.

Health literacy is the degree to which individuals understand the new technology and its implications, and this often needs to be addressed for the introduction of a new medical technology to be successful. From the Health Minister tasked with supporting the development of a new facility, to the patient wanting to understand the treatment they are receiving, the health literacy requirements need to be tailored to address the specific needs of each group.

Success of a new treatment programme can rely on the development of an appropriate level of understanding for each group involved, and without this the new interventions may be at risk of failing, despite successful technical skill transfer. The experience of the Transplant Links (TLC) charity group in addressing health literacy challenges related to the introduction of kidney transplantation in LMIC countries, and the measures taken to overcome them, are described here as an example of those that may be encountered in the introduction of other complex medical interventions.

Renal Transplantation

The global burden of renal failure is enormous (Jha et al, 2013). Despite this, there is very little general understanding of what it means to have kidney failure, compared with the understanding of other chronic illnesses such as diabetes or cancer. In high-income countries, large kidney transplant programmes attempt to address the overwhelming need of end-stage kidney failure, although there is a constant shortage of organs. Attempts have been made to overcome this through the development of live-donor transplant programmes, and extension of criteria for acceptance of kidneys from deceased donors, in the knowledge that a kidney transplant offers better outcomes than dialysis, which is the only other alternative (Nieto, Inston, & Cockwell, 2016).

Renal transplantation is an example of a complex medical intervention which is now commonplace in many countries and offers clear clinical and financial advantages over peritoneal and haemodialysis. However, life on a kidney dialysis machine is expensive and open-ended. Quality of life is poor, with most patients on haemodialysis requiring three sessions per week for four hours at a time for the rest of their lives. Patients often describe it as existing rather than living. The financial burden of the treatment in LMIC countries frequently has to be taken on by the patients and their families, with many patients succumbing to their condition when their funds run out. Often, access to such services for children is non-existent, meaning that many young patients simply die. In many such countries with a public health service, healthcare managers are increasingly concerned about the financial burden of dialysis, and the escalating need for more facilities to be made available (Muller, 2016). The concern is intensified as the global incidence of renal failure and its risk factors such as diabetes and hypertension continue to rise, and are more prevalent in African and Caribbean communities (Bamgboye, 2006). Many countries are therefore reviewing kidney transplantation as a route to cost-effectively improving quality of life, life expectancy and the burden on the health service.

The introduction of ethical live donor kidney transplantation has created opportunities for kidney transplantation services in many countries. This is particularly so in places where a deceased donor programme would be culturally unacceptable and/or logistically too challenging and where the legal infrastructure may prohibit it without complicated and lengthy legal amendments. Live donor transplantation also creates an opportunity to develop technical skills required for kidney transplantation because the surgery is planned, allowing advanced planning for personnel who wish to be in attendance. With support of specialist overseas colleagues through Transplant Links (TLC), these skills can be developed through long-term partnerships and mentoring, and offer the potential to pave the way for development of a deceased donor programme at a later stage (Ready, Nath, Milford, Adu, & Jewitt-Harris, 2016).

Health Literacy and Renal Transplantation

Despite the huge and expanding burden of renal failure, the level of health literacy related to it and transplantation is poor in countries with advanced facilities to treat it (Dageforde, & Cavanaugh, 2013), creating a significant challenge in addressing it in countries that don't have those facilities but need to develop an understanding to progress.

Transplant Links (TLC) is a UK registered charitable organisation whose goal is the development of ethical, sustainable kidney transplantation programmes in LMIC countries (Transplant Links Community, 2017). The skill transfer required to achieve this takes place through partnership with each country over several years until sustainability is reached.

Figure 1. Surgical teaching in transplantation in the Caribbean (©2016, A Jewitt-Harris, used with permission)

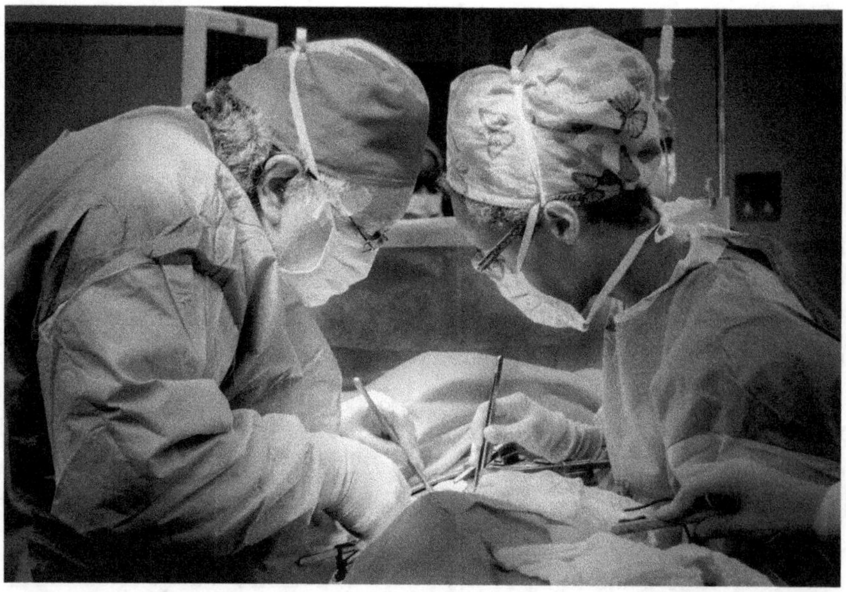

TLC has developed over ten years' experience in supporting the development of kidney transplant centres in Africa, Asia and the Caribbean (Ready et al, 2016). TLC has a small management team with a large group of volunteer specialist healthcare professionals who give up their time to work with partner countries over several years to support the development of transplant programmes. Volunteers include transplant surgeons, nephrologists, nurses, anaesthetists, operating theatre technicians and other associated specialties as required. A bespoke approach is taken to the support of each partner country to align with their specific development needs. Addressing the health literacy issues in each TLC partner country is fundamental to the success of the project at a variety of levels.

TLC surgical volunteer teams are often needed to undertake live-donor transplants within the partner countries, supported by operating theatre specialists and transplant nephrologists and nurses. Through repeated visits long-term skill development is supported so that demonstration of skills is eventually replaced by mentoring and support. Key programmes supported by TLC have included Trinidad and Tobago, Ghana, Nigeria, Nepal, Kenya, Jamaica, and Barbados. Each partner country approached TLC with a view to setting up a national transplant service, and developing the infrastructure required, and to obtain the advice, support and specialist skill transfer needed to make this possible. The first country to be supported by TLC was Trinidad and Tobago where the programme is operating independently and over 160 transplants have now been carried out (firstly live donor, then more recently also deceased donor), and support from TLC is now only needed for the more complicated and paediatric cases (Ready et al, 2016).

The stakeholders in any radical change in medical practice are wide-ranging and all require consideration regarding improving health literacy. When the TLC project began, it was assumed that the necessity for health literacy development would principally apply to patients and potential donors but it quickly became apparent that a much broader approach to addressing health literacy concerns was required for developing programmes to succeed and be sustained.

In all TLC partner countries, the challenges are many and varied ranging from political, to managerial, financial, institutional, logistical, medical, cultural and educational. The latter presents challenges at several levels. Health literacy relating to transplantation may be poor not only for patients and their potential live donors and their families but potentially also for the supporting healthcare staff, hospital management, local media and healthcare politicians. The groundwork needed to address this is pivotal, by both the TLC team and partner colleagues before transplants can be planned. Challenges are increased by the influence of local cultural understandings and customs, which in the field of transplantation can be significant and multi-layered. The myths and misunderstandings that are common in the UK in transplantation are usually supplemented in TLC partner countries and hindered by the lack of long-term media coverage and education on the subject. This finding is not surprising given the lack of previous availability of the specialty but does create a challenging starting point, where incorrect assumptions about pre-existing levels of knowledge may create further challenges. In some countries, for example, TLC has been surprised to learn that renal failure is regarded as the work of a demon, and patients have reported that they have been rejected by family members to avoid the effects of the demon.

Lack of transplantation health literacy in associated medical professions in partner countries is addressed through direct contact, teaching and mentoring by the TLC team. Volunteer transplant professionals are tasked with educating their peers in each country and supporting them in dealing with the transplant-specific health literacy needs of colleagues, patients, and families.

Addressing the transplantation health literacy of patients and potential donors has been challenging, as myths and misunderstandings in transplantation are common worldwide, and limited health literacy is already known to be common in kidney patients (Demian, Shapiro, & Thornton, 2016). Transplant recipients with low health literacy have been found to have higher creatinine levels (Gordon, & Wolf, 2009), indicative of a poorer outcome. The need to overcome this is vital given the importance of immunosuppression (anti-rejection medicine) adherence, essential to prevent rejection of the transplanted organ and known to be influenced by health literacy. In transplantation, the understanding of the donor, recipient and their families can affect the path of events and dictate the outcome of the transplant.

At the outset, TLC team members attempted to identify common misunderstandings in kidney transplant patients and donors in the UK and expected these to be similar, or possibly increased, in countries where transplantation is not part of daily life. These misunderstandings were uncovered through conversations with British patients and their donors and with transplant coordinators and consultant nephrologists and transplant surgeons. They frequently encounter misunderstandings through their daily work, and these provided a starting point to address the specific health literacy need overseas.

Several themes emerged that were frequently encountered. A commonly reported basic misunderstanding relates to poor knowledge of anatomy and even the number of kidneys that are normally present. Patients and donors are often not aware that it is normal to have two kidneys and that a person can function normally with one. Without this basic knowledge, people cannot identify themselves as potential live donors or recipients. Where the kidneys are located within the body, how they connect to the bladder and what they do seems poorly understood. Those with kidney disease often don't realise that the old diseased kidneys are usually left in place and that the transplanted kidney is placed in the groin rather than near the other diseased kidneys. This can totally alter their perception of what the surgery will involve.

With regards to an understanding of the transplant process, misunderstandings relating to matching a donor kidney with a recipient are common. There is often surprise that donors do not have to be the same gender, or be genetically related. The early concept that a close match was mandatory for a transplant to take place is still widely thought of as relevant today (and is possibly confused by the use of a matching system to allocate organs through the deceased donation system).

The benefits of transplantation are often not well understood. The fact that life expectancy, morbidity, and quality of life are all improved through transplantation is often not apparent to patients and their relatives, who may perceive the risk of a transplant as being greater. They are also often unaware that anti-rejection medicine must be taken for the life of the kidney, and that without it, rejection can happen at any time. Rejection is often perceived to be an all-or-nothing situation that only occurs immediately post-transplant, and depends on whether the body will "accept" or "reject" the kidney. While rejection is more common in the early phase after transplantation, it is an issue in the longer-term. This fact is frequently poorly understood as is the recognition that the long-term use of anti-rejection medicines (known as immunosuppressants) is something of a pharmaceutical juggling act; therapeutic drugs being maintained to avoid rejection while avoiding over-immunosuppression and the risk of infection or cancer.

Potential live donors are frequently unaware that they can return to a normal healthy life after donating a kidney, can have a family as normal and will not need lifelong medication. The TLC team have even experienced cases in partner countries where the donor thought they would have to go on dialysis (and in the event of a parent donating to their child, have been willing to do so). Both patients and potential donors are also sometimes unaware that a kidney transplanted from a live donor has a greater chance of working well than a kidney from a deceased donor.

These are complicated concepts and the need for the patient and the donor to engage with them is essential for the success of the transplant. A potential transplant recipient must understand the delicate balance of their immunosuppressive medication, and the need for the levels of the medication to remain within a therapeutic window, for the transplant to be successful and for side effects to be minimised. Even an understanding of the timing of the blood tests to check the levels of the anti-rejection medicine is necessary for these tests to be meaningful in the management of their dosing.

In the UK, the general concepts around organ donation and transplantation have been present in popular media for decades. These have included campaigns for organ donation on high profile television programmes such as "That's Life" to storylines in soap operas, such as "Coronation Street" that involve key characters needing a kidney for transplantation. Despite stories about transplantation becoming part of normal life in the UK, health literacy relating to the subject remains sparse and often confusing. Addressing this in partner countries where transplantation has never been part of everyday experience is even more challenging, but crucial to the success of the project. It is very different from many other developing surgical technologies, where the success of a new procedure may rely entirely on the skill transfer to the local surgeon, and the patient may indeed know no or very little difference in the technique used. With transplantation, there is a political, ethical, medical, logistical, surgical and consequently educational minefield to cross.

Addressing Health Literacy Needs

Health literacy is a positive predictor of transplant outcomes (Kazley, Hund, Simpson, Chavin, & Baliga. 2015). It is important in kidney transplantation for many reasons in addition to the adherence to medications which prevent graft loss. It is also crucial for understanding symptoms of rejection and infection, how to care for a transplant (cardiovascular risk, hydration, diabetes, blood pressure), successful pregnancy outcomes and how to live well with a transplant.

For TLC, the starting point in addressing the need for patient and donor education was a review of materials already available for patients and donors in the UK and to then make appropriate adaptations. However, the lack of availability of general educational materials that were not institution or nation-specific created the need from the outset for the development of new educational items for potential recipients and donors, family members and parents of paediatric patients. New materials were developed incorporating the feedback and input of local doctors and nurses from partner countries, paying attention to frequently asked questions by local patients and relatives.

The TLC educational materials are in a constant state of development, incorporating unexpected questions, and adjusting to respond to cultural and regional differences, and use of language. Posters for dialysis centres have been very useful, aimed at patients and their relatives, dispelling specific local myths about being a donor. Information leaflets (in print and online) outlining the steps before, during and after transplantation have been developed and adjusted to each country's specific needs.

The role of the nurses cannot be underestimated in the long-term development of an educational relationship with the patients, their donors, and families. Teaching seminars with nursing staff have been a core part of the TLC programme, ensuring their full understanding, and of the common misunderstandings and concerns of patients. Demian et al. (2016) describe health literacy in transplantation as a modifiable risk factor with educational interventions as crucial in addressing risks. The TLC experience is that the relationship with nurses is key to the delivery of such interventions.

Figure 2. Transplant Links educational materials for patients, donors, and families

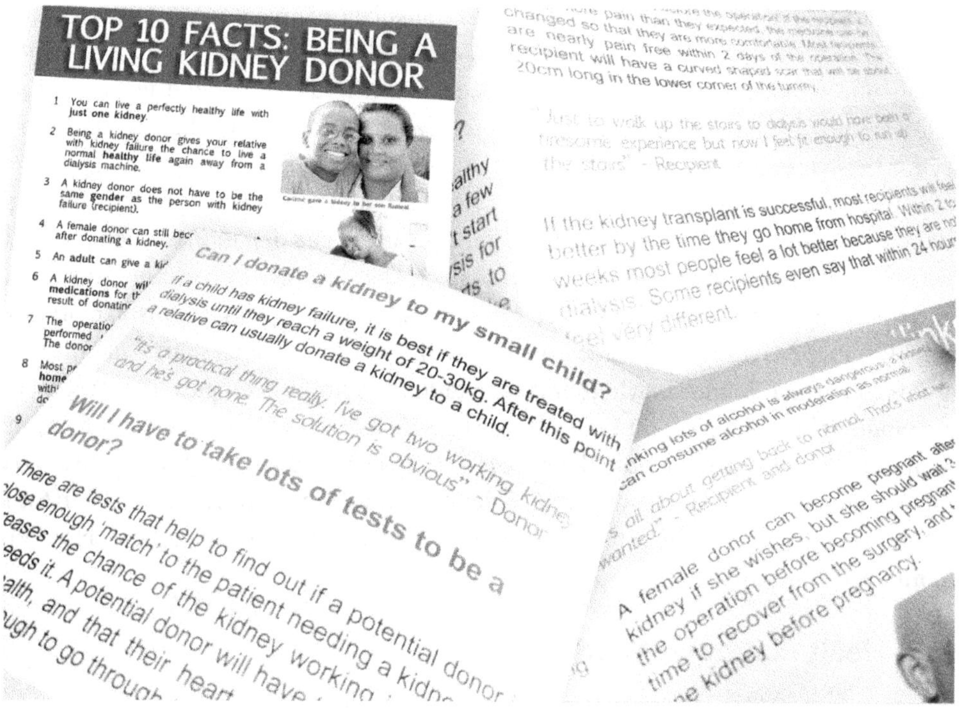

The challenge is increased by other culturally related factors such as patients' relationships with doctors. In the UK, questions from patients to doctors are frequent and encouraged, but in some TLC partner countries, there is a culturally embedded greater reluctance to ask, despite great care being taken to create the space to do so. In one example, in Nigeria, a young man was donating a kidney to his sibling. He listened carefully to the surgeon's unambiguous account of what would happen in the operation. It was not till afterwards that he plucked up the courage to ask "will I be asleep?". It was a stark reminder of the information that is taken for granted as understood, and the need to place information clearly in context. The assumption that everyone would understand that they will be under anaesthetic for the operation, in this case, could have created significant distress for the potential donor, and may even put them off coming forward, without such misunderstandings being addressed.

The transplant literacy of healthcare professionals associated with the introduction of a new programme must also be addressed at many levels to ensure that the process is successful. What might initially be seen as a minor procedural matter, such as the request to have ice available in the operating theatre, is soon recognised as vital when it becomes clear that it is needed to preserve the kidney between the donor and recipient operations, and failure to do so may forever affect the performance of that kidney.

The excitement created by the first transplant in a country is usually encouragement for learning in advance of the procedure, but it is often only 'in the doing' that learning happens. A stark example was during Ghana's first ever transplant, where a young man received a kidney from his sibling. The operating theatre nurse had prepared for weeks for the operations, and her professionalism and capability was outstanding. It was not until the recipient operation was carried out though, and the donated kidney was presented to the surgeon, that the nurse realised what a transplant actually meant and exclaimed: "but only Jesus Christ himself can do that!". While this amused all, and lightened the atmosphere, it illus-

Figure 3. Ghana's first ever transplant (©2008, J Jewitt-Harris)

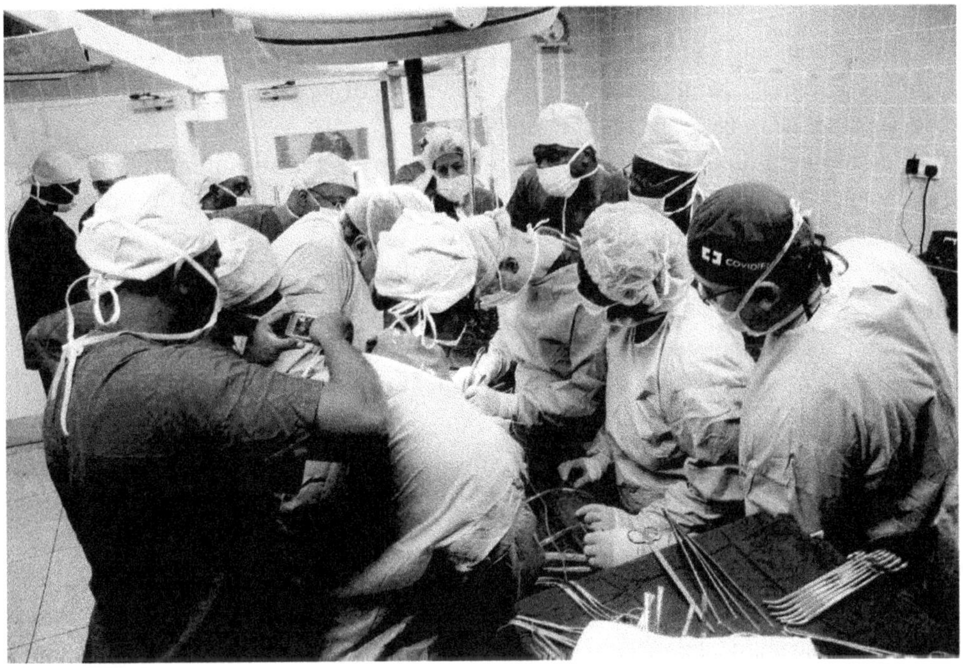

trated how transplantation in many countries is so outside of the normal that it takes time to filter into the everyday of even the healthcare professionals involved, and that there is a conceptual and education hurdle to overcome before it does.

Cultural differences in communications may create additional barriers to improving local health literacy. In countries such as Ghana, it is well known that communications are often indirect and there is a reluctance to give feedback that may be considered negative in any way by its recipient. Silence is common if there is discomfort about a question that has been asked or concern that the answer will not be the one that is desired. This makes producing information leaflets difficult, as the feedback of patients and nurses is crucial in developing materials that are informative and meaningful, and that use accessible language. When producing draft educational materials for local adaptation, feedback was often difficult to obtain, even though the draft needed to be adapted to make it locally useable. This is an interesting challenge. In these situations, the TLC team often seek the assistance of local healthcare workers many of who have spent time training or working in the UK. Such personnel are often more comfortable with giving "negative" feedback (despite assurance that it is not regarded as negative) as well as imparting their understanding of how the information would be interpreted locally, and could be best adapted.

In contrast, in Jamaica, feedback is more direct, and comments on the very British phraseology in some of the draft materials was useful to make changes that communicate clearly with local patients and have a feeling of local relevance. Other cultural differences in Jamaica impacted on the relationships developed with local healthcare professionals, and the subsequent development of useful materials. For example, the formality of addressing colleagues in Jamaican hospitals was not something the TLC volunteers had anticipated, and the use of first names may not be appropriate, and possibly even be offensive, if used too early in a professional relationship. Building of relationships is fundamental to improving health literacy and all other aspects of the projects in all TLC partner countries. Assumptions made about the way to behave created challenges, and attention to cultural differences in behaviour, etiquette, philosophy for life, and ways of living have had to be understood in both directions for progress to be made and literacy to be improved. Religious and spiritual considerations may also be important in some countries, as well as an understanding of other local concerns such as the role of witchcraft in developing renal failure, and the use of spiritual healing and herbal medicines.

Use of images or photographs within the educational materials is also culturally embedded. Different meanings can be taken from images, and working with local staff, particularly the nurses, who develop the closest relationships with the patients and donors, was essential to try to ensure the most useful, acceptable and informative images were incorporated into educational materials. Smiling for the camera is not always regarded as a positive thing, and in some instances, may be seen as unprofessional. Similarly, hand gestures in photographs often have different meanings in different cultures.

The lack of health literacy in kidney transplantation also needs addressing beyond medical professionals and patients. Detailed summaries of the field of kidney transplantation, and its benefits over dialysis must also be provided to healthcare managers and politicians, and lengthy conversations have often been required to elaborate on the intricacies which are broad ranging and essential for an understanding of the value and challenges of developing a programme.

Health literacy development beyond the hospital is challenging. The introduction of complex medical technologies requires support at governmental level. The support of Health Ministers as well as regional and local healthcare management has been essential to the success of developing transplant programmes, and local financing of the projects, and requires a significant investment in time in the early stages of a new project. Health Ministers and their colleagues sometimes have a background in healthcare but this is not always the case, and it has often been important to ensure that they receive the information about a proposed transplantation project in a clear and detailed way, making no assumptions. The TLC team has found that it is preferable to furnish the local doctors with the proposal documents and encourage them to adapt them as they feel appropriate and present them to politicians, with the stated full support of TLC, as opposed to TLC sending them directly.

Well written articles about the work of TLC and transplantation, in newspapers and magazines, have often been beneficial supplementary materials to append to proposal documents. The work of a good journalist is invaluable in getting the concepts across in a clear and concise way. TLC documents are frequently prepared by doctors who, despite best efforts and intentions, are notorious for using medical language and assuming knowledge. Any good relevant articles written by journalists will have the benefit of clarifying as well as endorsing the goals of the project and achieving the goal of enhancing the transplant literacy of the decision makers. In all cases, there is no substitute for the development of good relationships with policy makers to support health literacy, and in all countries, the progress of TLC projects has been enhanced where this has been possible, and misunderstandings are readily addressed.

The health literacy of sponsors of charitable projects including the TLC programmes equally needs attention. Sponsorship is increasingly difficult to secure - and sustain - and the development of an understanding of the field of transplantation for key decision makers is crucial to this. Sponsors may not be just financial but also political, managerial or charitable including patient groups. All sponsors need to understand from the outset that the very positive long-term goal of a national sustainable kidney transplant programme may have some negative hurdles along the way such as transplants not working, being cancelled, or being delayed. These are all normal occurrences in any transplant programme, but may need managing and careful communication to maintain relationships, engagement and long-term support.

Ethics and Health Literacy

Health literacy in the context of transplantation extends to an understanding of the ethical framework in which a transplant can take place. The ethical understandings and assumptions around organ donation are complicated and deeply embedded in local culture. The rigour with which concerns relating to organ trafficking are upheld in the UK is often not matched elsewhere. On one occasion, a senior ministerial official who was very supportive of the development of an ethical kidney transplant programme in his country, asked as we were leaving a meeting "where can I buy a kidney for my friend?". While this seemed to be an extraordinary and inappropriate question to the TLC team, it was seemingly asked in complete innocence, and with surprise at the TLC team's response.

In some partner countries, the legal and ethical framework for transplantation requires development so that live donor transplantation can proceed. In these situations, again, the need to develop materials (presentations, documents, and films) pitched at the right level for the audience are essential for addressing the health literacy needs of those involved. In the UK, live-donor transplantation takes place under the framework of the Human Tissue Act 2004, and the guidelines for this are often used in partner countries to develop a framework for a committee approach to ensuring the ethical process is maintained. Committee members may include patients, legal representatives, and other non-medical professionals, all of whom will be required to take on an advanced level of understanding of the subject to make appropriate and impactful decisions.

A crucial aspect of the ethical and health literacy challenge is the need to ensure the full understanding of the donor who is undergoing an operation for the benefit of the health of another person. It is even more important that they understand the implications when they are putting themselves at risk for the interests of another. The donor goes through many steps to ensure that they are healthy and to minimise the risk to them, as well as to optimise the chances of success of the transplant. Informed consent of the donor is crucial, and opportunities for asking questions and raising concerns must be created. The committee approach to ethical donation is a further opportunity for donors to raise their concerns, away from the pressures inherent in the pre-transplant assessment process. The TLC team impresses upon everyone involved in the many steps of the process that the understanding of the donor is mandatory, and as in the UK, the opportunity to ask questions and to withdraw from donation remains open.

The Patient's Voice

In all aspects of health literacy relating to kidney transplantation and the introduction of any new complex medical treatment, the voice of the patients is paramount. There is no better advocate, or more convincing influencer and educator, than a patient who can put across their experience to others. This can take place in many situations, from a press conference to a conversation with a fellow patient in an outpatients department, and opportunities to encourage and nurture it are welcomed.

In Jamaican newspapers, the voice of the patients who were the first to have successful transplants as part of the TLC project was a significant step in improving health literacy about kidney transplantation at the same time as gaining political support for the project.

Within a newspaper article was a quote that demonstrated a clear understanding of kidney failure and the benefits of transplantation. It stated,

Figure 4. Good media coverage as a source of helpful health information

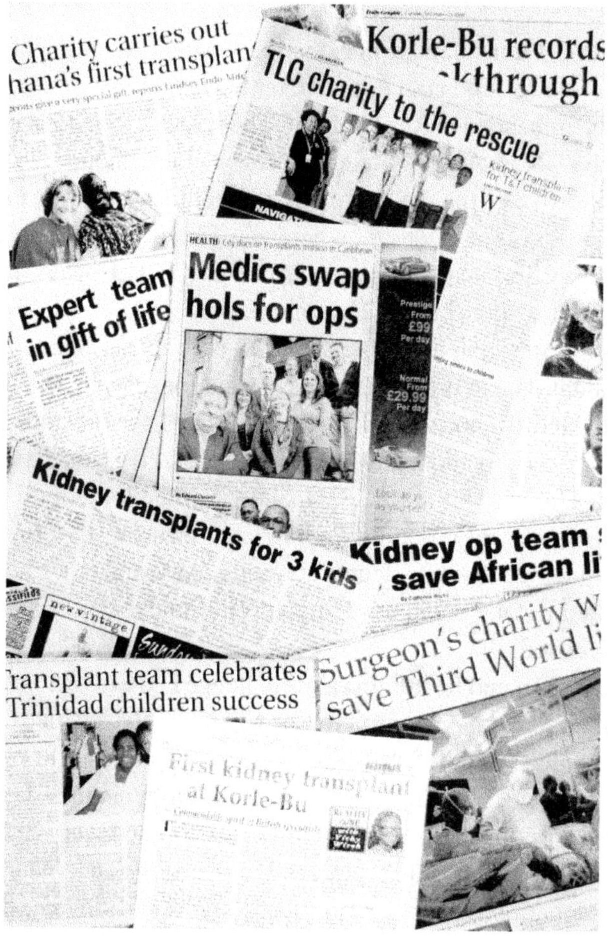
Charity carries out
hana's first transplan
Korle-Bu records
-k through
TLC charity to the rescue
Medics swap hols for ops
Expert team in gift of life
Kidney transplants for 3 kids
Kidney op team
save African li
ransplant team celebrates
Trinidad children success
Surgeon's charity w
save Third World li
First kidney transplant
at Korle-Bu

"One of three patients who received kidney transplants last year, Shaneik Lawson, expressed appreciation for the programme and stressed the need for its continuation to help others like her get a second chance at living a normal life, free of the stress of multiple dialysis treatments every week for the rest of their lives" (Pickering. 2014)

Journalists in all countries have been supported through the proactive provision of detailed press releases from TLC in association with partner hospitals outlining the project and providing supporting background material to avoid assumptions and misunderstandings where possible and increasing the chances that the outcome is appropriately informative as well as of public interest. Appearances on television and radio have also supported the development of public understanding. This is usually most effective when local patients and doctors are interviewed, but has also been usefully supported by TLC team members in some circumstances where a third party voice adds to the strength of the messages. A wife who successfully donated a kidney to her husband, in an interview said: "There's nothing I love more than to hear the sound of my husband peeing with my kidney". In one sentence, she conveyed so much about the role of the donor, the reality of a successful outcome, and the fact that genetically unrelated, across gender donation is possible.

Patient groups have a powerful collective voice and are a great asset in supporting the development of educational materials for future patients and donors. TLC have sought the assistance of patients and donors in maintaining the ongoing development of materials through asking them about their experience, and clarifying what they did or didn't know or expect, what they wish they had known before the procedure, and what information might help future patients and donors. The materials developed for patients and donors can also be beneficial for giving an insight to those who are involved in the system and may need their understanding of the field to be enhanced. These individuals may include administrators, volunteers, and ethics committee members.

Many additional approaches have been taken by the TLC team to broaden the understanding of transplantation for all involved. These have included online articles and interviews in the forms of diaries, videos and newsletters, each adding a different angle to create engagement with the project, and increase understanding.

The TLC experience across a variety of countries and cultures has resulted in development of teaching materials for a variety of audiences, continually adapted to the needs of each partner country. The potential to partner with local media, as well as the use of new technologies presents opportunities to create accessible materials to continue to improve health literacy in this and other medical fields. The development of new technologies is expected to make a significant difference to the way in which TLC can improve health literacy in kidney transplantation with its partner countries. Novel ways of illustrating complex technologies, apps, animations, podcasts and videos are increasingly more able to be accessed across the globe, and offer real opportunities to improve health literacy in this field, particularly now that mobile phones are so widely available in many partner countries.

Figure 5. Transplant Links educational video explaining how the kidney works

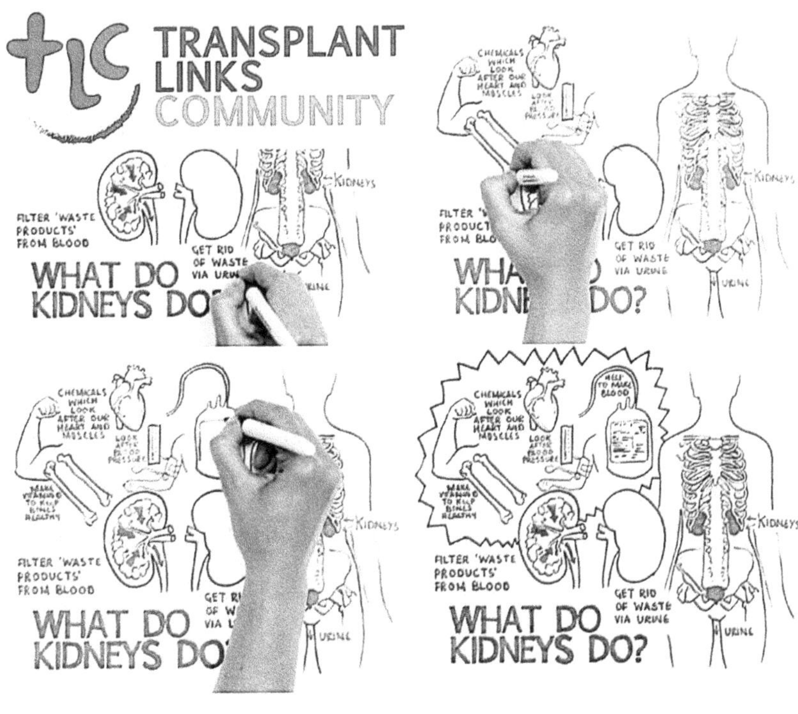

CONCLUSION

In summary, the success of the introduction of new complex medical interventions relies not just on the transfer of medical skills, but also on careful attention to the health literacy of all those involved in the process. The TLC experience demonstrates some of the challenges and the actions taken to address them, and the need to remain constantly vigilant and open minded about the unexpected, as well as constantly mindful of the role of culture and experience in creating an environment receptive to a new technology. In assessing the potential to support the introduction of new technologies, consideration must be given to health literacy concerns from the outset, and to the time, effort and expense required to investigate, address and maintain these factors.

The introduction of complex medical technologies in LMIC countries is a growing challenge. Infrastructure development in many countries whose GDP is increasing and whose access to healthcare is improving is often not matched by skill development across the range of healthcare professionals to provide complex services. The challenges are manifold and include addressing the level of health literacy of patients, their families, and of the many tiers of involvement within the community as well as within hospital management and healthcare professionals. The success of a new technology relies on skill and knowledge transfer to the professionals involved, supplemented by an awareness and willingness to seek out and address health literacy issues.

Transplant Links experience in dealing with health literacy challenges as part of the introduction of kidney transplantation provides an example of the many difficulties that may be anticipated with similar programmes. However, it also illustrates approaches through which they may be addressed and particularly the need to work with the material that is available and accessible and the need to constantly adapt this to meet local requirements. Above all, it illustrates the pivotal reliance on team working and communication between all involved.

ACKNOWLEDGMENT

With thanks to Aimee Jewitt-Harris and Laura Ludman for assistance with text, photography and the management of TLC; and to all TLC volunteers who have given their time to support this work and share their knowledge and skills. Please visit www.transplantlinks.org for further information.

REFERENCES

Bamgboye, E. (2006). End-stage renal disease in sub-saharan Africa. Ethnicity and Disease, 16, S2-5 – S2-9

Dageforde, L., & Cavanaugh, K. (2013). Health Literacy: Emerging Evidence and Applications in Kidney Disease Care. *Advances in Chronic Kidney Disease*, *20*(4), 311-319.

Demian, M., Shapiro, R., & Thornton, W. (2016). An observational study of health literacy and medication adherence in adult kidney transplant recipients. *Clinical Kidney Journal*, *9*(6), 858–865. doi:10.1093/ckjfw076 PMID:27994867

Gordon, E.J., & Wolf, M.S. (2009). Health literacy skills of kidney transplant recipients. *Progress in Transplantation, 19*(1), 25-34.

Jha, V., Garcia-Garcia, G., Iseki, K., Li, Z., Naicker, S., Plattner, B., ... Yang, C. W. (2013). Chronic kidney disease: Global dimension and perspectives. *Lancet, 382*(9888), 260–272. doi:10.1016/S0140-6736(13)60687-X PMID:23727169

Kazley, A., Hund, J., Simpson, K., Chavin, K., & Baliga, P. (2015). Health literacy and kidney transplant outcomes. *Progress in Transplantation, 25*(1), 85-90.

Muller, E. (2016). Transplantation in Africa – an overview. *Clinical Nephrology, 86*(13), 90-95.

Nieto, T., Inston, N., & Cockwell, P. (2016). Renal transplantation in adults. *British Medical Journal, 355*, i6158. doi:10.1136/bmj.i6158 PMID:27903494

Pickering, C. (2014). Ferguson to implement kidney transplant policy. *WiredJa Online News.* Retrieved from http://www.wiredja.com/sci-tech-health/health/kidney-transplant-policy-coming

Ready, R., Nath, J., Milford, D., Adu, D., & Jewitt-Harris, J. (2016). Establishing sustainable kidney transplantation programmes in developing world countries: A 10-year experience. *Kidney International, 90*(5), 916–920. doi:10.1016/j.kint.2016.08.024 PMID:27742191

Transplant Links Community. (2017). Retrieved from http://www.transplantlinks.org

KEY TERMS AND DEFINITIONS

Deceased Donor: A person who has died and whose organs are to be donated for transplantation.

Dialysis: A procedure for treating kidney failure through connection to a blood filtration machine.

Kidney Transplantation: The process of removal of a kidney from one person with normal kidney function and implanting into another to treat their kidney failure.

Live-Donor Transplant: The removal of one kidney from a healthy live person to donate to another person to treat their kidney failure.

Renal Failure: Cessation of the normal functioning of kidneys.

Skill Transfer: Sharing of specialist knowledge and procedures.

Stakeholders: Those with a vested interest in a project or activity.

Sustainable: With the potential to be independently maintained over a long period of time.

Chapter 14
Living Organ Donation Role of Ethics for Improved Clinical Practice

Pierpaolo Di Cocco
Imperial College Healthcare NHS Trust, UK

ABSTRACT

Solid organ transplantation represents one of the most important achievements in history of medicine. Over the last decades, the increasing number of transplants has not been of the same extent of the number of patients in the waiting lists. Live donation has been implemented in order to reduce the gap between supply and demand. From an ethical standpoint, the donation process from a live donor seems to violate the traditional first rule of medicine—primum non nocere because inevitably exposes healthy persons to a risk in order to benefit another person. In the chapter will be presented the crucial role of ethics and specific ethical issues in the different forms of live donation, such as financial incentives for living donation, reimbursement in unrelated live donation, minor sibling-to-sibling organ donation. The ethical aspects of live donor organ transplantation are continuously evolving; in order to make this strategy more beneficial and lifesaving, everyone involved in the process should make every possible effort with in mind the best interests of the patients.

INTRODUCTION

The success of solid organ transplantation as a treatment of end stage organ failure expanded its indications resulting in an increased demand for organs. Despite efforts and numerous strategies applied by the transplant and medical community at large, the gap between demand and supply is widening. As a result, many institutions expanded their live donor programs, including primarily kidney, but also liver and bone marrow, partial pancreas, single or double lung (from 1 or 2 donors) and small bowel. From an historical perspective, the first successful transplant operation involved a live donor kidney transplant between identical twin brothers, carried out by Joseph Murray in 1954, in Boston (Merril et al., 1956); since then, live donation has had variable application in clinical practice. Up until the late 1980s, con-

DOI: 10.4018/978-1-5225-4074-8.ch014

tinuous improvements on immunosuppressive therapy (particularly the introduction of the cyclosporin), and on patient management (pre-, intra- and post-operative), made transplantation from deceased donors a successful therapeutic option; live donor transplantation (mainly kidney) was not performed in the western society, but continued in the developing countries because of lack of legal and societal regulations to use organs from deceased donors. After this era, the rapidly increasing number of patients on the transplant waiting list and the insufficient donor availability forced many centers in Europe and USA to utilize live donors. In the USA, for example, out of 30.974 organ transplants performed in 2015, 24.986 were from deceased donors and 5.989 from live donors. Currently the number of live donor transplants in the USA represents nearly 24% of all transplants (UNOS, 2016). Similar trends are taking place in Europe and Canada. "In the UK, latest statistics show that 42% of all organ donors are living donors and living donor transplantation represents 22% of total transplant activity" (NHS Blood and Transplant, n.d.)

LIVE DONATION: ETHICAL STANDPOINT

Since its inception in the clinical practice more than 60 years ago, live donation has raised a wide range of complex ethical issues for all health professionals involved in the process. This chapter summarizes key ethical principles; a detailed description of the theoretical and philosophical background to the subject can be found in several reviews in the literature (Price, 2009; Price, 2000a; plant et al., 2002; Ross et al., 2002; Kahn & Matas, 2002; Truog, 2005). Organ donation by living donors starts as an amazing act of altruism and presents a unique ethical dilemma, in that physicians must pose at risk a healthy person to save or improve the life of a patient. From the donor perspective, the donation process from a live donor seems to violate the traditional first rule of medicine—*primum non nocere* (above all, do no harm)—because inevitably exposes healthy persons to a risk during the removal of an organ or part of it in order to benefit another person. From the recipient perspective, not only patient survival is markedly prolonged, but also the quality and productivity of life is considerably improved, with decreased cost of health care for the society. For example, the expected survival of a patient with end-stage renal disease treated with kidney transplantation, at 1, 5, 10 years is 20–40% higher than treatment with dialysis. Also, the cost of dialysis is 3 times the cost of kidney transplantation over a 5-year period (Keown, 2001; Eggers, 1998; Hunsicker, 1999; Caplan & Coehlo, 1998). For the above-mentioned reasons, the live donation process has to follow ethically accepted rules and guidelines. The ethical principals include respect for the donor's autonomy, donor selection and full, voluntary, informed consent (Pruett et al., 2006).

Donor Autonomy

In live donation, the donor comes forward as a consequence of its voluntary decision (Hou, 2000). This reflects the ethical basis of a liberal society in which a consenting adult has a right to make decisions about his or her own body and to refuse medical treatment, even life sustaining. Traditionally a consenting adult has a right of access to a medical procedure only in cases where a physician is willing to cooperate (Levinsky, 1984); this is also the ethical basis of living, genetically related and unrelated, donations. The physician, serving the patient best interest, still poses limitations on the autonomy of the donor (Spital, 2001). It has obviously been considered unacceptable the donation of life saving organs; in other words, to date, there has been no petition to court from a potential live donor to be allowed to donate the heart. In this regard, libertarian theorists are debating weather this prohibition should be absolute (Veatch &

Ross, 2015). It is unethical for physicians to conduct deliberately harmful interventions, this is the case reported in the literature of a father willing to donate his second kidney to his daughter. Although the procedure would have not killed the donor, it would have left him in need of renal replacement therapy; the surgeon refused to perform the operation and the ethics committee affirmed his right to refuse, therefore the procedure was not performed (Ross, 2000). The potential donor must be reassured that the freedom to withdraw from the donation process at any time exists with a supportive environment and the transplant team in assistance (Abecassis et al., 2000). All medical or other reasons for not proceeding with donation will be kept confidential (Nuffield Council on Bioethics, 1995).

Donor Selection

Whereas donor autonomy is essential, it is not sufficient to proceed to donation (Spital, 2001). Medical evaluation and team approval are fundamental; in other words a donor's desire and willingness to proceed should not trump medical judgment and the decision-making process has to be balanced (Spital, 2001). The process of donor selection leads to the exclusion of individuals who are legally incompetent or who lack the capacity for autonomous decision-making capacity. A transplant team may also refuse to accept a donor who exhibits comorbidities (i.e. diabetes, hypertension), advanced age, or the potential for complications during surgery (Hou, 2000). For physicians, the prevailing ethical principle, according to the Hippocratic oath, is to "do no harm"; in live donation transplant, surgeons seem to violate this principle causing potential harm to a healthy person for the benefit of the recipient. This is true if we consider the donation process only from the recipient perspective (Nuffield Council on Bioethics, 1995; Reese et al., 2006; Spital, 2004). In agreement with Spital, a physician taking care of an organ donor must believe that the benefits for the patient outweigh the risks (Spital, 2004) and must act solely as that "patient's advocate" and in the patient's best interest (Spital, 2004; Kasiske, et al., 1996). Physicians cannot accomplish this goal if, when trying to decide whether to recommend a procedure for one patient, they are asked to balance the risks for that person against the benefits for another. Such an approach would pose a clear conflict of interest, the recognition of which has led to the sensible recommendation that potential donors and recipients be evaluated by separate physicians (Pruett et al., 2006; Spital, 2004). Furthermore, separate teams enhance confidentiality, as information and record storage is maintained and appropriate information shared by the separate teams. The main barrier of separate teams appears to be the need of sufficient staff specialized in living-donor transplantation (Kasiske et al., 1996). As reported in the literature, the benefits for live donors are mainly psychological (Spital, 2004; Pierce & Pierce, 1973; Majeske et al., 1996); the magnitude of these benefits depends on individual patient and should have a predominant role during the donor assessment (Spital, 2004). During donor assessment, considering the donor benefits will allow to respect individual values, avoiding conflicts of interest, and to act in the best donor's interest directs. The likelihood of recipient benefit is important information not because it balances donor risk but because it affects the probability that the volunteer will benefit (Spital, 2004). The common ethical problem related to the uncertainty regarding the magnitude of risk for live donors (Reese et al., 2006), it is usually resolved communicating in a transparent way to the potential donor that the uncertainty comes from limited medical knowledge, as it is often the case in medicine (Majeske et al., 1996). In agreement with Elliott (1995), the most challenging and fundamental ethical problem for transplant physicians evaluating potential donors is the "chance of harm to a healthy donor." If the transplant physician feels unable to accept a potential donor, he or she should inform that donor of the reasons for rejection and offer a referral for a second opinion (Mazaris & Papalois, 2006).

In a nutshell: What are the responsibilities of the transplant team towards the potential donors? The transplant team is responsible for a complete and thorough evaluation of potential donors from medical, psychological, and social perspective and their overall fitness to become live donors (Pruett et al., 2006; Simmons et al., 1987; Smith et al., 1986) – table 1

Informed Consent

Once the donor selection is completed, an informed consent is essential (Ingelfinger, 1972). As stated earlier, the potential donor must have a cognitive capacity sufficient to make a voluntary decision to donate (Ingelfinger, 1972; Valapour, 2008). The donor must receive and understand relevant and sufficient information about the procedure, associated risks and possible consequences. The disclosure should include information about the associated risks, including, but not limited to, the risk of death, reported worldwide and at the center where the procedure is proposed; medical morbidities; changes in health and organ function; impact upon insurability and employability; potential effects on family and social life; and the psychological impact of donation and nondonation. The responsibility of health and social systems in the management of medical conditions discovered during the evaluation process. The discovery of any conditions in the recipient that may impact upon expected outcome and, therefore, the donor's decision to donate. Information regarding alternative treatments for the recipient must be presented, most importantly, the chances for deceased organ transplantation.

The essential components of informed consent are the following (Ingelfinger, 1972): competence, disclosure, understanding, freedom to choose, and consent. Understanding and freedom to choose has generated much concern regarding the validity of the live donor's consent (Ingelfinger, 1972; Valapour, 2008). There has long been concern that living organ donors may not (want to) fully understand what they are agreeing to do. Numerous authors believe that the majority of potential live donors decide to proceed with organ donation based on the potential to provide significant benefit to the recipient (moral reasoning) rather than on careful weighing of the risks and benefits of donation to themselves (deliberative reasoning) (Fellner & Marshall, 1970; Fellner & Marshall, 1968; Simmons et al., 1987). In their pioneering works, Fellner and Marshall found that many kidney donors decide to donate very quickly, before learning and considering all relevant information (Fellner & Marshall, 1970; 1968). These data show that potential donors often make decisions with limited understanding; an observation that led the authors to conclude that for many organ donors informed consent is a myth (Fellner & Marshall, 1970).

Table 1. Responsibilities of the donor team

Pre-Donation	Donation (Positive Outcome)	Non-Donation (Negative Outcome)
• Information about organ donation at multiple points during the evaluation process	• Provision of medical care for the donor until complete recovery	• Confidentiality
• Thorough assessment by dedicated donor team	• Long-term follow-up	• Supportive environment
• Psychological support	• Report of complications and outcomes to registries	
• Implementation of procedural safeguards to enhance donor understanding, safety, and autonomous decision-making		

In the study of Simmons et al (1987), 78% of the donors interviewed knew right away they would donate and 62% made an immediate choice. When the health of a loved one is at stake, if there is a reasonable chance for benefit, many people will want to donate almost regardless of the risks involved. These volunteers seem to base their decisions primarily on care and concern rather than on a careful review of the pros and cons of donating (Price, 2000b). Based on these observations, a legitimate question is the following: is the consent in live donation truly and fully informed? Some authors believe that a fully informed consent may not always be achieved when moral reasoning prevail, but should be considered equally valid (Valapour, 2008; Price, 2000b; Simmons et al., 1987; Spital, 2001). The observation that the vast majority of kidney donors are glad they donated and would do it again supports this position (Fellner & Marshall, 1968; Ubel & Mahowald, 1995, Fehrman-Ekuholm et al., 2000).

Despite all the above-mentioned considerations and potential limitations, it is our job to educate all potential donors as much as possible, in fact only a thoroughly informed donor can make a truly voluntary decision (Faden & Beauchamp, 1986; Somerville, 1979; Stansfield, 1979; Couch & Eliott, 1999). A strictly informed consent, carried out by a multidisciplinary team, with the support of experienced donor counsellors in issues related to living donor transplantation and medical ethics, is essential to ensure voluntary and autonomous choice in any form of live donation (directed, nondirected or altruistic live organ donation) (Spital, 2001; Ubel & Mahowald, 1995).

ROLE OF ETHICS IN THE DIFFERENT FORMS OF LIVE DONATION

In live donation can be distinguished three broad categories: directed donation to a relative, a loved one or friend; nondirected donation, in which the donor, sometimes called "Good Samaritan donor" gives an organ to the general pool; and directed donation to a stranger, whereby donors choose to give to a specific person with whom they have no prior emotional connection. Each type of donation prompts distinct ethical concerns. With directed donation to a relative, loved ones or friends, one ethical concern is related to the potential intense pressure, leading those who are reluctant to feel coerced (Price, 2000b; Spital, 2001; Faden & Beauchamp, 1986; Somerville, 1979; Stansfield, 1979; Crouch & Eliott, 1999). If they say no, how could they face their ill relatives, their families, and themselves? The voluntary decision of some potential donors might be influenced by a sense of duty or guilt (Simmons et al., 1987). Equally important, on the other hand, is when people feel compelled to donate regardless of the consequences to themselves, which is not unusual mostly in case of parental donation (Crouch & Eliott, 1999). In these cases, simply obtaining the informed consent is insufficient — physicians are obligated to prevent people from making potentially life-threatening sacrifices, serving the best interest of their patient.

Nondirected Donation

Nondirected donation raises different ethical concerns. The pure altruism that motivates a person to become a live donor for a stranger calls for careful scrutiny. One recent case involved a man who seemed pathologically obsessed with giving away everything, from his money to his organs (Parker, 2004). After donating one kidney to a stranger, he wondered how he might give away all his other organs in an attempt of "medically assisted" suicide. A thorough psychological assessment is of paramount importance (Matas et al., 2000). Is the person trying to compensate for depression or low self-esteem, seeking media attention, or harboring hopes of becoming involved in the life of the recipient? Transplantation teams have an obligation to assess potential donors in all these dimensions and prohibit donations that arouse serious concern (Truogg, 2005; Spital 2001; Matas et al., 2000; Spital, 1998).

Directed Donation

Directed donation to a stranger raises slightly different ethical questions; this type of donation usually occurs when a patient advertises for an organ publicly, on television or billboards or over the Internet. The practice of media appeals is not illegal, but it raises questions of fairness (Veatch & Ross, 2015); despite it is not encouraged by the transplant community, it is growing in popularity (Veatch & Ross, 2015; Gunby, 1983; Living Kidney Donors Network, 2018). Patients with stories more appealing for the media and more means to advertise tend to have an advantage compared to others, which could need the most. The most ethically problematic cases are those in which the recipient is chosen on the basis of race, religion, or ethnic group. In one case, for example, the family of a brain-dead Florida man agreed to donate his organs — but insisted that because of the man's racist beliefs, the recipients must be white. Although the organs were allocated accordingly, Florida subsequently passed a law prohibiting patients or families from placing such restrictions on donation (Gunby, 1983). Even when the motives for choosing a recipient may be unethical, however, there might be reasons for allowing the donation to proceed. Consider the case of direct donation on religious ground, a Jewish man in New York learned of a Jewish child in Los Angeles who needed a kidney transplant (Veatch & Ross, 2015). The man wanted to help someone of his own faith and decided he was willing to donate a kidney to help this particular child. Despite his discriminatory preference, one might view the donation as permissible, since at least some patients would benefit (the child would receive a kidney, and the patients below on the waiting list would move up) without causing any harm. Once established, it will be very difficult to prohibit discriminatory preferences, since donors can simply specify that the organ must go to a particular person, without saying why. The other substantial cause for concern about this type of donation is its potential for making possible an organ sale, which is prohibited by law. Since 1982, the first reported case of direct organ donation to stranger (Gunby, 1983), the number of media appeals has increased enormously; the creation of the website MatchingDonors.com in 2004 has certainly increased the magnitude of the phenomenon. Potential ethical concerns of the website are future exploitation of the recipient and the promotion of the interests of some groups at the expenses of others. According to Dees and Singer, it could potentially undermine the whole transplant allocation system and lead to commodification (Living Kidney Donors Network, 2018).

EXPANDING LIVING DONORS: PAIRED LIVE-DONOR EXCHANGES

Some living donors are unable to donate to an emotionally related recipient (typically due to ABO incompatibilities, positive T-cell cross-match or size miss-match). One option is the use of desensitization protocols (Becker et al., 2013). An alternative option involves the paired-exchange program, which is an exchange of donors between pairs (Rapaport, 1986; Ross et al., 1997; Park et al., 1999; McLellan, 2003). In addition, instead of occurring as a direct exchange between donor pairs, kidney donations could be made via an exchange donor pool (McLellan, 2003; Ferrari et al., 2015; Kranenburg et al., 2004; Veale & Hil, 2011). In 'conventional' kidney paired live donation of two or more pairs, transplants are simultaneously performed (synchronous donation) to guarantee that all recipients receive a transplant and eliminate the risk of any donor reneging and leaving a recipient with no transplants after their co-registered donor has donated their kidney (Rees et al., 2009). Since a synchronous donation could be technically challenging, the incorporation of non-directed anonymous donors, also known as Good Samaritan (Spital, 1998), into the pool can initiate a chain of transplants without obligatory matching of a paired recipient (Rees et al., 1009; Roodnat et al., 2010; Mongomery et al., 2006). Such chains are usually terminated with the last paired registered donor donating to a waitlist recipient (Montgomery et al., 2006).

In pair-exchange programs, the psychologic pressure on the donor may be greater than that on the recipient, because the donor is asked to give a kidney to a stranger rather than to a loved one. Nonetheless, potential donors can understand that their donation will indirectly benefit their loved ones (Park et al., 1999). Another ethical aspect of such a program is the possibility of coercion to donate, because a reluctant donor cannot use an excuse such as ABO incompatibility to obviate donation. Thus, a meticulous psychologic evaluation of the donor should be conducted to ensure the donor's willingness (Mazaris & Papalois, 2006; Simmons et al., 1987).

ORGAN TRAFFICKING AND TRANSPLANT TOURISM

The international trade in human organs represents a deplorable type of medical mal-practice, mostly involving human kidneys, where organs are bought from the poor for transplantation into the wealthy clientele.

The United Nations consider organ trafficking only a part of a larger crime, human trafficking with the purpose of forced labor, prostitution and any other form of exploitation (Council of Europe and United Nations, 2009). It is estimated that since 1980, several thousands of patients from the Middle East, the Far East and Europe have received kidneys sold in India, Iraq, Philippines, Iran and elsewhere (Shimazono, 2007; Budiani-Saberi, 2008). This phenomenon, according to some authors, could represent around 10% of all live donations (International Summit on Transplant Tourism and Organ Trafficking, 2008). It has been pointed out that organ sale has negative impact not only on all aspects of transplantation, undermining the cardinal principal of live donation, altruism, but also the medical profession and the moral and ethical values of the society (Steering Committee of the Istanbul Summit, 2008; Delmonico, 2008a; The Declaration of Istanbul on Organ Trafficking and Transplant Tourism, 2008a; The Declaration of Istanbul on Organ Trafficking and Transplant Tourism, 2008b; Delmonico, 2008b; Yang et al., 2007; Danovich et al., 2013; Salomon et al., 2015; Glazier et al., 2014; Sun et al., 2006).

In 2004, the World Health Organization called on member states "to take measures to protect the poorest and vulnerable groups from transplant tourism and the sale of tissues and organs, including attention to the wider problem of international trafficking in human tissues and organs" (Shimazono, 2007). As a result, the Transplantation Society and the International Society of Nephrology held a consensus conference in Istanbul in April 2008. The result of these deliberations was the "Istanbul Declaration on Organ Trafficking and Transplant Tourism," with the aim to address organ trafficking and transplant tourism with a consensus meeting, including medical staff, social scientists, government officials and ethicists (Steering Committee of the Istanbul Summit, 2008; Delmonico, 2008a; The Declaration of Istanbul on Organ Trafficking and Transplant Tourism, 2008a; The Declaration of Istanbul on Organ Trafficking and Transplant Tourism, 2008b; Delmonico, 2008b) (table 2).

Table 2. Key principles highlighted in the document "Declaration of Istanbul"

• Governments working to screen, prevent and treat organ failure
• Legislation to standardize living donation
• Equitable allocation of organs within countries without racial or financial prejudice
• Optimizing patient health
• Regions working to provide sufficient organs for residents within the country
• Prohibition of organ trafficking and transplant tourism

Most transplant professionals believe that organ sale is an affront not only to altruism, but also to basic human dignity for the following main reasons: (a) it promotes coercion and exploitation of the poor. (b) It promotes poor quality of care to the donor and recipient as documented in several reports. (c) It benefits ruthless entrepreneurs, greedy doctors who care for their egos and financial gain. (d) It is against the patient's right for autonomy, the potential donor comes forward as a consequence of its voluntary decision (Yang et al., 2007, Saloman et al., 2015; Glazier et al., 2014; Sun et al., 2006; Ambagtsheer et al., 2016).

Despite numerous efforts in fighting organ trafficking, it is alarming the conclusion of Ambagtsheer et al. (2016), in a recent paper, that "the scientific literature does not reflect a large number of patients buying organs." Considering the difficulties in defeating this phenomenon, some professionals in the transplant community believe that an organ sale, regulated by an independent organization, does have several major advantages. Cameron and Hoffenberg (1999) recommended a payment system through nationally established organ sharing networks in order to ensure quality of care and to promote the equity of distribution. Radcliffe-Richards et al. (1998) also suggest that a national organization be established to regulate the sale of organs or provide educational and appropriate consultation to patients. The same organization will regulate and control organ vending, proper selection, payment of fees and provision of necessary care which will prevent the current exploitation, the risk of removing organs, both for the donor and the recipient, and provide screening and counseling, together with reliable payment and financial advice. As an example, the Iranian model of compensated living kidney donation has apparently led to the elimination of their national kidney transplant waiting list (Ghods & Nasrollahzadeh, 2005). The proposal of legalizing the living donor markets would require changes to the law in most of the countries, where this practice is currently illegal (Shimazono, 2007). The first question we must ask is if this change would be ethical.

FINANCIAL INCENTIVES FOR LIVING DONATION

Pradel et al. showed that a proportion of recipients would not accept kidneys from potential live donors, if the donation would impose a financial burden on the donor (Pradel et al., 2003). It is increasingly recognized the importance to make the donation process at least financially neutral for the donor and there are currently proposals and systems in place to reach this goal (Unrelated Live Transplant Regulatory Authority, 1998; Steiner & Gert, 2000; Delmonico et al., 2002; Gill et al., 2017). Some programs in United States offer small financial incentives to the donors to be used for expenses such as food, housing, and transportation (Gridelli & Remuzzi, 2000; Yen, 2000).

It is also possible that noneconomic rewards might promote donation even further (Gridelli & Remuzzi, 2000). A medal or certificates for a generous and altruistic action, the recognition of donors in an official ceremony with media attention, have all been proposed. Other rewards could be free medical follow-up and health insurance. Providing medical follow-up for donors is also important to identify possible long-term risks and to ensure the early diagnosis and treatment of any conditions that are either donation related or may compromise post donation kidney function (Gill et al., 2017; Gabolde et al., 2001).

MINOR DONORS

Live donation from minors continues to raise ethical concerns. Important questions to be answered are: Should minors be allowed to be live donors? If yes, what should be the minimum age? Is the child assent required? What is the role of the court? (Spital, 1997; Ross et al., 2008a; Delmonico & Harmon, 2002). Surveys of US transplant centers have demonstrated that although great controversy regarding the acceptable age for kidney donors exists, the acceptance of children as living kidney donors is decreasing and most kidneys transplanted to children come from their parents (Ross et al., 2008a; Delmonico & Harmon, 2002). There is currently lack of stringent criteria regarding the participation of minors as donors from international data (Delmonico & Harmon, 2002; Delmonico & Council of the Transplantation Society, 2005; American Academy of Pediatrics & Committee on Bioethics, 1995). The Amsterdam Consensus Panel, an international panel of experts in transplantation, accepted a proposal that minors should not be allowed to donate (Delmonico & Council of the Transplantation Society, 2005). In contrast, the US Live Organ Donor Consensus Group and the American Academy of Pediatrics stated that minors could ethically serve as live donors but only in exceptional circumstances when specific criteria are fulfilled (Veatch & Ross, 2015; Ross et al., 2008a; American Academy of Pediatrics & Committee on Bioethics, 1995) (table 3).

From the legal standpoint, parental permission is all that is required for consent to clinical treatment (with a few exceptions), whereas parental permission and the child's assent are necessary for research purposes. Ethically, there are guidelines that promote obtaining both parental permission and the child's assent for both clinical and research purposes (Ross et al., 2008a; American Academy of Pediatrics & Committee on Bioethics, 1995). The American Academy of Pediatrics suggests that in case of live donation both parental permission and the child's assent are required (American Academy of Pediatrics & Committee on Bioethics, 1995). The scenario is even more complex in case of very young children and cognitively disabled children who are not able to give assent (Ross et al., 2008a, American Academy of Pediatrics & Committee on Bioethics, 1995). In the early court cases regarding kidney donation, some

Table 3. Criteria to be met in order to consider children as solid-organ live donors

• Donor and recipient are both highly likely to benefit
• Surgical risk for the donor is extremely low
• All other deceased and living donor options have been exhausted
• Assent of the minor (established by an independent advocacy team)
• Emotional and psychological risks to the donor are minimized

courts expressed concern about individuals with cognitive disabilities serving as organ donors (In re Richardson, 1973 as cited in Ross et al., 2008b; Justia US Law, 1975).

The evaluation of children as live donors requires a rigorous consideration of risk/benefit ratio. Some of the benefits include: preventing the trauma caused by the death of a very close relative such as a sibling, avoiding future guilt secondary to the refusal to donate, increasing self-esteem from donation, and maintaining the integrity of the family (Ross et al., 2008a). Potential complications can be medical and psychological in nature. Risks of surgery and anesthesia themselves can lead to significant morbidity, including postoperative bleeding and infections. The calculated risk of mortality from kidney donation is approximately 2 in 10 000 (American Academy of Pediatrics & Committee on Bioethics, 1995) and is up to 10-fold greater for a left lateral segment living liver donation (with the right-lobe having a greater risk than left-lobe) (Middleton et al., 2006). The true rate of morbidity and mortality for other solid-organ donations is difficult to establish (eg, lung, pancreas, and small bowel) because of the small numbers of reported cases in the literature and the lack of living-donor registries (Ross et al., 2007). Kidney donation poses a risk of chronic renal disease (Ellison et al., 2002) and potential risks to the remaining kidney (i.e. trauma, the development of a neoplasm or infection), could have a negative impact his or her future, degree of physical activity, or career choice (Salvatierra, 2001). Psychological risks as lower self-esteem, depression, sense of neglect and guilt and blame if the transplant fails and/or the recipient dies, can significantly affect daily life and the emotional and intellectual development (Holm, 2004). In assessing minors as potential organ donors it is important to evaluate the potential coercive nature of the request, which very often comes from their parents. How can children refuse when their parents are asking them to donate? (Ross et al., 2008a; Hamburger & Crosnier, 1968). And parents of a child who requires a kidney transplant and a healthy sibling (a potential donor), on the other hand, may experience a conflict of interest (Ross et al., 2008a; Hamburger & Crosnier, 1968). A multidisciplinary team (physicians, surgeons, skilled mental health professionals and the donor advocacy team) should ensure that the donation is a voluntary act and that the minor understands its risks and benefits (Ross et al., 2008a). If the minor is unwilling or is emotionally or cognitively unable to understand the risks and benefits or the procedures involved, the team should recommend against the donation (Ross et al., 2008a).

Even more complex is to set an age limit for live donation; some authors suggest that the decision to donate should depend on psychologic maturity rather than age (Hamburger & Crosnier, 1968). As a result, some US states have begun to legally accept the consent of minors older than 14 years for organ and tissue donation. In Alabama, for example, minors of that age can consent to bone marrow donation, and in Michigan (with court approval), they can serve as a kidney donor for an immediate family member (Ross et al., 2008a). Although children younger than 10 years rarely serve as living organ donors, there are cases reported (Lewis, 1974). Live donation from minors it is not prohibited but considered only under exceptional circumstances when strict criteria are met. Long-term follow-up data on live donation for minors should be collected to help determine the actual benefits and risks of donation, both medically and psychologically, in order to modify and improve the current guidelines (Ross et al., 2008a; Delmonico & Harmon, 2002; Delmonico & Council of the Transplantation Society, 2005; American Academy of Pediatrics & Committee on Bioethics, 1995; Ladd, 2004; Jansen, 2004).

CONCLUSION

The current scenario faced by clinical organ transplantation, a widening gap between demand and supply, translates in long waiting times and many deaths among potential transplant recipients. The donation from live donors, in an attempt to increase the number of transplants, has many medical advantages and can be further enhanced by appropriate public education. It is considered a truly heroic act, a 'gift of life' to a fellow human purely on humanitarian grounds. There is debate regarding the institution of a tightly regulated living organ market with compensation for the donor; this proposal is controversial and raises a number of moral and ethical issues. A new model considering economic and noneconomic rewards may be ethically acceptable and could increase the number of live donations. Finally, for clinical organ and tissue transplantation to be fully beneficial and life saving, everyone involved in the process, including physicians and medical institutions, must only respect and consider the best interest of the patient. The unique ethical concerns can be addressed with reflection on practice and open debate in a transparent process.

ACKNOWLEDGMENT

This research received no specific grant from any funding agency in the public, commercial, or not-for-profit sectors.

REFERENCES

Abecassis, M., Adams, M., Adams, P., Arnold, R. M., Atkins, C. R., Barr, M. L., ... Youngner, S. (2000). Consensus statement on the live organ donor. *Journal of the American Medical Association*, *284*(22), 2919–2926. doi:10.1001/jama.284.22.2919 PMID:11187711

Ambagtsheer, F., de Jong, J., Bramer, W. M., & Weimar, W. (2016). On Patients Who Purchase Organ Transplants Abroad. *American Journal of Transplantation*, *16*(10), 2800–2815. doi:10.1111/ajt.13766 PMID:26932422

American Academy of Pediatrics, Committee on Bioethics. (1995). Informed consent, parental permission, and assent in pediatric practice. *Pediatrics*, *95*, 314–317. PMID:7838658

Becker, L. E., Susal, C., & Morath, C. (2013). Kidney transplantation across HLA and ABO antibody barriers. *Current Opinion in Organ Transplantation*, *18*, 445–454. PMID:23838650

Budiani-Saberi, D. A., & Delmonico, F. L. (2008). Organ trafficking and transplant tourism: A commentary on the global realities. *American Journal of Transplantation*, *8*(5), 925–929. doi:10.1111/j.1600-6143.2008.02200.x PMID:18416734

Cameron, J. S., & Hoffenberg, R. (1999). The ethics of organ transplantation reconsidered: Paid organ donation and the use of executed prisoners as donors. *Kidney International*, *55*(2), 724–732. doi:10.1046/j.1523-1755.1999.00286.x PMID:9987097

Caplan, A. L., & Coehlo, O. H. (1998). *The Ethics of Organ Transplantation: The Current Debate*. New York: Prometheus Books.

Council of Europe and United Nations. (2009). *Trafficking in Organs, Tissues and Cells and Trafficking in Human Beings for the Purpose of the Removal of Organs, Joint Council of Europe/United Nations Study*. Retrieved from http://ec.europa.eu/anti-trafficking/sites/antitrafficking/files/council-un_study_on_trafficking_in_organs_2009_en_1.pdf

Crouch, R. A., & Elliott, C. (1999). Moral agency and the family: The case of living related organ transplantation. *Cambridge Quarterly of Healthcare Ethics*, *8*(3), 275–287. doi:10.1017/S096318019980303X PMID:10388928

Danovitch, G. M., Chapman, J., Capron, A. M., Levin, A., Abbud-Filho, M., Al Mousawi, M., ... Delmonico, F. L. (2013). Organ trafficking and transplant tourism: The role of global professional ethical standards-the 2008 Declaration of Istanbul. *Transplantation*, *95*(11), 1306–1312. doi:10.1097/TP.0b013e318295ee7d PMID:23644753

Delmonico, F. (2005). A report of the Amsterdam Forum on the Care of the Live Kidney Donor: Data and medical guidelines. *Transplantation*, *79*, S53–S66. doi:10.1097/01.TP.0000157343.27949.9F PMID:15785361

Delmonico, F. L. (2008a). The declaration of Istanbul on organ trafficking and transplant tourism. *Indian Journal of Nephrology*, *18*(3), 135–140. PMID:20142924

Delmonico, F. L. (2008b). The development of the Declaration of Istanbul on Organ Trafficking and Transplant Tourism. *Nephrology, Dialysis, Transplantation*, *23*(11), 3381–3382. doi:10.1093/ndt/gfn552 PMID:18922862

Delmonico, F. L., Arnold, R., Scheper-Hughes, N., Siminoff, L. A., Kahn, J., & Youngner, S. J. (2002). Ethical incentives--not payment--for organ donation. *The New England Journal of Medicine*, *346*(25), 2002–2005. doi:10.1056/NEJMsb013216 PMID:12075064

Delmonico, F. L., & Harmon, W. E. (2002). The use of a minor as a live kidney donor. *American Journal of Transplantation*, *2*(4), 333–336. doi:10.1034/j.1600-6143.2002.20407.x PMID:12118854

Eggers, P. W. (1998). Effect of transplantation on the Medicare End Stage Renal Disease Program. *The New England Journal of Medicine*, *38*, 223–229. PMID:3275896

Elliott, C. (1995). Doing harm: Living organ donors, clinical research and The Tenth Man. *Journal of Medical Ethics*, *21*(2), 91–96. doi:10.1136/jme.21.2.91 PMID:7608947

Ellison, M. D., McBride, M. A., Taranto, S. E., Delmonico, F. L., & Kauffman, H. M. (2002). Living kidney donors in need of kidney transplants: A report from the organ procurement and transplantation network. *Transplantation*, *74*(9), 1349–1351. doi:10.1097/00007890-200211150-00025 PMID:12451277

Faden, R. R., & Beauchamp, T. L. (1986). *A history and theory of informed consent*. New York: Oxford University Press.

Fehrman-Ekuholm, I., Brink, B., Ericsson, C., Elinder, C. G., Dunér, F., & Lundgren, G. (2000). Kidney donors don't regret: Follow-up of 370 donors in Stockholm since 1964. *Transplantation*, *69*, 2067–2071. PMID:10852598

Fellner, C. H., & Marshall, J. R. (1968). Twelve kidney donors. *Journal of the American Medical Association*, *206*(12), 2703–2707. doi:10.1001/jama.1968.03150120037007 PMID:4880430

Fellner, C. H., & Marshall, J. R. (1970). Kidney donors: The myth of informed consent. *The American Journal of Psychiatry*, *126*(9), 1245–1251. doi:10.1176/ajp.126.9.1245 PMID:4905016

Ferrari, P., Weimar, W., Johnson, R. J., Lim, W. H., & Tinckam, K. J. (2015). Kidney paired donation: Principles, protocols and programs. *Nephrology, Dialysis, Transplantation*, *30*(8), 1276–1285. doi:10.1093/ndt/gfu309 PMID:25294848

Gabolde, M., Herve, C., & Moulin, A. M. (2001). Evaluation, selection, and follow-up of live kidney donors: A review of current practice in French renal transplant centers. *Nephrology, Dialysis, Transplantation*, *16*(10), 2048–2052. doi:10.1093/ndt/16.10.2048 PMID:11572895

Ghods, A. J., & Nasrollahzadeh, D. (2005). Transplant tourism and the Iranian model of renal transplantation program: Ethical considerations. *Experimental and Clinical Transplantation*, *3*, 351. PMID:16417442

Gill, J. S., Delmonico, F. L., Klarenbach, S., & Capron, A. M. (2017). Providing coverage for the unique life-long health care needs of living kidney donors within the framework of financial neutrality. *American Journal of Transplantation*, *17*(5), 1176–1181. doi:10.1111/ajt.14147 PMID:27888569

Glazier, A. K., Danovitch, G. M., & Delmonico, F. L. (2014). Organ transplantation for nonresidents of the United States: A policy for transparency. *American Journal of Transplantation*, *14*(8), 1740–1743. doi:10.1111/ajt.12770 PMID:24840545

Gridelli, B., & Remuzzi, G. (2000). Strategies for making more organs available for transplantation. *The New England Journal of Medicine*, *343*(6), 404–410. doi:10.1056/NEJM200008103430606 PMID:10933740

Gunby, P. (1983). Media-abetted liver transplants raise questions of "equity and decency". *Journal of the American Medical Association*, *249*(15), 1973–1974. doi:10.1001/jama.249.15.1973 PMID:6339755

Hamburger, J., & Crosnier, J. (1968). Moral and ethical problems in transplantation. In F. Rapaport & J. Daussert (Eds.), *Human transplantation*. New York: Grunn and Stratton.

Holm, S. (2004). The child as organ and tissue donor: Discussions in the Danish council of ethics. *Cambridge Quarterly of Healthcare Ethics*, *13*(02), 156–160. doi:10.1017/S0963180104132076 PMID:15124403

Hou, S. (2000). Expanding the kidney donor pool: Ethical and medical considerations. *Kidney International*, *58*(4), 1820–1836. doi:10.1046/j.1523-1755.2000.00345.x PMID:11012922

Hunsicker, L. G. (1999). Survival advantage for renal transplantation. *The New England Journal of Medicine*, *341*(23), 1762–1763. doi:10.1056/NEJM199912023412310 PMID:10580078

Ingelfinger, F. J. (1972). Informed (but uneducated) consent. *The New England Journal of Medicine, 287*(9), 465–466. doi:10.1056/NEJM197208312870912 PMID:5044921

International Summit on Transplant Tourism and Organ Trafficking. (2008). The Declaration of Istanbul on organ trafficking and transplant tourism. *Kidney International, 74*(7), 854–859. doi:10.1038/ki.2008.388 PMID:18810784

Jansen, L. A. (2004). Child organ donation, family autonomy, and intimate attachments. *Cambridge Quarterly of Healthcare Ethics, 13*(02), 133–142. doi:10.1017/S0963180104132040 PMID:15124400

JustiaU. S. Law. (1975). *In Re Guardianship of Pescinski.* Retrieved from https://law.justia.com/cases/wisconsin/supreme-court/1975/668-6.html

Kahn, J., & Matas, A. J. (2002). What's special about the ethics of living donors? *Transplantation, 74*(3), 421–422. doi:10.1097/00007890-200208150-00026

Kasiske, B., Ravenscraft, M., Ramos, E. L., Gaston, R. S., Bia, M. J., & Danovitch, G. M. (1996). The evaluation of living renal transplant donors: Clinical practice guidelines. *Journal of the American Society of Nephrology, 7*, 2288–2313. PMID:8959619

Keown, P. (2001). Improving the quality of life: The new target for transplantation. *Transplantation, 7*, S67–S74. PMID:11833144

Kranenburg, L. W., Visak, T., Weimar, W., Zuidema, W., de Klerk, M., Hilhorst, M., ... Busschbach, J. J. (2004). Starting a crossover kidney transplantation program in the Netherlands: Ethical and psychological considerations. *Transplantation, 78*(2), 194–197. doi:10.1097/01.TP.0000129259.02340.F7 PMID:15280677

Ladd, R. E. (2004). The child as living donor: Parental consent and child assent. *Cambridge Quarterly of Healthcare Ethics, 13*(02), 143–148. doi:10.1017/S0963180104132052 PMID:15124401

Levinsky, N. (1984). The doctor's master. *The New England Journal of Medicine, 311*(24), 1573–1575. doi:10.1056/NEJM198412133112412 PMID:6438510

Lewis, M. (1974). Kidney donation by a 7-year-old identical twin child: Psychological, legal, and ethical considerations. *Journal of the American Academy of Child and Adolescent Psychiatry, 13*(2), 221–245. doi:10.1016/S0002-7138(09)61313-3 PMID:4596778

Living Kidney Donors Network. (2018). *Matching Recipient and Donors.* Retrieved from http://lkdn.org/matching_recip_donors.html

Majeske, R. A., Parker, L. S., & Frader, J. E. (1996). In search of an ethical framework for consideration of decisions regarding live donation. In B. Spielman (Ed.), *Organ and Tissue Donation: Ethical, Legal, and Policy Issues.* Carbondale, IL: Southern Illinois University Press.

Matas, A. J., Garvey, C. A., Jacobs, C. L., & Kahn, J. P. (2000). Nondirected donation of kidneys from living donors. *The New England Journal of Medicine, 343*(6), 433–436. doi:10.1056/NEJM200008103430611 PMID:10933745

Mazaris, E., & Papalois, V. (2006). Ethical Issues in Living Donor Kidney Transplantation. *Experimental and Clinical Transplantation*, *2*, 485–497. PMID:17238845

McLellan, F. (2003). US surgeons do first "triple-swap" kidney transplantation. *Lancet*, *362*(9382), 456. doi:10.1016/S0140-6736(03)14106-2 PMID:12931692

Merrill, J. P., Murray, J. E., Harrison, J. H., & Guild, W. R. (1956). Successful homotransplantation of human kidneys between identical twins. *Journal of the American Medical Association*, *160*(4), 277–282. doi:10.1001/jama.1956.02960390027008 PMID:13278189

Middleton, P. F., Duffield, M., Lynch, S. V., Padbury, R. T., House, T., Stanton, P., ... Maddern, G. (2006). Living donor liver transplantation: Adult donor outcomes—a systematic review. *Liver Transplantation*, *12*(1), 24–30. doi:10.1002/lt.20663 PMID:16498709

Montgomery, R. A., Gentry, S. E., Marks, W. H., Warren, D. S., Hiller, J., Houp, J., ... Segev, D. L. (2006). Domino paired kidney donation: A strategy to make best use of live non-directed donation. *Lancet*, *368*(9533), 419–421. doi:10.1016/S0140-6736(06)69115-0 PMID:16876670

NHS Blood and Transplant. (n.d.). *Living Donation Guidance and Resources on Living Donation and Trandplantation*. Retrieved from http://www.odt.nhs.uk/living-donation/

Nuffield Council on Bioethics. (1995). *Human Tissue Ethical and Legal Issues*. London: Nuffield Council on Bioethics.

Park, K., Moon, J. I., Kim, S. I., & Kim, Y. S. (1999). Exchange donor program in kidney transplantation. *Transplantation*, *67*(2), 336–338. doi:10.1097/00007890-199901270-00027 PMID:10075605

Parker, I. (2004). The gift: Zell Kravinsky gave away millions: but somehow it wasn't enough. *The New Yorker*, *2*, 54-63.

Pierce, E. G., & Pierce, R. A. (1973). The agony and the ecstasy. *Transplantation Proceedings*, *5*, 1067–1068. PMID:4579042

Plant, W. D., Akyol, M. A., & Rudge, C. J. (2002). *The ethical dimension to organ transplantation in transplantation surgery* (J. L. R. Forsythe, Ed.; 2nd ed.). WB Saunders London.

Pradel, F. G., Mullins, C. D., & Bartlett, S. T. (2003). Exploring donors' and recipients' attitudes about living donor kidney transplantation. *Progress in Transplantation (Aliso Viejo, Calif.)*, *13*(3), 203–210. doi:10.1177/152692480301300307 PMID:14558635

Price, D. (2000a). *Legal and ethical aspects of organ transplantation*. Cambridge University Press.

Price, D. (2000b). Informed consent. In *Legal and Ethical Aspects of Organ Transplantation*. Cambridge, UK: Cambridge University Press.

Price, D. (2009). *Human tissue in transplantation and research: A model legal and ethical donation framework*. Cambridge University Press. doi:10.1017/CBO9781139195652

Pruett, T. L., Tibell, A., Alabdulkareem, A., Bhandari, M., Cronin, D. C., Dew, M. A., ... Delmonico, F. L. (2006). The ethics statement of the Vancouver Forum on the Live Lung, Liver, Pancreas, and Intestine Donor. *Transplantation*, *81*(10), 1386–1387. doi:10.1097/01.tp.0000214976.36526.e3 PMID:16732173

Radcliffe-Richards, J., Daar, A. S., Guttmann, R. D., Hoffenberg, R., Kennedy, I., Lock, M., … Tilney, N. (1998). The case for allowing kidney sales. International Forum for Transplant Ethics. *Lancet*, *27*, 1950-2.

Rapaport, F. T. (1986). The case for a living emotionally related international kidney donor exchange registry. *Transplantation Proceedings*, *18*, 5–9. PMID:11649919

Rees, M. A., Kopke, J. E., Pelletier, R. P., Segev, D. L., Rutter, M. E., Fabrega, A. J., ... Montgomery, R. A. (2009). A nonsimultaneous, extended, altruistic-donor chain. *The New England Journal of Medicine*, *360*(11), 1096–1101. doi:10.1056/NEJMoa0803645 PMID:19279341

Reese, P. P., Caplan, A. L., Kesselheim, A. S., & Bloom, R. D. (2006). Creating a medical, ethical, and legal framework for complex living kidney donors. *Clinical Journal of the American Society of Nephrology; CJASN*, *1*(6), 1148–1153. doi:10.2215/CJN.02180606 PMID:17699340

Roodnat, J. I., Zuidema, W., van de Wetering, J., de Klerk, M., Erdman, R. A., Massey, E. K., ... Weimar, W. (2010). Altruistic donor triggered domino-paired kidney donation for unsuccessful couples from the kidney-exchange program. *American Journal of Transplantation*, *10*(4), 821–827. doi:10.1111/j.1600-6143.2010.03034.x PMID:20199504

Ross, L. F. (2000). Donating a second kidney: A tale of family and ethics. *Seminars in Dialysis*, *13*(3), 201–203. doi:10.1046/j.1525-139x.2000.00054.x PMID:10833782

Ross, L. F., Glannon, W., & Josephson, M. A. (2002). Should all living donors be treated equally? *Transplantation*, *74*(3), 418–421. doi:10.1097/00007890-200208150-00025 PMID:12177627

Ross, L. F., Rubin, D. T., Siegler, M., Josephson, M. A., Thistlethwaite, J. R. Jr, & Woodle, E. S. (1997). Ethics of a paired-kidney-exchange program. *The New England Journal of Medicine*, *336*(24), 1752–1755. doi:10.1056/NEJM199706123362412 PMID:9180096

Ross, L. F., Siegler, M., & Thistlethwaite, J. R. Jr. (2007). We need a registry of living kidney donors. *The Hastings Center Report*, *7*, 1. PMID:18179104

Ross, L. F., & Thistlethwaite, J. R. Jr. (2008a). Minors as Living Solid-Organ Donors. *Pediatrics*, *122*(2), 454–461. doi:10.1542/peds.2008-1525 PMID:18676567

Ross, L. F., & Thistlethwaite, J. R. (2008b). Minor as Living Solid-Organ Donors. *Pediatrics*, *122*(2), 454–461. doi:10.1542/peds.2008-1525 PMID:18676567

Salomon, D. R., Langnas, A. N., Reed, A. I., Bloom, R. D., Magee, J. C., & Gaston, R. S(2015). AST/ASTS workshop on increasing organ donation in the United States: Creating an "arc of change" from removing disincentives to testing incentives. *American Journal of Transplantation*, *15*(5), 1173–1179. doi:10.1111/ajt.13233 PMID:25833653

Salvatierra, O. Jr. (2001). Transplant physicians bear full responsibility for the consequences of kidney donation by a minor. *American Journal of Transplantation*, *2*(4), 297–298. doi:10.1034/j.1600-6143.2002.20402.x PMID:12118849

Shimazono, Y. (2007). *The state of the international organ trade: a provisional picture based on integration of available information.* Retrieved from http://www.who.int/bulletin/volumes/85/12/06-039370/en/

Simmons, R. G., Marine, S. K., & Simmons, R. L. (1987). *Gift of Life. The Effect of Organ Transplantation on Individual, Family, and Societal Dynamics*. New Brunswick, NJ: Transaction Books.

Simmons, R. G., Marine, S. K., & Simmons, R. L. (1987). *Gift of life: the effect of organ transplantation on individual, family, and societal dynamics* (2nd ed.). New Brunswick, NJ: Transaction Publishers.

Smith, M. D., Kappell, D. F., Province, M. A., Hong, B. A., Robson, A. M., Dutton, S., ... Cameron, E. (1986). Living-related kidney donors: A multicenter study of donor education, socioeconomic adjustment, and rehabilitation. *American Journal of Kidney Diseases, 8*(4), 223–233. doi:10.1016/S0272-6386(86)80030-0 PMID:3532770

Somerville, M. (1979). *The duty to inform the patient or research subject for the purpose of obtaining "informed" consent. Consent to medical care*. Ottawa, Canada: Law Reform Commission of Canada.

Spital, A. (1997). Should children ever donate kidneys? Views of U.S. transplant centers. *Transplantation, 64*(2), 232–236. doi:10.1097/00007890-199707270-00009 PMID:9256179

Spital, A. (1998). When a stranger offers a kidney: Ethical issues in living organ donation. *American Journal of Kidney Diseases, 32*(4), 676–691. doi:10.1016/S0272-6386(98)70037-X PMID:9774135

Spital, A. (2001). Ethical Issues in Living Organ Donation: Donor Autonomy and Beyond. *American Journal of Kidney Diseases, 38*(1), 189–195. doi:10.1053/ajkd.2001.25213 PMID:11431202

Spital, A. (2001). Ethical issues in living related donors. In W. Shelton & J. Balint (Eds.), *The Ethics of Organ Transplantation*. New York, NY: Elsvier Science. doi:10.1016/S1479-3709(01)80008-X

Spital, A. (2004). Donor benefit is the key to justified living organ donation. *Cambridge Quarterly of Healthcare Ethics, 13*(01), 105–109. doi:10.1017/S0963180104131174 PMID:15045922

Stansfield, M. P. (1979). Malpractice: Toward a viable disclosure standard for informed consent. *Oklahoma Law Review, 32*, 868–890. PMID:11665171

Steering Committee of the Istanbul Summit. (2008). Organ trafficking and transplant tourism and commercialism: The Declaration of Istanbul. *Lancet, 372*(9632), 5–6. doi:10.1016/S0140-6736(08)60967-8 PMID:18603141

Steiner, R. W., & Gert, B. (2000). Ethical selection of living kidney donors. *American Journal of Kidney Diseases, 36*(4), 677–686. doi:10.1053/ajkd.2000.17611 PMID:11007668

Stothers, L., Gourlay, W. A., & Liu, L. (2005). Attitudes and predictive factors for live kidney donation: A comparison of live kidney donors versus nondonors. *Kidney International, 67*(3), 1105–1111. doi:10.1111/j.1523-1755.2005.00176.x PMID:15698451

Sun, C. Y., Lee, C. C., Chang, C. T., Hung, C. C., & Wu, M. S. (2006). Commercial cadaveric renal transplant: An ethical rather than medical issue. *Clinical Transplantation, 20*(3), 340–345. doi:10.1111/j.1399-0012.2006.00491.x PMID:16824152

The Declaration of Istanbul on Organ Trafficking and Transplant Tourism. (2008b). Istanbul Summit April 30-May 2. *Nephrology, Dialysis, Transplantation, 23*, 3375. PMID:18922861

The Declaration of Istanbul on Organ Trafficking and Transplant Tourism. (2018). Retrieved from http://www.declarationofistanbul.org/

The Declaration of Istanbul on organ trafficking and transplant tourism. (2008a). *Transplantation, 86*(8), 1013-1018. Retrieved from https://journals.lww.com/transplantjournal/Fulltext/2008/10270/The_Declaration_of_Istanbul_on_Organ_Trafficking.1.aspx

Truog, R. D. (2005). The ethics of organ donation by living donors. *The New England Journal of Medicine, 353*(5), 444–446. doi:10.1056/NEJMp058155 PMID:16079366

Ubel, P. A., & Mahowald, M. B. (1995). Ethical and legal issues regarding living donors. In W. T. Reich (Ed.), *Encyclopedia of Bioethics*. New York: Simon Schuster Macmillan.

United Nations Office on Drugs and Crime. (2015). *Trafficking in Persons for the Purpose of Organ Removal*. Retrieved from https://www.unodc.org/documents/human-trafficking/2015/UNODC_Assessment_Toolkit_TIP_for_the_Purpose_of_Organ_Removal.pdf

UNOS. (2016). *Increasing the number of Transplants in the United States: 2016 in review*. Retrieved from https://unos.org/about/annual-report/2016-annual-report/

Unrelated Live Transplant Regulatory Authority (ULTRA). (1998). Retrieved from http://www.advisorybodies.doh.gov.uk/ultra/index.htm

Valapour, M. (2008). The live organ donor's consent: Is it informed and voluntary? *Transplantation Reviews, 22*(3), 196–199. doi:10.1016/j.trre.2008.02.004 PMID:18631878

Veale, J., & Hil, G. (2011). The National Kidney registry: 175 transplants in 1 year. *Clinical Transplantation*, 255–278. PMID:22755419

Veatch, R. M., & Ross, L. F. (2015). *Transplantation ethics* (2nd ed.). Washington, DC: Georgetown University Press.

Wolters, H. H., Heidenreich, S., & Senninger, N. (2003). Living donor kidney transplantation: Chance for the recipient--financial risk for the donor? *Transplantation Proceedings, 35*(6), 2091–2092. doi:10.1016/S0041-1345(03)00675-4 PMID:14529850

Yang, R. C., Thiessen-Philbrook, H., Klarenbach, S., Vlaicu, S., & Garg, A. X. (2007). Insurability of living organ donors: A systematic review. *American Journal of Transplantation, 7*(6), 1542–1551. doi:10.1111/j.1600-6143.2007.01793.x PMID:17430400

Yen, H. (2000). PA plans financial aid for organ donors. *Philadelphia Inquirer*.

Chapter 15
Health Literacy:
The Way Forward to Increase the Rates of Deceased Organ Donation

Maria Theodosopoulou
Imperial College London, UK

Frank J. M. F. Dor
Imperial College Healthcare NHS Trust, UK

Daniel Casanova
University of Cantabria, Spain

Georgios Baskozos
Oxford University, UK

Vassilios Papalois
Imperial College Healthcare NHS Trust, UK

ABSTRACT

Organ shortage is a worldwide persisting problem, as patients on waiting lists increase while actual donors cannot meet the demand for organs. Cultural and religious concerns, gaps of information, lack of medical procedure awareness and of understanding transplant-related terminology are some reasons why people refuse to donate organs. The medical, ethical, social, cultural, religious aspects of deceased organ donation (DOD) bring out the need for a systematic agenda of lifelong learning public awareness raising and health literacy on this issue. This chapter presents findings of a comparative research project in three European countries about how people learn about DOD and their suggestions for systematically promoting health literacy. A total sample of 1309 medical students, renal patients, and hospital administrative staff participated in a survey regarding attitudes, knowledge, sources of information, and communication about DOD. In addition, 51 participants took part in focus groups elaborating on their experiences and suggestions regarding health literacy about DOD.

DOI: 10.4018/978-1-5225-4074-8.ch015

INTRODUCTION

The concept of health literacy has evolved by leaps and bounds during the last years. The range of definitions and conceptual frameworks have expanded considerably more than the first notion of HL, as it was presented by Simmons in 1974, which focused on health education on schools. Multiple researchers and organizations explore various issues of health literacy, such as knowledge and understanding regarding specific health issues, antecedents, prevalence, health promotion, disease prevention, and promotion of well-being.

How does health literacy work? Efforts to answer this question include smaller and larger scale projects. Literacy skills are essential for understanding health information, yet the 1992 National Adult Literacy Survey (NALS) in the United States found that 90 million Americans have limited literacy skills, which entails difficulty understanding information in complex texts, such as informed consent forms (Institute of Medicine, 2004). The 2003 NALS showed that the health literacy skills of 14% of the respondents were below a basic level, 22% were at a basic level, 53% were at intermediate, while 12% were at proficient level. According to the European Health Literacy Survey (Sørensen et al, 2013) found that about 47% fall into the categories of low and inadequate health literacy. In the UK, Rowlands et al (2014) found that 43-61% of the population have levels of low health literacy.

More specifically, patients with limited health literacy may have difficulty understanding key concepts and terms about their condition. A survey in 11 countries (Cajita et al, 2017) with 1365 patients suffering from heart conditions, showed that 33% of the overall participants had inadequate health literacy. Although the health literacy levels varied between the countries, lower educational levels were generally associated with lower health literacy levels. An Australian cross-sectional study (Lambert et al, 2015) with 366 patients with chronic kidney disease either at predialysis, or dialysis, and with transplanted patients explored and compared their health literacy needs using the Health Literacy Management Scale (HeLMS). According to their results, about 25% of patients on dialysis or having received a transplant have difficulties understanding health information. Transplanted patients seem to have the highest proportion of health literacy needs, while about 40% of all the patients in the study have difficulties with their attitudes towards health. Another study (Gordon & Wolf, 2009) focusing on the knowledge deficits of patients who underwent kidney transplant showed that they had limited knowledge regarding graft survival and the risk of adverse outcomes. The majority of these recipients (81%) had difficulty to understand one or more common terms used in transplants, such as sensitization, blood urea nitrogen, and urethra, while about 25% of the participants had poor understanding of terms, such as immunosuppression and toxicity.

Other problematic areas for patients with limited health literacy skills seem to be their attitudes towards their disease, adherence to medication, and self-management. According to Miller's (2016) meta-analysis of studies about patient populations with chronic conditions, medication compliance needs less health literacy skills than complex treatment management behaviors. In addition, health literacy interventions had a positive impact on patients' treatment compliance by 16% in comparison to patients who had not attended such interventions. Among the most effective interventions were found to be the use of audio-visual and online educational materials, web-based applications, handouts, and social support resources. Another study (Demian et al, 2016) in Canada explored the health literacy skills of 96 patients using the Health Literacy Questionnaire, as well as their compliance to medication. Transplant patients who scored lower on the health literacy scale also showed less adherence to immunosuppressant medications. Another area in need of health literacy efforts is end-of-life care and decision-making. Brach et al (2012) considered clear and precise communication about end-of-life situations, which usually create confusion to individuals, as one of the ten attributes of healthcare organizations.

This chapter focuses on health literacy regarding Deceased Organ Donation (DOD). By definition health literacy relates to the living not the dying and is concerned with health promotion, disease prevention and management, patient adherence, patient well-being and effective health communication. "DOD,is a complex end-of-life decision, and we will present why DOD is a topic which requires special attention at the very top of the health literacy research agenda, as the gift of life that a deceased donor links together in a unique way the concepts of life and death, health and disease. We will clarify various aspects of the concept of DOD related to knowledge and comprehension of complex medical conditions, such as brain death, ethical dilemmas faced by the family of the potential donor, cultural, religious, emotional, and social issues which influence individual decisions with extending to their own family and patients on waiting lists. We will also present the findings of a research project in the UK, the Netherlands, and Spain exploring health literacy on DOD.

BACKGROUND

Organ Donation Rates

The advancements in medicine over the last decades, make transplants a life-saving solution, prolonging the life of the patients, and enhancing the quality of their life and, indirectly, of their family. However, worldwide, the demand for organs outnumbers the supply, as increasingly more people are added every year in the organ waiting lists. According to the Organ Procurement and Transplantation Network (OPTN, 2015) in the USA in 2015, there were 122,071 patients on the waiting list, while 30,975 transplants took place with organs by 15,068 donors. In 2013, in Europe (European Union, 2014) there were 86,000 patients on organ waiting lists, and 6,000 of thoses died while waiting for an organ.

The deceased organ donation (DOD) rates vary among countries. In Europe, according to data regarding 2016 by the International Registry in Organ Donation and Transplantation (IRODAT, 2017) Spain has the highest rate (43.4 per million of population). In the UK, the organ donation rate is 21.4 per million of population and according to National Health System (NHS, 2016), 6,476 patients were on waiting lists, while 3,527 transplants were performed. Organ shortage could be better understood by looking at three factors, which influence the actual number of organ donations, that is legislation, circumstances of death, and family consent.

Consent Systems

Legislation regarding DOD can be distinguished between presumed consent – or 'opting out' and explicit consent – or 'opting in'. Presumed consent

permits material to be removed from the body of a deceased person for transplantation and, in some countries, for anatomical study or research, unless the person had expressed his or her opposition before death by filing an objection with an identified office, or an informed party reports that the deceased definitely voiced an objection to donation. (WHO, 2009)

It is based upon the principle that donation serves the society and it is morally imperative to give consent (Dalal, 2015).

On the other hand, in countries with explicit consent:

cells, tissues or organs may be removed from a deceased person if the person had expressly consented to such removal during his or her lifetime; depending upon domestic law, such consent may be made orally or recorded on a donor card, driver's license or identity card or in the medical record or a donor registry. When the deceased has neither consented nor clearly expressed opposition to organ removal, permission should be obtained from a legally specified surrogate, usually a family member. (WHO, 2009)

Much debate focuses on whether presumed consent system could improve the rates of organ donation. Gevers et al (2004), argued that the consent system does not impact donation rates, since family consent is almost always asked, while Mossialos et al (2009) studying the attitudes towards DOD in 15 European countries, found that the willingness to be donors was higher in countries with the opting-out system.

Circumstances of Death

DOD may take place after the death of the patient is determined either by circulatory or neurologic criteria. Donation after circulatory death (DCD), previously known as donation after cardiac arrest or non-heartbeating donation (NHS Blood and Transplant, n.d.b), refers to the permanent absence of respiration and circulation (Thuong et al, 2016). In 1995, the Maastricht classification distinguished four categories of donors after cardio-respiratory arrest, which refer to the circumstances of the cardiac arrest and the initial therapeutic procedure (Thuong et al, 2016). These categories were determined based on medical, technical and ethical issues, and improvements of the categories are proposed. Variations on DCD programs across European countries depend on legislative and technical issues, but according to data of the Council of Europe (Dominguez-Gil et al, 2011), Belgium, the Netherlands, the UK, France, and Spain achieved high rates of DCD donors in the period 2008-2009. The promising results of DCD call on more action to be taken by more countries to develop DCD programs.

Neurologic criteria confirm donation after Brainstem Death (DBD), which:

is possible from patients whose death has been confirmed using neurological criteria (also known as brain-stem death or brain death). Neurological criteria for the diagnosis and confirmation of death applies in circumstances where brain injury is suspected to have caused irreversible loss of the capacity for consciousness and irreversible loss of the capacity for respiration before terminal apnoea has resulted in hypoxic cardiac arrest and circulatory standstill. This diagnosis is only possible in patients who are on mechanical ventilation. (NHS Blood and Transplant, n.d.a)

The first description of brain death, referred to as 'irreversible coma' was made by Mollaret and Goulon in 1957 in France, but it was in 1968 that the ad hoc committee of Harvard Medical School examined its medical and ethical aspects (Drake et al, 2017). The concept of brain death is well established in the medical community, but still more education on it is essential, as even, medical students may have gaps in their knowledge regarding brain death, even though this shortage did not interfere with their positive attitudes to DOD (Essman & Thornton, 2006). Even more problematic can be the general public's comprehension of it (Lewis & Caplan, 2016). A study of references regarding brain death in top ten Google websites and YouTube videos showed that the information provided in 40% of the websites and 60% of the videos analysed was inaccurate and did not agree with the scientific guidelines (Jones et al, 2018). Education of the public by the scientific community is essential, so that the concept and its definition can be better understood and a more concrete sense of trust of the public towards the medical community is built.

Family Consent

A family's right to finally decide whether to donate or not the organs of the deceased in some cases leads to an overrule of the decision or wishes of the deceased. The right to overrule is a topic raising both supportive and opposing arguments (Shaw et al, 2017). Some arguments in favour of the right of family to overrule their next of kin decision take into consideration the emotional distress that family members experience when they have to acknowledge both the death of their relative and, at the same time, give consent for organ donation. This perspective considers DOD not entirely as an individual decision, but the implications it has on the family of the potential donor. Another argument focuses on the potential of a family to present information on the change of the decision of their relative, which they feel that they need to respect. It is also argued that not allowing this right may severely undermine the public's trust in the healthcare system.

Conversely, those who oppose family members making decision about DOD argue that this heavy burden of the final decision should not be placed on the family, as they are not ready to cope with such an emotionally laden situation. It is also considered as disregarding the decision and wishes of the deceased. Other opposing arguments highlight the implications of an overrule to patients on waiting lists and the regret of that decision that family members may experience.

The consent rates vary considerably across countries. The refusal rate in Spain is 15.6% (IRODAT, 2016), while UK has one of the highest rates, as four in ten families refuse to give consent (NHS Activity Report 2015-2016). Possible explanations of those variations can be traced both to the different national organizational systems of organ transplantation, as well as to the lack of understanding of the donation process, personal, cultural, religious reasons. Hulme et al (2016) studying factors influencing the consent rate in the UK distinguish between easily and less easily modifiable factors. The approach of communicating with the family is found to be a significant factor and easily modifiable factor. Among the clinical staff approaching the family the role of Specialist Nurses in Organ Donation (SN-ODs) is highlighted. SN-ODs are trained on how to help families cope with the emotionally charged situations surrounding their relative's death and wishes about organ donation. The active communication role of SN-ODs with the family, as opposed to their mere presence among the specialist, is found to have a positive impact on consent, especially in the cases of circulatory death of the potential donor. On the other hand, factors such as the patient's ethnical background, death circumstances, and end-of-life wish regarding DOD are considered to be important to the consent but need more effort to be modified, as they rely on promoting family discussions and engaging more people from ethnic minorities.

The family's decision can be influenced by various factors. A systematic review of 34 qualitative studies in 13 countries (Ralph et al, 2014) showed that the rationale behind a family's decision to give or refuse consent seems to fall under 7 categories:

- Understanding of death (such as brain death, medical terms);
- Finding meaning (such as giving life to others, relief);

- Fear and suspicion (such as mistrust of healthcare system);
- Decisional conflict (such as the burden of the decision, religious beliefs);
- Vulnerability (such as feeling the need of more information and support);
- Respect of the wish of the deceased;
- Need of closure (such as wanting to know the positive outcomes of the transplant, having second thoughts about their decision).

Families are often unaware that one day they might find themselves in a situation when they need to give consent for their relatives. Findings from an online survey of 1549 adults in England (Webb et al, 2015) demonstrated that more than half did not know that they would need to give a consent, if the potential donor was already in the organ donor register. It was also found that about 47% had discussed their wishes about donation with their family, but even participants with positive attitudes towards DOD, did not think that they would give consent unless they knew the wish of their next of kin. A comparative study between the presumed consent systems of 25 countries and the explicit consent of 29 countries (Rosenblum et al, 2012) showed that there are discrepancies between the legislation and the practice as far as the impact of next-of-kin's decision on organ donation is concerned. Next of kin were approached in all the countries with explicit consent, while next of kin could object a donation in 21 out of the 25 countries with presumed consent. Positive attitudes towards DOD are not always translated in concrete decisions, such as registering as a donor or giving consent for next of kin, and the need for encouraging meaningful discussions about their wishes and decisions regarding DOD becomes more and more obvious.

KNOWLEDGE AND ATTITUDES ABOUT DOD

Understanding DOD and making decisions, such as registering as a donor or giving consent, are influenced by accurate knowledge about different aspects of it, as well as attitudes. Multiple sources of information exist regarding DOD: awareness campaigns, national websites about organ donation, information through school curricula, and healthcare professionals are some sources of reliable information motivating the public and explaining facts and procedures, such as transplantable organs, waiting lists, registering, consent, as well as stories about experiences of recipients and persons who gave consent for their next-of-kin.

However, not all portrayals of DOD are based on scientific evidence, but rather on fictional consumer scenarios, which do not target health promotion and education of the public, but instead feed on myths around DOD. A common example of inaccurate messages, which may be conveyed through films or television series, is the idea of manipulating DOD procedures in favour of some patients over others, especially in the categories of relatives, rich, famous and the celebrities, thus encouraging mistrust towards the medical system (Harbaugh et al, 2011; Quick, 2009; Morgan et al., 2007, 2005, 2002). On the contrary, scientifically accurate messages are shown to increase awareness and encourage discussions of donation wishes within families (Khalil and Rintamaki, 2014).

All major religions -Christianity, Judaism, Islam, Buddhism, Hinduism, Sikhism- accept DOD (Bendorf et al, 2013). However, there are voices within religions, which vary in their approach to DOD decision-making. As organ transplants are a recent 20th century medical development, they are not specifically cited as such in scriptures and holy texts. Therefore, interpretations of the religious texts and teachings serve as a basis for religious standings on DOD. Public statements and official documentation by religious leaders about the importance of organ donations, such as Pope Benedict XVI being a registered organ donor or the 1996 Muslim Law in the UK Council that organ donation is compatible with Islam, are some examples of the advocacy provided by faith leaders (Oliver et al, 2012). However, among some of their followers there is unawareness and confusion about the standing of their faith on this issue (Rykhoff et al, 2010; Cantarovich et al, 2007). As Randhawa and Neuberger (2011) emphasize, a more vigorous collaboration and dialogue among faith leaders, communities, healthcare professionals, and policy makers needs to take place on a continuous and systematic base, including outreach events at community and national level as well as a systematic agenda of lifelong education about organ donation starting early at schools.

A Cross-Cultural Perspective on DOD

Based on the findings from a research project that took place in the UK, the Netherlands, and Spain exploring the attitudes, knowledge, sources of information, and communication of wishes about DOD. More specifically, we will focus on the sources participants of the project used to learn about DOD, as well as suggestions on how these sources could be further utilised.

Sample of the research project included medical students, transplanted and non-transplanted renal patients, and hospital administrative staff at Hammersmith Hospital and Imperial College in London, Erasmus University and Medical Centre in Rotterdam, and University of Cantabria in Santander. The project followed two lines of research. The first line was the collection of quantitative data from the three sites. A survey was completed by 1309 participants, which covered areas regarding attitudes and knowledge about DOD, as well as communication patterns of wishes regarding this issue. More specifically, there were 359 participants from the UK (149 medical students, 64 administrative staff, and 146 kidney patients, 627 participants from the Netherlands (202 medical students, 285 administrative staff, and 140 kidney patients, and 323 participants from Spain (194 medical students, 52 administrative staff, and 77 kidney patients).

The second line of research focused on the collection of qualitative data through 9 focus group discussions in the three sites, in which a total of 51 individuals participated (18 from the UK, 16 from the Netherlands, and 17 from Spain). These discussions provided the participants with the opportunity to explain their points of view experiences and arguments, as well as express their opinion on how health literacy on DOD could be systematically promoted as part of a lifelong learning health literacy agenda.

Learning About DOD

All the groups of the UK sample, selected the same top three popular sources of getting information about DOD. 16% patients, 12% staff, and 11% students learnt through stories of recipients, 12% patients and staff, and 11% students through medical documentaries. Family and friends was the most popular among students (13%), as well as for 11% patients and 12% staff.

In the Dutch sample, the stories of organ recipients served as a basic source of information for 17% patients, 12% staff, and 13% students. For medical students, information received at school (14%) and family and friends (13%) contributed also to their awareness. Family (12%) and medical documentaries (11%) were selected by staff. Documentaries were also a source of information for patients, as well as brochures and the official website of NTS, each of which collected 10% of preference.

Learning from other recipients was also very important for Spanish patients (19%) and administrative staff (17%). Patients also relied on awareness campaigns (13%), family and friends (12%), and stories in newspapers and magazines (8%). Awareness campaigns were a very significant source of information for hospital administrative staff (25%), as well as learning through their colleagues (10%). Spanish students reported as their top three sources of information as: family and friends (12%), medical television shows (12%), and awareness campaigns (11%).

During the focus group discussions, the participants talked more extensively about the various ways they heard about DOD. Patient stories, learning at school, discussing with family, relatives and friends, as well as media were the main sources of information. It was a common sense in all the discussions that the stories of patients were not only informative, but also inspirational. Patients were able to explain what being ill meant to them and how it impacted their daily life and the life of their family. *'in Spain, I think, it influenced a lot, at that time, to put a face to the people with transplants' (administrative hospital staff, Spain).* Their narrative uses clear language to describe first hand experiences about the changes of their life due to disease, their hopes, fears and frustrations, the adjustment to new situations following the transplant. The authenticity of these narratives brings the listener closer to the humane sides of organ donation rather than its scientific ones. *'It's the patients talking in front of you with the symptoms' (female medical student, UK).* Patients not always help by sharing their stories, but often help by answering questions of people who either are outside the scope of issues regarding organ donation and transplantation or other patients who would like to know what lies ahead and how others coped with a similar situation. *'You get to meet them, you talk to them and that was very important' (male transplanted patient, UK).*

Family for many participants is a safe place where they share opinions, wishes and decisions about DOD. However, some participants gave reasons why the issue may not be discussed. One such example is thinking that it was not an urgent matter to discuss, while another is that people are not ready to talk about it.

The experience of older participants regarding school was that it did not provide them any information about DOD. Younger participants, though, mention about being informed during assemblies, speaking about it in Biology class or in a discussion about ethics during the Religious Education class. However, many participants feel that children and parents need to learn about DOD, so that they do not only get aware about it but be comfortable to discuss about it.

Media coverage of DOD varies across the countries. In Spain, some participants spoke about regular reports in the news about transplants, organ donation rates, and stories about patients, as well as memorable awareness campaigns *'they made a video with children that were in hospital and they danced and it was very emotional' (female medical student, SP).* In the Netherlands, the impact of media on raising awareness was discussed, as people would remember stories. As one participant, who had appeared on television to talk about organ donation said people were emotionally engaged by what they learnt through him. It was argued, though, that the topic is not covered on a regular basis in the media *'Like once in a couple of years' (male medical student, NL).* The feeling that awareness is not promoted enough through the social media, was expressed among some participants in the UK, *'You don't get so much about organ transplant stuff in the social media' (female medical student, UK).*

SOLUTIONS AND RECOMMENDATIONS

Systematic public dialogue about DOD is needed; discussion to embrace the levels and groups that compose the habitat of DOD. Taking into account the recommendations of the focus groups participants, we briefly present some suggestions on how the public can become more health literate about DOD. Families and communities, healthcare professionals, patients, mass and social media, at local, regional national, and international levels need to talk to each other, listen each other's points of view, and act together.

Within families, discussion is important as it informs about wishes and decisions, but also makes it easier for the other family members to give consent, if needed. It is difficult to respect people's wishes when they have not been expressed, because according to the participants, the relatives are too emotionally charged to make decisions. People who expect that their wishes about DOD may stumble upon their family's concerns need to have more guidance on how to support their decisions and how to overcome possible conflicts. The public needs to be better informed about the processes in which family plays role in DOD. Kits, like the one produced in NHS, gives some pointers on how a discussion within family can be initiated.

Community networks help shape attitudes about DOD. In many communities there is a lack of dialogue or awareness raising about that issue and this inertia could show, among others, a deeper lack of interest in the subject, lack of knowledge, or even disagreement to the idea of DOD. However, initiatives which involve community members would be opportunities to engage more members s to share their questions, perspectives, and concerns would help shape a bottom-up culture of learning about DOD from where people are and what they would like to learn instead of what they should learn.

The healthcare sector also needs to become more closely acquainted with the different needs of different populations. Understanding concerns and locating areas of misinformation are critical to establishing common codes of communication between the healthcare community and the public. Simple language which explains, yet not oversimplifies, processes, clear description of the steps along the way that healthcare teams, potential donors, their family, potential recipients have to take, are only a few ways to establish transparency and promote reflection in this complex issue.

One of the suggestions by participants of all groups in all three countries was the active involvement of patients in awareness campaigns. This engagement would help the public not only to learn about a health issue, but, more importantly, realise the importance of learning and deciding about an important, but not much discussed health issue. Patient stories are a primary source of information which seems to be more relatable than secondary sources focusing on data about DOD. Patients can portray in an authentic way their emotional and physical condition. Giving a face to complex medical issues also involves the families of donors who have given consent, as they could have a more central role in explaining to the public their own journey along accepting the loss of their next of kin and giving consent. *'I think the person who can transmit it the best is the patient and the family' (medical student, Spain).* The problems of patients waiting for a transplant could be better understood by giving the opportunities of presenting the spectrum of various patients. As it is not only the general public which should be more health literate about DOD, but also the patients in need of a transplant, the patients would also like to hear about experiences of multiple patients, so that the diversity of the population in need of transplant is more accurately represented.

Another suggestion of the participants was that information should be balanced, containing both informational and emotional elements. While the emotional elements can motivate people to act, there is also a need for people to be informed on relevant processes, such as waiting lists, and convinced about the transparency of the organ donation system.

Awareness raising, information and education about DOD need to be available on a continuous basis. It is a matter on which education needs to take the lead to open conversations within the family, among friends and colleagues, instead of being seen as a strictly individual issue. Widely available information and frequent reminders keep the issue in sight and helps the public realise that it is a topic relevant to all and thinking and deciding about it is should not be postponed. It is certainly very important having the topic in the spotlight during certain days, such as Organ Donation Week, but it is also important to bring it up on a regular basis.

The media has a significant role to play in informing, educating and motivating the public. Regular updates about the progress of DOD, as well as advocacy by high-profile people are some ways to keep the topic in the public arena. Communication approaches should be tailored to the needs of different target groups, taking into consideration factors, such as age, ethnical background, involvement in the issue. The accurate depiction of facts and processes are of paramount importance and every effort should be paid for a closer collaboration of the scientific community with the entertainment industry, so that the storylines relating to DOD project a true portrayal. Social media also has a vital role to play in engaging the public, not only to become aware about organ donation, but also to take action, such as motivating them to register as organ donors, express their decision to friends and family. Media and social media have an overarching attribute, which makes the messages cross over borders and bridge distance and time. The democracy of social media gives a platform to everybody interested to express themselves. Highly recognizable persons as well as non-famous persons take the opportunities to speak about DOD, with some of their interventions becoming viral.

FUTURE RESEARCH DIRECTIONS

Optimizing health literacy about DOD is an endeavour, which requires the collaboration of different fields, such as medicine, education, psychology, religion. Exploring the various ways through which people learn and designing environments which foster dialogue about DOD are aspects which need to be further studied. Educating people on such a complex and sensitive issue requires building trust so that people who have concerns may feel freely to express them. Organ donation rates are especially low among ethnic minorities, although more and more patients from these minorities are on the waiting lists for organ transplant. Looking at health literacy and its links with civic, cultural and science literacies (Zarcadoolas et al, 2005) would help us design culturally sensitive interventions and assess their impact. Qualitative research studies are especially valuable on this field, as they give more opportunities to participants to talk about their experiences, fears, concerns, and wishes. Most importantly, through qualitative research, they talk about what they would like to learn, what they believe is currently lacking regarding the available information, and the sources they would like to get this information from. Starting from the needs of people, then health education on DOD could be differentiated more effectively according to the different target groups it addresses.

CONCLUSION

DOD is at the crossroads of medicine, lifelong learning, law, ethics, culture, and religion. Trying to capture the nature of the topic looking at it only from a single discipline perspective fails to grasp the complexity of matters related to life and death, health and disease. There is a need for a case based interdisciplinary dialogue and problem-solving research approach that brings together all stakeholder networks related to DOD (hospitals, healthcare professionals and policy makers, patient groups, educators, schools, media and the general public) as a matter of lifelong health literacy -starting early from school and ending at a patient's bedside in an ICU (Intensive Care Unit) or A&E (Accident & Emergency) hospital department. After all, according to ancient Greek philosopher Protagoras '*Man is the measure of all things in life*'.

REFERENCES

Bendorf, A., Pusell, B., Kelly, P., & Kerridge, I. (2013). Socioeconomic, demographic and policy comparisons of living and deceased kidney transplantation rates across 53 countries. *Nephrology (Carlton, Vic.)*, *18*(9), 633–640. doi:10.1111/nep.12101 PMID:23692370

Brach, C., Keller, D., Hernandez, L. M., Baur, C., Parker, R., Dreyer, B., ... Schillinger, D. (2012). *Ten Attributes of Health Literate Health Care Organizations*. Washington, DC: National Academy of Sciences.

Cajita, M. I., Denhaerynck, K., Dobbels, F., Berben, L., Russell, C. L., Davidson, P. M., ... Maddicks-Law, J. (2017). Health literacy in heart transplantation: Prevalence, correlates and associations with health behaviors - findings from the international BRIGHT study. *The Journal of Heart and Lung Transplantation*, *36*(3), 272–279. doi:10.1016/j.healun.2016.08.024 PMID:27773449

Cantarovich, F., Heguilen, R., Filho, M. A., Duro-Garcia, V., Fitzgerald, R., Mayrhofer-Reinhartshuber, D., ... Esnault, V. L. M. (2007). An international opinion poll of well-educated people regarding awareness and feelings about organ donation for transplantation. *Transplant International*, *20*(6), 512–518. doi:10.1111/j.1432-2277.2007.00473.x PMID:17355245

Dalal, A. R. (2015). Philosophy of organ donation: Review of ethical facets. *World Journal of Transplantation*, *5*(2), 44–51. doi:10.5500/wjt.v5.i2.44 PMID:26131406

Demian, M. N., Shapiro, R. J., & Thornton, W. L. (2016). An observational study of health literacy and medication adherence in adult kidney transplant recipients. [doi]. *Clinical Kidney Journal*, *9*(6), 858–865. doi:10.1093/ckjfw076 PMID:27994867

Domínguez-Gil, B., Haase-Kromwijk, B., Van Leiden, H., Neuberger, J., Coene, L., Morel, P., ... Matesanz, R. (2011). Current situation of donation after circulatory death in european countries. *Transplant International*, *24*(7), 676–686. doi:10.1111/j.1432-2277.2011.01257.x PMID:21504489

Drake, M., Bernard, A., & Hessel, E. (2017). Brain death. *The Surgical Clinics of North America*, *97*(6), 1255–1273. doi:10.1016/j.suc.2017.07.001 PMID:29132508

Essman, C., & Thornton, J. (2006). Assessing medical student knowledge, attitudes, and behaviors regarding organ donation. *Transplantation Proceedings*, *38*(9), 2745–2750. doi:10.1016/j.transproceed.2006.08.127 PMID:17112821

European Union. (2014). *Journalist Workshop on Organ donation and transplantation.* Retrieved 24/06/17 from https://ec.europa.eu/health//sites/health/files/blood_tissues_organs/docs/ev_20141126_factsfigures_en.pdf

Gevers, S., Janssen, A., & Friele, R. (2004). Consent systems for post mortem organ donation in europe. *European Journal of Health Law, 11*(2), 175–186. doi:10.1163/1571809041457422 PMID:15387424

Gordon, E. J., & Wolf, M. S. (2009). Health literacy skills of kidney transplant recipients. *Progress in Transplantation (Aliso Viejo, Calif.), 19*(1), 25–34. doi:10.1177/152692480901900104 PMID:19341060

Harbaugh, C., Afana, M., Burdick, S., East, J., Kodali, S., Lee, J., ... Mathur, A. K. (2011). Portrayal of organ donation and transplantation on american primetime television. *Clinical Transplantation, 25*(4), 375–380. doi:10.1111/j.1399-0012.2011.01427.x PMID:21410759

Hulme, W., Allen, J., Manara, A. R., Murphy, P. G., Gardiner, D., & Poppitt, E. (2016). Factors influencing the family consent rate for organ donation in the UK. *Anaesthesia, 71*(9), 1053–1063. doi:10.1111/anae.13535 PMID:27440055

Institute of Medicine. (2004). *Health literacy: A prescription to end confusion* (L. Nielsen-Bohlman, A. M. Panzer, & D. A. Kindig, Eds.). Washington, DC: The National Academies Press.

International Registry in Organ Donation and Transplantation (IRODAT). (2017). Retrieved from http://www.irodat.org/img/database/pdf/NEWSLETTER2017_firstedition.pdf

Jones, A. H., Dizon, Z. B., & October, T. W. (2018). Investigation of public perception of brain death, using the internet. *Chest.* doi:10.1016/j.chest.2018.01.021 PMID:29382473

Khalil, G. E., & Rintamaki, L. S. (2014). A televised entertainment-education drama to promote positive discussion about organ donation. *Health Education Research, 29*(2), 284–296. doi:10.1093/her/cyt106 PMID:24399264

Kutner, M., Greenburg, E., Jin, Y., & Paulsen, C. (2006). *The health literacy of America's adults: Results from the 2003 National Assessment of Adult Literacy. NCES 2006-483. U.S. Department of Education.* Washington, DC: National Center for Education Statistics.

Lewis, A., & Caplan, A. (2016). Brain death in the media. *Transplantation, 100*(5), e24. doi:10.1097/TP.0000000000001147 PMID:27116579

Manara, A. R., Murphy, P. G., & O'Callaghan, G. (2012). Donation after circulatory death. *BJA: British Journal of Anaesthesia, 108*(suppl_1), i121. doi:10.1093/bja/aer357

Miller, T. A. (2016). Health literacy and adherence to medical treatment in chronic and acute illness: A meta-analysis. *Patient Education and Counseling, 99*(7), 1079–1086. doi:10.1016/j.pec.2016.01.020 PMID:26899632

Morgan, S., & Miller, J. (2002). Communicating about gifts of life: The effect of knowledge, attitudes, and altruism on behavior and behavioral intentions regarding organ donation. *Journal of Applied Communication Research, 30*(2), 163–178. doi:10.1080/00909880216580

Morgan, S. E., Harrison, T. R., Long, S. D., Afifi, W. A., Stephenson, M. S., & Reichert, T. (2005). Family discussions about organ donation: How the media influences opinions about donation decisions. *Clinical Transplantation*, *19*(5), 674–682. doi:10.1111/j.1399-0012.2005.00407.x PMID:16146561

Morgan, S. E., Movius, L., & Cody, M. J. (2009). The power of narratives: The effect of entertainment television organ donation storylines on the attitudes, knowledge, and behaviors of donors and nondonors. *Journal of Communication*, *59*(1), 135–151. doi:10.1111/j.1460-2466.2008.01408.x

Mossialos, E., Costa-i-Font, J., & Rudisill, C. (2008). Does organ donation legislation affect individuals' willingness to donate their own or their relative's organs?: Evidence from European Union survey data. *BMC Health Services Research*, *8*(1), 48. doi:10.1186/1472-6963-8-48 PMID:18304341

NHS Blood and Transplant. (n.d.a). *Donation After Brainstem Death*. Retrieved https://www.odt.nhs.uk/deceased-donation/best-practice-guidance/donation-after-brainstem-death/

NHS Blood and Transplant. (n.d.b). *Donation After Circulatory Death*. Retrieved https://www.odt.nhs.uk/deceased-donation/best-practice-guidance/donation-after-circulatory-death/

NHS Blood and Transplant Organ Donation and Transplantation 2013-2014. (n.d.). Retrieved https://nhsbtmediaservices.blob.core.windows.net/organ-donation-assets/pdfs/activity_report_2013_14.pdf

Oliver, M., Ahmed, A., & Woywodt, A. (2012). Donating in good faith or getting into trouble? religion and organ donation revisited. *World Journal of Transplantation*, *2*(5), 69–73. doi:10.5500/wjt.v2.i5.69 PMID:24175198

Organ Procurement and Transplantation Network (OPTN). (n.d.). Retrieved September, 2017, from https://optn.transplant.hrsa.gov/

Quick, B. L., Kim, D. K., & Meyer, K. (2009). A 15-year review of ABC, CBS, and NBC news coverage of organ donation: Implications for organ donation campaigns. *Health Communication*, *24*(2), 137–145. doi:10.1080/10410230802676516 PMID:19280457

Ralph, A., Chapman, J. R., Gillis, J., Craig, J. C., Butow, P., Howard, K., ... Tong, A. (2014). Family perspectives on deceased organ donation: Thematic synthesis of qualitative studies. *American Journal of Transplantation*, *14*(4), 923–935. doi:10.1111/ajt.12660 PMID:24612855

Randhawa, G., & Neuberger, J. (2011). Role of religion in organ donation - development of the United Kingdom faith and organ donation action plan. *Transplantation Proceedings*, *48*(3), 689–694. doi:10.1016/j.transproceed.2015.10.074 PMID:27234715

Rosenblum, A. M., Horvat, L. D., Siminoff, L. A., Prakash, V., Beitel, J., & Garg, A. X. (2012). The authority of next-of-kin in explicit and presumed consent systems for deceased organ donation: An analysis of 54 nations. *Nephrology, Dialysis, Transplantation*, *27*(6), 2533–2546. doi:10.1093/ndt/gfr619 PMID:22121233

Rowlands, G., Protheroe, J., Price, H., & Rafi, I. (2014). *Health literacy report from an RCGP-led health literacy workshop*. London: Royal College of General Practitioners.

Rykhoff, M. E., Coupland, C., Dionne, J., Fudge, B., Gayle, C., Ortner, T. L., ... Wrobleska, M. (2010). A clinical group's attempt to raise awareness of organ and tissue donation. *Progress in Transplantation (Aliso Viejo, Calif.)*, *20*(1), 33–39. doi:10.1177/152692481002000106 PMID:20397344

Shaw, D., Georgieva, D., Haase, B., Gardiner, D., Lewis, P., Jansen, N., ... Ploeg, R. (2017). Family over rules? an ethical analysis of allowing families to overrule donation intentions. *Transplantation*, *101*(3), 482–487. doi:10.1097/TP.0000000000001536 PMID:27764030

Sørensen, K., Van den Broucke, S., Pelikan, J. M., Fullam, J., Doyle, G., Slonska, Z., ... Brand, H. (2013). Measuring health literacy in populations: Illuminating the design and development process of the european health literacy survey questionnaire (HLS-EU-Q). *BMC Public Health*, *13*(1), 1–22. doi:10.1186/1471-2458-13-948 PMID:24112855

Thuong, M., Ruiz, A., Evrard, P., Kuiper, M., Boffa, C., Akhtar, M. Z., ... Ploeg, R. (2016). New classification of donation after circulatory death donors definitions and terminology. *Transplant International*, *29*(7), 749–759. doi:10.1111/tri.12776 PMID:26991858

Webb, G., Phillips, N., Reddiford, S., & Neuberger, J. (2015). Factors affecting the decision to grant consent for organ donation: A survey of adults in England. *Transplantation*, *99*(7), 1396–1402. doi:10.1097/TP.0000000000000504 PMID:25675195

World Health Organization WHO. (2009). *Guiding principles on human cell, tissue and organ transplantation*. World Health Organization.

Zarcadoolas, C., Pleasant, A., & Greer, D. S. (2005). Understanding health literacy: An expanded model. *Health Promotion International*, *20*(2), 195–203. doi:10.1093/heapro/dah609 PMID:15788526

Compilation of References

(2016).. . *Following an Educational Intervention Using the Integrated Model for Behavior Change.*, *86*(11), 813–822.

Abecassis, M., Adams, M., Adams, P., Arnold, R. M., Atkins, C. R., Barr, M. L., ... Youngner, S. (2000). Consensus statement on the live organ donor. *Journal of the American Medical Association*, *284*(22), 2919–2926. doi:10.1001/jama.284.22.2919 PMID:11187711

Abel, T. (2008). Cultural capital and social inequality in health. *Journal of Epidemiology and Community Health*, *62*(7), e13–e13. doi:10.1136/jech.2007.066159 PMID:18572429

Abrams, M. A., Kurtz-Rossi, S., Riffenburgh, A., & Savage, B. A. (2014). *Building health literate organizations: A guidebook to achieving organizational change*. Retrieved May 11, 2017 from http://www.healthliterateorganization.org

Ackerman, I. N., Bennell, K. L., & Osborne, R. H. (2011). Decline in Health-Related Quality of Life reported by more than half of those waiting for joint replacement surgery: A prospective cohort study. *BMC Musculoskeletal Disorders*, *12*(1), 108–108. doi:10.1186/1471-2474-12-108 PMID:21605398

Ad Hoc Committee on Health Literacy for the Council on Scientific Affairs, American Medical Association. (1999). Health literacy report of the council on scientific affairs. *Journal of the American Medical Association*, *281*(6), 552–557. doi:10.1001/jama.281.6.552 PMID:10022112

Adams, K., & Corrigan, J. M. (2003). *Priority areas for national action: Transforming health care quality*. Washington, DC: National Academies Press.

Adoption of Electronic Health Record Systems among U.S. Non Federal Acute Care Hospitals: 2008-2014. (n.d.). Retrieved from https://www.healthit.gov/sites/default/files/databrief/2014HospitalAdoptionDataBrief.pdf

Aetna. (2015). *Mental Health, wellness, and corporate America*. Retrieved from https://news.aetna.com/2015/03/mental-health-wellness-corporate-america/

Aetna. (n.d.). *Survey finds Americans' health literacy lacking*. Retrieved from https://news.aetna.com/2015/04/survey-finds-americans-health-literacy-lacking/

Affordable Care Act (ACA). (2015). *Affordable Care Act and Title X Program*. Retrieved from: http://www.hhs.gov/opa/affordable-care-act/index.html

Agarwal, R., & Khuntia, J. (2010). *Personal Health Information and the Design of Consumer Health Information Technology: Background Report*. Prepared by Insight Policy Research under Contract No. HHSA290200710072T for the Agency for Healthcare Research and Quality U.S. Department of Health and Human Services. Retrieved from https://healthit.ahrq.gov/sites/default/files/docs/citation/AHRQ_Personal_Health_InfoFinalReport_FINAL508compliant.pdf

Agency for Health Care Research and Quality (AHRQ). (2011). *Health Literacy Interventions and Outcomes: an Update of the Literacy and Health Outcomes Systematic Review of Literature*. Author.

Agency for Healthcare Research and Quality (AHRQ). (2014). *Voluntary Patient Safety Event Reporting (Incident Reporting)*. Retrieved from: http://psnet.ahrq.gov/primer.aspx?primerID=13

Agency for Healthcare Research and Quality. (2010). *Health Literacy Universal Precautions Toolkit*. Rockville, MD: US Department of Health and Human Services. Retrieved June 10, 2017, from http://www.ahrq.gov/qual/literacy/

Agency for Research and Quality Indicators. (2006). *Patient Safety Indicators*. Retrieved from: https://www.qualityindicators.ahrq.gov/Downloads/Modules/PSI/V30/2006-Feb-PatientSafetyIndicators.pdf

Agency for Research and Quality Indicators. (n.d.a). *Inpatient Quality Indicators Overview*. Retrieved from: www.ualityindicators.ahrq.gov/Modules/iqi_resources.aspx

Agency for Research and Quality Indicators. (n.d.b). *Prevention Quality Indicators Overview*. Retrieved from: www.qualityindicators. ahrq.gov/Modules/pqi_resources.aspx

Ahier, B. (2014). *Healthcare Analytics: Realizing the Value of Health IT*. Retrieved from: https://www.healthcatalyst.com/analytics-realizing-the-value-of-health-it

Ahmed, R., & Bates, B. R. (2016). To accommodate, or not to accommodate: Exploring patient satisfaction with doctors accommodative behaviour during clinical encounter. *Journal of Communication in Healthcare*, *9*(1), 22–32. doi:10.1080/17538068.2015.1126936

Ajzen, I. (1992). *Persuasive communication theory in social psychology: A historical perspective*. Amherst, MA: University of Massachusetts.

Alberti, R. E., & Emmons, M. L. (2008). *Your perfect right: Assertiveness and equality in your life and relationships*. Atascadero, CA: Impact Publishers.

Alrubaiy, L., Hutchings, H. A., & Williams, J. G. (2014). Assessing patient reported outcome measures: A practical guide for gastroenterologists. *United European Gastroenterology Journal*, *2*(6), 463–470. doi:10.1177/2050640614558345 PMID:25452841

Altin, S. V., Finke, I., Kautz-Freimuth, S., & Stock, S. (2014). The evolution of health literacy assessment tools: A systematic review. *BMC Public Health*, *14*(1), 1207. doi:10.1186/1471-2458-14-1207 PMID:25418011

Altin, S., & Stock, S. (2015). Health literate healthcare organizations and their role in future healthcare. *The Journal of Nursing Care*, *4*(2). doi:10.4172/2167-1168.1000238

Ambagtsheer, F., de Jong, J., Bramer, W. M., & Weimar, W. (2016). On Patients Who Purchase Organ Transplants Abroad. *American Journal of Transplantation*, *16*(10), 2800–2815. doi:10.1111/ajt.13766 PMID:26932422

American Academy of Pediatrics, Committee on Bioethics. (1995). Informed consent, parental permission, and assent in pediatric practice. *Pediatrics*, *95*, 314–317. PMID:7838658

American Heritage Dictionary of the English Language. (2012). (4th ed.). Retrieved April 25, 2017 from http://www.wordnik.com/words/tapestry

Ancker, J.S., Senathirajah, Y, Kukafka, R., Starren, B. (2006). Design Features of Graphs in Health Risk Communication: A Systematic Review. *Journal of the American Medical Informatics Association, 13*(6).

Ancker, J. S., & Kaufman, D. (2007). Rethinking health numeracy: A multidisciplinary literature review. *Journal of the American Medical Informatics Association*, *14*(6), 713–721. doi:10.1197/jamia.M2464 PMID:17712082

Andrade, I., Silva, C., & Martins, A. C. (2017). Application of the Health Literacy INDEX on the development of a manual for prevention of falls for older adults. *Patient Education and Counseling, 100*(1), 154–159. doi:10.1016/j.pec.2016.07.036 PMID:27516436

Andreassen, H. K., Bujnowska-Fedak, M. M., Chronaki, C. E., Dumitru, R. C., Pudule, I., Santana, S., ... Wynn, R. (2007). European citizens' use of E-health services: A study of seven countries. *BMC Public Health, 7*(1), 53. doi:10.1186/1471-2458-7-53 PMID:17425798

Andrus, M. R., & Roth, M. T. (2002). Health Literacy: A Review. *Pharmacotherapy, 22*(3), 282–302. doi:10.1592/phco.22.5.282.33191 PMID:11898888

Annarumma, C., Palumbo, R., & Cavallone, M. (2016). Empowering patients by empowering health care organizations: a comparative study. In *Proceedings of 19th Toulon-Verona International Conference*. University of Huelva.

Annarumma, C., & Palumbo, R. (2016). Contextualizing health literacy to health care organizations: Exploratory insights. *Journal of Health Management, 18*(4), 611–624. doi:10.1177/0972063416666348

APA Practice Organization. (2014). *The Health Information Technology For Economic and Clinical Health Act (HITECH Act).* Retrieved from:httptp://www.apapracticecentral.org/advocacy/technology/hitech-act.aspx

Arachne: GreekMythology.com. (2017, July 11). Retrieved from https://www.greekmythology.com/Myths/Mortals/Arachne/arachne.html

Arafat, S. M. Y. (2017a). Abnormal Health Believes with Frequent Presentations: Ethnographic Observation from Primary Care of Bangladesh. *International Journal of Perceptions in Public Health, 1*(2), 85–86.

Arafat, S. M. Y. (2017b). Mental Health Promotion or Public Mental Health: The Time Demanded Area. *Journal of Behavioral Health, 6*(1), 1–3. doi:10.5455/jbh.20161121095655

Arafat, S. M. Y., & Ahmed, S. (2017). Burden of Misconception in Sexual Health Care Setting: A Cross-Sectional Investigation among the Patients Attending a Psychiatric Sex Clinic of Bangladesh. *Psychiatry Journal, 2017*, 4. doi:10.1155/2017/9827083 PMID:28740851

Ardey, R., & Ardey, R. (2015). Patient Perceptions and Expectations From Primary Health-care Providers in India. *Journal of Family Medicine and Primary Care, 4*(1), 53–63. doi:10.4103/2249-4863.152254 PMID:25810990

Arocha, J. F., & Hoffman-Goetz, L. (2008). Improving Internet-based health knowledge through attention to literacy. In A. Kushniruk & E. Borycki (Eds.), *Human, social, and organizational aspects of health information systems* (pp. 331–346). Hershey, PA: IGI Global. doi:10.4018/978-1-59904-792-8.ch020

Asaria, M. (2017) *The economics of health inequality in the English NHS – the long view* (Centre for Health Economics Research Paper 142). University of York.

Atienza, A. A., Zarcadoolas, C., Vaughon, W., Hughes, P., Patel, V., Chou, W. Y. S., & Pritts, J. (2015). Consumer attitudes and perceptions on mHealth Privacy and Security: Findings from a Mixed-Methods Study. *Journal of Health Communication*, 1-7.

Auerbach, A. D., Kripalani, S., Vasilevskis, E. E., Sehgal, N., Lindenauer, P. K., Metlay, J. P., ... Fletcher, G. (2016). Preventability and causes of readmissions in a national cohort of general medicine patients. *JAMA Internal Medicine, 176*(4), 484–493. doi:10.1001/jamainternmed.2015.7863 PMID:26954564

Backes, A. C., & Kuo, G. M. (2012). The association between functional health literacy and patient-reported recall of medications at outpatient pharmacies. *Research in Social & Administrative Pharmacy, 8*(4), 349–354. doi:10.1016/j.sapharm.2011.08.001 PMID:22133649

Bailey, S. C., Brega, A. G., Crutchfield, T. M., Elasy, T., Herr, H., Kaphingst, K., ... Schillinger, D. (2014). Update on health literacy and diabetes. *The Diabetes Educator*, *40*(5), 581–604. doi:10.1177/0145721714540220 PMID:24947871

Bailey, S. C., Fang, G., Annis, I. E., O'Conor, R., Paasche-Orlow, M. K., & Wolf, M. S. (2015). Health literacy and 30-day hospital readmission after acute myocardial infarction. *BMJ Open*, *5*(6), e006975. doi:10.1136/bmjopen-2014-006975 PMID:26068508

Baker, D. W. (2006). The meaning and the measure of health literacy. *Journal of General Internal Medicine*, *21*(8), 878–883. doi:10.1111/j.1525-1497.2006.00540.x PMID:16881951

Baker, D. W., Gazmararian, J. A., Williams, M. V., Scott, T., Parker, R. M., Green, D., ... Peel, J. (2002). Functional health literacy and the risk of hospital admission among Medicare managed care enrollees. *American Journal of Public Health*, *92*(8), 1278–1283. doi:10.2105/AJPH.92.8.1278 PMID:12144984

Baker, D. W., Parker, R. M., Williams, M. V., & Clark, W. S. (1998). Health literacy and the risk of hospital admission. *Journal of General Internal Medicine*, *13*(12), 791–798. doi:10.1046/j.1525-1497.1998.00242.x PMID:9844076

Baker, D. W., Parker, R. M., Williams, M. V., Pitkin, K., Parikh, N., Coates, W., & Imara, M. (1996). The health care experience of patients with low literacy. *Archives of Family Medicine*, *5*(6), 329–334. doi:10.1001/archfami.5.6.329 PMID:8640322

Baker, D. W., Wolf, M. S., Feinglass, J., & Thompson, J. A. (2007). Health literacy and mortality among elderly persons. *Archives of Internal Medicine*, *167*(14), 1503–1509. doi:10.1001/archinte.167.14.1503 PMID:17646604

Bamgboye, E. (2006). End-stage renal disease in sub-saharan Africa. Ethnicity and Disease, 16, S2-5 – S2-9

Bandura, A. (1986). *Social foundations of thought and action: A social cognitive theory*. Englewood Cliffs, NJ: Prentice Hall.

Bandura, A. (1993). Perceived self-efficacy in cognitive development and functioning. *Educational Psychologist*, *28*(2), 117–148. doi:10.120715326985ep2802_3

Bandura, A. (1994). Self-efficacy. In V. S. Ramachaudran (Ed.), *Encyclopedia of Human Behavior* (Vol. 4, pp. 71–81). New York, NY: Academic Press.

Bandura, A. (1999). Social cognitive theory of personality. In L. A. Pervin & O. P. John (Eds.), *Handbook of personality: Theory and research* (pp. 154–196). New York: The Guilford Press.

Bandura, A., Adams, N. E., & Beyer, J. (1977). Cognitive processes mediating behavioral change. *Journal of Personality and Social Psychology*, *35*(3), 125–139. doi:10.1037/0022-3514.35.3.125 PMID:15093

Barnett, S. G., & Kaske, B. (2012). Impact of a health literacy presentation during an introductory pharmacy practice experience. *Currents in Pharmacy Teaching and Learning*, *4*(1), 39–45. doi:10.1016/j.cptl.2011.10.001

Barrio, C., Palinkas, L., Yamada, A. M., Fuentes, D., Criado, V., Garcia, P., & Jeste, D. (2008). Unmet needs for mental health services for Latino older adults: Perspectives from consumers, family members, advocates, and service providers. *Community Mental Health Journal*, *44*(1), 57–74. doi:10.100710597-007-9112-9 PMID:18026876

Basch, E., Dueck, A. C., Rogak, L. J., Minasian, L. M., Kelly, W. K., O'Mara, A. M., ... Schrag, D. (2017). Feasibility assessment of patient reporting of symptomatic adverse events in multicenter cancer clinical trials. *JAMA Oncology*, *3*(8), 1043. doi:10.1001/jamaoncol.2016.6749 PMID:28208174

Bass, P. F., Wilson, J. F., & Griffith, C. H. (2003). A Shortened Instrument for Literacy Screening. *Journal of General Internal Medicine*, *18*(12), 1036–1038. doi:10.1111/j.1525-1497.2003.10651.x PMID:14687263

Batterham, R., Hawkins, M., Collins, P., Buchbinder, R., & Osborne, R. (2016). Health literacy: Applying current concepts to improve health services and reduce health inequalities. *Public Health Journal, 132*, 3–12. doi:10.1016/j.puhe.2016.01.001 PMID:26872738

Becker, L. E., Susal, C., & Morath, C. (2013). Kidney transplantation across HLA and ABO antibody barriers. *Current Opinion in Organ Transplantation, 18*, 445–454. PMID:23838650

Begoray, D. L., Wharf-Higgins, J., & MacDonald, M. (2009). High school health curriculum and health literacy: Canadian student voices. *Global Health Promotion, 16*(4), 35–42. doi:10.1177/1757975909348101 PMID:20028667

Belfast Healthy City. (2014). *Health Literacy workshop Report*. Belfast, Ireland: Author.

Belfast Healthy City. (2017). *Health Literacy Case Studies*. Retrieved June 15, 2017, from http://www.belfasthealthycities.com/health-literacy-case-studies

Bendorf, A., Pusell, B., Kelly, P., & Kerridge, I. (2013). Socioeconomic, demographic and policy comparisons of living and deceased kidney transplantation rates across 53 countries. *Nephrology (Carlton, Vic.), 18*(9), 633–640. doi:10.1111/nep.12101 PMID:23692370

Benson, B. J. (2014). Domain of competence: Interpersonal and communication skills. *Academic Pediatrics, 14*(2S), S55–S65. PMID:24602649

Bentkover, J., & Ph, D. (2012). Executive Master of Healthcare Leadership, Brown University. *Leadership is Central to Healthcare System Reform*. Retrieved from: http://www.beckershospitalreview.com/hospital-management-administration/leadership-is-central-to-healthcare-system-reform.html

Berenson, R., Paulus, R., & Kalman, N. (2012). Medicare's Readmissions-Reduction Program - A Positive Alternative. *The New England Journal of Medicine, 366*(15), 1364–1366. doi:10.1056/NEJMp1201268 PMID:22455754

Bergner, M., Bobbitt, R. A., Carter, W. B., & Gilson, B. S. (1981). The Sickness Impact Profile: Development and final revision of a health status measure. *Medical Care, 19*(8), 787–805. doi:10.1097/00005650-198108000-00001 PMID:7278416

Berkman, N. D., Davis, T. C., & McCormack, L. (2010). Health literacy: What is it? *Journal of Health Communication, 15*(Suppl 2), 9–19.

Berkman, N. D., Davis, T. C., & McCormack, L. (2010). Health literacy: What is it? *Journal of Health Communication, 15*(S2), 9–19. doi:10.1080/10810730.2010.499985 PMID:20845189

Berkman, N. D., Dewalt, D. A., Pignone, M. P., Sheridan, S. L., Lohr, K. N., Lux, L., ... Bonito, A. J. (2004). *Literacy and Health Outcomes: AHRQ Evidence Report Summaries.* Agency for Healthcare Research and Quality.

Berkman, N. D., Sheridan, S. L., Donahue, K. E., Halpern, D. J., & Crotty, K. (2011). Low health literacy and health outcomes: An updated systematic review. *Annals of Internal Medicine, 155*(2), 97–107. doi:10.7326/0003-4819-155-2-201107190-00005 PMID:21768583

Berry, J. (2016). *Does Health Literacy Matter?* Retrieved on 24 May 2017 from https://www.england.nhs.uk/blog/jonathan-berry/

Bickmore, T. W., & Paasche-Orlow, M. K. (2012). The role of information technology in health literacy research. *Journal of Health Communication, 17*(Sup3), 23-29. doi:10.1080/10810730.2012.712626

Bihari, M. (2014*). Mandated Benefits - Understanding Mandated Health Insurance Benefits: Health Benefit Mandates Are Controversial*. Retrieved from: http://healthinsurance.about.com/od/reform/a/mandated_benefits_overview.htm

Bittner, A., Jonietz, A., Bittner, J., Beickert, L., & Harendza, S. (2015). Translating medical documents into plain language enhances communication skills in medical students: A pilot study. *Patient Education and Counseling*, *98*(9), 1137–1141. doi:10.1016/j.pec.2015.05.024 PMID:26095344

Black, J. L., Macinko, J., Dixon, L. B., & Fryer, G. E. Jr. (2010). Neighborhoods and obesity in New York City. *Health & Place*, *16*(3), 489–499. doi:10.1016/j.healthplace.2009.12.007 PMID:20106710

Black, N., Varaganum, M., & Hutchings, A. (2014). *Relationship between patient reported experience (PREMs) and patient reported outcomes (PROMs) in elective surgery. BMJ Quality & Safety.*

Bleach, S. (2005). *Medical Errors: Five Years After the IOM Report. Issue Brief.* Retrieved from: http://www.commonwealthfund.org/usr_doc/830_Bleich_errors.pdf

Bledsoe, C. H., Casterline, J. B., Jonson-Kuhn, J. A., & Haaga, J. G. (1999). *Critical Perspectives on Schooling and Fertility in the Developing World.* Washington, DC: National Academy Press.

Blumenthal, D. (2010). Launching HITECH. *The New England Journal of Medicine*, 362–385. PMID:20042745

Blumer, H. (1969). *Symbolic interactionism: Perspective and method.* Englewood Cliffs, NJ: Prentice-Hall.

Bodenheimer, T., Lorig, K., Holman, H., Grumbach, K. (2002). Patient self-management of chronic disease in primary care. *Journal of the American Medical Association, 288*(19), 2469-2475.

Boston University. (n.d.). *Health Literacy Tool Shed.* Retrieved February 12, 2017, from http://healthliteracy.bu.edu/

Brach, C. (2017). The journey to become a health literate organization: A snapshot of health system improvement. *Studies in Health Technology and Informatics, 240*, 203-237. Retrieved from http://www.ncbi.nlm.nih.gov/pmc/articles/PMC5666686/

Brach, C., Keller, D., Hernandez, L. M., Baur, C., Parker, R., & Dreyer, B. … Schillinger, D. (2012). *Ten Attributes of Health Literate Health Care Organizations.* Washington, DC: National Academy of Sciences. Retrieved April 26, 2017 from http://iom.edu/~/media/Files/Perspectives-Files/2012/ Discussion-Papers/BPH_Ten_HLit_Attributes.pdf

Brach, C., Dreyer, B., & Schillinger, D. (2013). Physicians' role in creating health literate organizations: A call to action. *Journal of Internal Medicine*, *29*(2), 273–275.

Brach, C., Dreyer, B., Schyve, P., Hernandez, L. M., Lemerise, A. J., & Parker, R. (2012). *Attributes of a Health Literate Organization.* Washington, DC: National Academy of Sciences.

Brach, C., Keller, D., Hernandez, L. M., Baur, C., Dreyer, B., & Schyve, P. (2012). *Ten attributes of health literate health care organizations.* Washington, DC: Institute of Medicine of the National Academies.

Brach, C., Keller, D., Hernandez, L. M., Baur, C., Parker, R., Dreyer, B., ... Schillinger, D. (2012). *Ten Attributes of Health Literate Health Care Organizations.* Washington, DC: National Academy of Sciences.

Brazier, J., Usherwood, T., Harper, R., & Thomas, K. (1998). Deriving a preference-based single index from the UK SF-36 Health Survey. *Journal of Clinical Epidemiology*, *51*(11), 1115–1128. doi:10.1016/S0895-4356(98)00103-6 PMID:9817129

Brega, A. G., Barnard, J., Mabachi, N. M., Weiss, B. D., DeWalt, D. A., Brach, C., . . . West, D. R. (2015). *AHRQ Health Literacy Universal Precautions Toolkit* (2nd ed.). AHRQ Publication No. 15-0023-EF. Rockville, MD. Agency for Healthcare Research and Quality.

Brega, A. G., Barnard, J., Mabachi, N. M., Weiss, B. D., DeWalt, D. A., Brach, C., . . . West, D. R. (2015). AHRQ Health Literacy Universal Precautions Toolkit. Prepared by Colorado Health Outcomes Program, University of Colorado Anschutz Medical Campus. AHRQ Publication No. 15-0023-EF. Rockville, MD: Agency for Healthcare Research and Quality.

Britto, M. T., Jimison, H. B., Munafo, J. K., Wissman, J., Rogers, M. L., & Hersh, W. (2009). Usability testing finds problems for novice users of pediatric portals. *Journal of the American Medical Informatics Association*, *16*(5), 660–669. doi:10.1197/jamia.M3154 PMID:19567793

Brown, D. R., & Topcu, M. (2003). Willingness to participate in clinical treatment research among older African Americans and Whites. *The Gerontologist*, *43*(1), 62–72. doi:10.1093/geront/43.1.62 PMID:12604747

Bryman, A. (2012). *Social Research methods*. Oxford, UK: Oxford University Press.

Budiani-Saberi, D. A., & Delmonico, F. L. (2008). Organ trafficking and transplant tourism: A commentary on the global realities. *American Journal of Transplantation*, *8*(5), 925–929. doi:10.1111/j.1600-6143.2008.02200.x PMID:18416734

Buffin, J., Jain, N., Little, R., & Warrens, A. N. (2015). A peer outreach initiative to increase the registration of minorities as organ donors. *Clinical Kidney Journal*. Retrieved on 11 June 2017 from https://www.ncbi.nlm.nih.gov/pmc/articles/PMC4581384/

Burchfield, S., Hua, H., Baral, D., & Rocha, V. (2002b). *A Longitudinal Study of the Effect of Integrated Literacy and Basic Education Programs on the Participation of Women in Social and Economic Development in Nepal*. Washington, DC: United States Agency for International Development Office of Women in Development.

Burchfield, S., Hua, H., Iturry, T. S., & Rocha, V. (2002a). *A Longitudinal Study of the Effect of Integrated Literacy and Basic Education Programs on the Participation of Women in Social and Economic Development in Bolivia*. Washington, DC: United States Agency for International Development Office of Women in Development.

Burnapp, L. (2017). *Organ donation transplantation acceptance, empowerment and choice in living donor kidney transplantation* (Unpublished internal report). NHS Blood & Transplant Advisory and Dissemination Board.

Cajita, M. I., Cajita, T. R., & Han, H.-R. (2016). Health Literacy and Heart Failure: A Systematic Review. *The Journal of Cardiovascular Nursing*, *31*(2), 121–130. doi:10.1097/JCN.0000000000000229 PMID:25569150

Cajita, M. I., Denhaerynck, K., Dobbels, F., Berben, L., Russell, C. L., Davidson, P. M., ... Maddicks-Law, J. (2017). Health literacy in heart transplantation: Prevalence, correlates and associations with health behaviors - findings from the international BRIGHT study. *The Journal of Heart and Lung Transplantation*, *36*(3), 272–279. doi:10.1016/j.healun.2016.08.024 PMID:27773449

Calvert, M., Blazeby, J., Altman, D. G., Revicki, D. A., Moher, D., Brundage, M. D., & CONSORT PRO Group. (2013). Reporting of patient-reported outcomes in randomized trials: The CONSORT PRO extension. *Journal of the American Medical Association*, *309*(8), 814–822. doi:10.1001/jama.2013.879 PMID:23443445

Cameron, I., & McBride, N. (1995). Creating health promoting schools: Lessons from the west Australian school health project. *Health Promotion Journal of Australia*, *5*, 4–10.

Cameron, J. S., & Hoffenberg, R. (1999). The ethics of organ transplantation reconsidered: Paid organ donation and the use of executed prisoners as donors. *Kidney International*, *55*(2), 724–732. doi:10.1046/j.1523-1755.1999.00286.x PMID:9987097

Cammaerts, B. (Ed.). (2003). Beyond the digital divide: reducing exclusion, fostering inclusion. Brussels: University Press.

Cantarovich, F., Heguilen, R., Filho, M. A., Duro-Garcia, V., Fitzgerald, R., Mayrhofer-Reinhartshuber, D., ... Esnault, V. L. M. (2007). An international opinion poll of well-educated people regarding awareness and feelings about organ donation for transplantation. *Transplant International*, *20*(6), 512–518. doi:10.1111/j.1432-2277.2007.00473.x PMID:17355245

Cantrill, S. (2010). Computers in Patient Care: The Promise and the Challenge. *Communications of the ACM*, *53*(9), 42–47. doi:10.1145/1810891.1810907

Caplan, A. L., & Coehlo, O. H. (1998). *The Ethics of Organ Transplantation: The Current Debate*. New York: Prometheus Books.

Carels, R. A., Selensky, J. C., Rossi, J., Solar, C., & Hlavka, R. (2017). A novel stepped-care approach to weight loss: The role of self-monitoring and health literacy in treatment outcomes. *Eating Behaviors*, *26*, 76–82. doi:10.1016/j.eatbeh.2017.01.009 PMID:28189945

Castro, C. M., Wilson, C., Wang, F., & Schillinger, D. (2007). Babel babble: Physicians' use of unclarified medical jargon with patients. *American Journal of Health Behavior*, *31*(Suppl. 1), S85–S95. doi:10.5993/AJHB.31.s1.11 PMID:17931142

Castro-Sánchez, E., Chang, P. W. S., Vila-Candel, R., Escobedo, A. A., & Holmes, A. H. (2016). Health literacy and infectious diseases: Why does it matter? *International Journal of Infectious Diseases*, *43*, 103–110. doi:10.1016/j.ijid.2015.12.019 PMID:26751238

Cegala, D. J. (2003). Patient communication skills training: A review with implications for cancer patients. *Patient Education and Counseling*, *50*(1), 91–94. doi:10.1016/S0738-3991(03)00087-9 PMID:12767592

Cegala, D. J. (2011). An exploration of factors promoting patient participation in Primary Care Medical Interviews. *Health Communication*, *26*(5), 427–436. doi:10.1080/10410236.2011.552482 PMID:21416422

Cella, D., Yount, S., Rothrock, N., Gershon, R., Cook, K., Reeve, B., ... Rose, M. (2007). The Patient-Reported Outcomes Measurement Information System (PROMIS): Progress of an NIH Roadmap cooperative group during its first two years. *Medical Care*, *45*(5Suppl 1), S3–s11. doi:10.1097/01.mlr.0000258615.42478.55 PMID:17443116

Center for Creative Leadership (CCL). (2015). *Nearly 70% of all change efforts fail. We can do better*. Retrieved from: http://www.ccl.org/leadership/landing/leadingContinousChange.aspx

Center for Health Care Strategies Inc. (2013). *What is Health Literacy?* Retrieved from https://www.chcs.org/media/CHCS_Health_Literacy_Fact_Sheets_2013.pdf

Centers for Disease Control and Prevention, Department of Health and Human Safety, National Institute for Occupational Safety and Health. (2008, July). *Exposure to stress: Occupational hazards in hospitals, 2008-136*. Retrieved from www.cdc.gov/niosh/docs/2008-136/pdfs/2008-136.pdf

Centers for Disease Control and Prevention. (2011). *Health communication basics*. Atlanta: Division of Public Affairs (DPA), Office of the Associate Director for Communication (OADC). Retrieved June 10, 2017, from http://www.cdc.gov/healthcommunication/healthbasics/whatishc.html

Centers for Disease Control and Prevention. (2013, November 22). Health Disparities & Inequalities Report. United States. Morbidity & Mortality Weekly Report (MMWR). *Supplement*, *62*(Supplement No. 3), 1–187.

Centers for Disease Control and Prevention. (2016). *Health literacy: Find training*. Retrieved from https://www.cdc.gov/healthliteracy/gettraining.html

Centers for Disease Control and Prevention. (2016). *Heart Disease Fact Sheet*. Retrieved from: https://www.cdc.gov/dhdsp/data_statistics/fact_sheets/docs/fs_heart_disease.pdf

Centers for Medicare and Medicaid Services.gov. (2016). *CMS Quality Strategy Update*. Retrieved from: www.cms.gov/Medicare/Quality-Initiatives-Patient-Assessment-Instruments/QualityInitiativesGenInfo/Downloads/CMS-Quality-Strategy.pdf

Chant, S., Jenkinson, T., Randle, J., & Russell, G. (2002). Communication skills: Some problems in nursing education and practice. *Journal of Clinical Nursing*, *11*(1), 12–21. doi:10.1046/j.1365-2702.2002.00553.x PMID:11845748

Charrow, R. P., & Charrow, V. R. (1979). Making legal language understandable: A psycholinguistic study of jury instructions. *Columbia Law Review*, *79*(7), 1306–1374. doi:10.2307/1121842

Chathoth, P., & Olsen, M. (2002, April-September). Organizational Leadership and Strategy in the Hospitality Industry. *Journal of Services Research*, *2*(1).

Chen, M., & Decary, M. (2017). *A Prototype of Seenso Self-care Hub*. Exhibition at The Canadian Conference on Medical Education 2017 (CCME 2017), Winnipeg, MA.

Chen, M., & Decary, M. (2017). Seenso Health – Medical Search Made Easier and Better, in Privacy. Medical Search Engine Exhibited at Consumer Electronics Show 2017 (CES 2017), Las Vegas, NV.

Chinn, D. (2011). Critical health literacy: A review and critical analysis. *Social Science & Medicine*, *73*(1), 60–67. doi:10.1016/j.socscimed.2011.04.004 PMID:21640456

Chronaki, C.E., Kouroubali, A., Esterle, L., Orphanoudaki, E., Roumeliotaki, T., Stathopoulou, A., & Tsiknakis, M. (2006). eHealth consumer trends survey in Greece: Results of the 1st phase. *FORTH-ICS TR-365*.

Clinicaltrials.gov. (2017). *Trends, Charts, and Maps*. Retrieved from https://www.clinicaltrials.gov/ct2/resources/trends

Clochesy, J. M. (2015). Wait, won't! Want: Barriers to health care as perceived by medically and socially disenfranchised communities. *Journal of Health and Human Services Administration*, *38*(2), 174–214. PMID:26442361

Cluss, P., Lorigan, D., Kinsky, S., Nikolajski, C., McDermott, A., & Bhat, K. B. (2016). School-Based Health Promotion Initiative Increases Children's Physical Activity. *American Journal of Health Education*, *47*(6), 343–354. doi:10.1080/19325037.2016.1219287

Cobley, P., & Schulz, P. J. (2013). *Theories and models of communication. Handbook of Communication Science* (Vol. 1). De Gruyer Mouton. doi:10.1515/9783110240450

Coeira, E., & Ong, M.-S. (2014). Systemwide communication. In L. R. Martin & M. R. DiMatteo (Eds.), *The Oxford handbook of health communication, behavior change, and treatment adherence* (pp. 155–176). Oxford, UK: Oxford University Press.

Coleman, C., Kurtz-Rossi, S., McKinney, J., Pleasant, A., Rootman, I., & Shohet, L. (2008). *The Calgary Charter on health literacy: Rationale and core principles for the development of health literacy curricula*. Retrieved from http://www.centreforliteracy.qc.ca/sites/default/files/CFL_Calgary_Charter_2011.pdf

Collins, S. R., Rasmussen, P. W., Doty, M. M., & Beutel, S. (2014). *Too High a Price: Out-of-Pocket Health Care Costs in the United States. Commonwealth Fund*. Retrieved from http://www.commonwealthfund.org/publications/issue-briefs/2014/nov/out-of-pocket-health-care-costs

Consumer Health Informatics Research resource. (2012). *Variable: Self efficacy*. Retrieved from http://chirr.nlm.nih.gov/self-efficacy.php

Contopoulos-Ioannidis, D. G., Karvouni, A., Kouri, I., & Ioannidis, J. P. A. (2009). Reporting and interpretation of SF-36 outcomes in randomised trials: Systematic review. *BMJ (Clinical Research Ed.)*, *338*(jan12 1), a3006. doi:10.1136/bmj.a3006 PMID:19139138

Cookson, R., Propper, C., Asaria, M., & Raine, R. (2016). *Socioeconomic inequalities in health care in England* (Centre for Health Economics Research Paper 129). University of York.

Copeland, W. (n.d.). *Electronic Data Interchange: Concepts and Effects.* Retrieved from: https://www.isoc.org/inet97/proceedings/C5/C5_1.HTM

Corbie-Smith, G., Thomas, S. B., Williams, M. V., & Moody-Ayers, S. (1999). Attitudes and beliefs of African Americans toward participation in medical research. *Journal of General Internal Medicine*, *14*(9), 537–546. doi:10.1046/j.1525-1497.1999.07048.x PMID:10491242

Corbin, C. B., McConnell, K., Le Masurier, G., Corbin, D., & Farrar, T. (2014). *Health opportunities through physical education.* Springfield, IL: Human Kinetics.

Cosmides, L., & Tooby, J. (1996). Are humans good intuitive statisticians after all? Rethinking some conclusions from the literature on judgment under uncertainty. *Cognition*, *58*(1), 1–73. doi:10.1016/0010-0277(95)00664-8

Coulombe, S. Tremblay, J., & Marchand, S. (2004). *Literacy scores, human capital and growth across fourteen OECD countries.* Statistics Canada Catalogue number 89-552-MIE200411.

Coulter, A., & Ellins, J. (2007). Effectiveness of strategies for informing, educating, and involving patients. *BMJ (Clinical Research Ed.)*, *335*(7609), 24–27. doi:10.1136/bmj.39246.581169.80 PMID:17615222

Council of Europe and United Nations. (2009). *Trafficking in Organs, Tissues and Cells and Trafficking in Human Beings for the Purpose of the Removal of Organs, Joint Council of Europe/United Nations Study.* Retrieved from http://ec.europa.eu/anti-trafficking/sites/antitrafficking/files/council-un_study_on_trafficking_in_organs_2009_en_1.pdf

Cronbach, L. J., & Meehl, P. E. (1955). Construct validity in psychological tests. *Psychological Bulletin*, *52*(4), 281–302. doi:10.1037/h0040957 PMID:13245896

Crouch, R. A., & Elliott, C. (1999). Moral agency and the family: The case of living related organ transplantation. *Cambridge Quarterly of Healthcare Ethics*, *8*(3), 275–287. doi:10.1017/S096318019980303X PMID:10388928

Curtis, J., Cheng, S., Rose, K., & Tsai, O. (2011). Promoting adoption, usability and research for personal health records in Canada: The MyChart experience. *Health Management Forum*, *24*(3), 149–154. doi:10.1016/j.hcmf.2011.07.004 PMID:22165576

D'Cruz, A. M., & Aradhya, M. R. S. (2013). Health literacy among Indian adults seeking dental care. *Dental Research Journal*, *10*(1), 20–24. PMID:23878559

Dageforde, L., & Cavanaugh, K. (2013). Health Literacy: Emerging Evidence and Applications in Kidney Disease Care. *Advances in Chronic Kidney Disease*, *20*(4), 311-319.

Dalal, A. R. (2015). Philosophy of organ donation: Review of ethical facets. *World Journal of Transplantation*, *5*(2), 44–51. doi:10.5500/wjt.v5.i2.44 PMID:26131406

Danovitch, G. M., Chapman, J., Capron, A. M., Levin, A., Abbud-Filho, M., Al Mousawi, M., ... Delmonico, F. L. (2013). Organ trafficking and transplant tourism: The role of global professional ethical standards-the 2008 Declaration of Istanbul. *Transplantation*, *95*(11), 1306–1312. doi:10.1097/TP.0b013e318295ee7d PMID:23644753

Davison, A., Kantor, R. N., Hannah, J., Herman, G., Lutz, R., & Salzillo, R. (1980). *Limitations of Readability Formulas in Guiding Adaptations of Texts. Technical Report (No. 162)*. Champaign, IL: Center for the Study of Reading.

Davis, T. C., Berkel, H. J., Holcombe, R. F., Pramanik, S., & Divers, S. G. (1998). Informed consent for clinical trials: A comparative study of standard versus simplified forms. *Journal of the National Cancer Institute*, *90*(9), 668–674. doi:10.1093/jnci/90.9.668 PMID:9586663

Davis, T., Crouch, M., Wills, G., Miller, S., & Abdehou, D. (1990). Gap between patient reading comprehension and the readability of patient education materials. *The Journal of Family Practice*, *31*(5), 533–538. PMID:2230677

Davis, T., Williams, M., Marin, E., Parker, R., & Glass, J. (2002). Health literacy And cancer communication. *CA: a Cancer Journal for Clinicians*, *52*(3), 134–149. doi:10.3322/canjclin.52.3.134 PMID:12018928

de Greeff, J. W., Hartman, E., Mullender-Wijnsma, M. J., Bosker, R. J., Doolaard, S., & Visscher, C. (2016). Effect of Physically Active Academic Lessons on Body Mass Index and Physical Fitness in Primary School Children. *The Journal of School Health*, *86*(5), 346–352. doi:10.1111/josh.12384 PMID:27040472

De Leeuw, E. (2009). Evidence for Healthy Cities: reflections on practice, method and theory. *Health Promotion International, 24*(suppl 1), i19–i36.

de Vet, H. C., Foumani, M., Scholten, M. A., Jacobs, W. C., Stiggelbout, A. M., Knol, D. L., & Peul, W. C. (2015). Minimally important change values of a measurement instrument depend more on baseline values than on the type of intervention. *Journal of Clinical Epidemiology*, *68*(5), 518–524. doi:10.1016/j.jclinepi.2014.07.008 PMID:25544741

Delmonico, F. (2005). A report of the Amsterdam Forum on the Care of the Live Kidney Donor: Data and medical guidelines. *Transplantation*, *79*, S53–S66. doi:10.1097/01.TP.0000157343.27949.9F PMID:15785361

Delmonico, F. L. (2008a). The declaration of Istanbul on organ trafficking and transplant tourism. *Indian Journal of Nephrology*, *18*(3), 135–140. PMID:20142924

Delmonico, F. L. (2008b). The development of the Declaration of Istanbul on Organ Trafficking and Transplant Tourism. *Nephrology, Dialysis, Transplantation*, *23*(11), 3381–3382. doi:10.1093/ndt/gfn552 PMID:18922862

Delmonico, F. L., Arnold, R., Scheper-Hughes, N., Siminoff, L. A., Kahn, J., & Youngner, S. J. (2002). Ethical incentives--not payment--for organ donation. *The New England Journal of Medicine*, *346*(25), 2002–2005. doi:10.1056/NEJMsb013216 PMID:12075064

Delmonico, F. L., & Harmon, W. E. (2002). The use of a minor as a live kidney donor. *American Journal of Transplantation*, *2*(4), 333–336. doi:10.1034/j.1600-6143.2002.20407.x PMID:12118854

Demian, M., Shapiro, R., & Thornton, W. (2016). An observational study of health literacy and medication adherence in adult kidney transplant recipients. *Clinical Kidney Journal*, *9*(6), 858–865. doi:10.1093/ckjfw076 PMID:27994867

Demissie, Z., & Brener, N. (2017). Demographic Differences in District-Level Policies Related to School Mental Health and Social Services-United States, 2012. *The Journal of School Health*, *87*(4), 227–235. doi:10.1111/josh.12489 PMID:28260247

Den Oudsten, B. L., Zijlstra, W. P., & De Vries, J. (2013). The minimal clinical important difference in the World Health Organization Quality of Life instrument--100. *Supportive Care in Cancer*, *21*(5), 1295–1301. doi:10.100700520-012-1664-8 PMID:23203652

Department of Community and Family Medicine. (2014). *What is Quality Improvement? How Do You Define Quality?* Retrieved from: http://patientsafetyed.duhs.duke.edu/module_a/introduction/define_quality.html

Department of Health and Human Services. (1998). *Informed consent checklist (1998)*. Retrieved from https://www.hhs.gov/ohrp/regulations-and-policy/guidance/checklists/index.html

Department of Health. (2017). *Making Life Better - Strategic Framework for Public Health*. Retrieved June 15, 2017, from https://www.health-ni.gov.uk/articles/making-life-better-strategic-framework-public-health

Department of Managed Health Care (DMHC). (2015). *DMHC regulates Health Plans and Helps health plan members and providers*. Retrieved from: http://www.dmhc.ca.gov

Desta, M., Deyessa, N., Fish, I., Maxwell, B., Zerihun, T., Levine, S., … Garland, A. F. (2017). *Teachers to Identify Mental Health Problems : A Task-Sharing Intervention in Ethiopia*. Academic Press.

DeWalt, D. A., & Hink, A. (2009). Health Literacy and Child Health Outcomes: A Systematic Review of the Literature. *Pediatrics*, *124*(Supplement), S265–S274. doi:10.1542/peds.2009-1162B PMID:19861480

DeWalt, D. A., & McNeill, J. (2013). *Integrating health literacy with health care performance measurement*. Washington, DC: Institute of Medicine.

Dickens, C., Lambert, B., Cromwell, T., & Piano, M. (2013). Nurse overestimation of patients' health literacy. *Journal of Health Communication*, *18*(sup1), 62–69. doi:10.1080/10810730.2013.825670 PMID:24093346

Dickson-Swift, V., Kenny, A., Farmer, J., Gussy, M., & Larkins, S. (2014). Measuring oral health literacy: A scoping review of existing tools. *BMC Oral Health*, *14*(148), 13. PMID:25472659

Diemer, F. S., Haan, Y. C., Nannan Panday, R. V., van Montfrans, G. A., Oehlers, G. P., & Brewster, L. M. (2017). Health literacy in Suriname. *Social Work in Health Care*, *56*(4), 283–293. doi:10.1080/00981389.2016.1277823 PMID:28271964

DiMatteo, M. R., Prince, L. M., & Taranta, A. (1979). Patients' perceptions of physicians' behavior: Determinants of patient commitment to the therapeutic relationship. *Journal of Community Health*, *4*, 280–290. PMID:469038

Dişsiz, G., & Yilmaz, M. (2016). Complementary and alternative therapies and health literacy in cancer patients. *Complementary Therapies in Clinical Practice*, *23*, 34–39. doi:10.1016/j.ctcp.2016.02.004 PMID:27157956

Diviani, N., van den Putte, B., Meppelink, C. S., & van Weert, J. C. M. (2016). Exploring the role of health literacy in the evaluation of online health information: Insights from a mixed-methods study. *Patient Education and Counseling*, *99*(6), 1017–1025. doi:10.1016/j.pec.2016.01.007 PMID:26817407

Doak, L., & Doak, C. (2002). *Pfizer Health Literacy Principles*. New York, NY: Pfizer, Inc.

Dodson, S., Good, S., & Osborne, R. (2015). *Health literacy toolkit for low and of middle-income countries: a series of information sheets to empower communities and strenghten health systems*. New Delhi.

Domínguez-Gil, B., Haase-Kromwijk, B., Van Leiden, H., Neuberger, J., Coene, L., Morel, P., ... Matesanz, R. (2011). Current situation of donation after circulatory death in european countries. *Transplant International*, *24*(7), 676–686. doi:10.1111/j.1432-2277.2011.01257.x PMID:21504489

Donovan, J. L., Hamdy, F. C., Lane, J. A., Mason, M., Metcalfe, C., Walsh, E., ... Neal, D. E. (2016). Patient-Reported Outcomes after Monitoring, Surgery, or Radiotherapy for Prostate Cancer. *The New England Journal of Medicine*, *375*(15), 1425–1437. doi:10.1056/NEJMoa1606221 PMID:27626365

Dorland's. (2014). *Dorland's medical dictionary*. Retrieved June 10, 2017, from https://www.dorlands.com/

Dowell, J., Jones, A., & Snadden, D. (2002). Exploring medication use to seek concordance with 'non-adherent' patients: A qualitative study. *The British Journal of General Practice*, *52*, 24–32. PMID:11791812

Drake, M., Bernard, A., & Hessel, E. (2017). Brain death. *The Surgical Clinics of North America, 97*(6), 1255–1273. doi:10.1016/j.suc.2017.07.001 PMID:29132508

Drapeau, V., Savard, B. A., Gallant, A., Nadeau, L., & Gagnon, J. (2016). The Effectiveness of A School-Based Nutrition Intervention on Children's Fruit, Vegetables, and Dairy Product Intake. *The Journal of School Health, 86*(5), 353–362. doi:10.1111/josh.12385 PMID:27040473

Dresser, M., Short, L., Wedemeyer, L., Bredow, V. L., Sacks, R., Larson, K., & Silver, L. D. (2012). Public Health Detailing of Primary Care Providers: New York City's Experience, 2003–2010. *American Journal of Public Health, 102*(S3), S342–S352. doi:10.2105/AJPH.2011.300622 PMID:22690970

Duffy, T. M., & Kabance, P. (1982). Testing a readable writing approach to text revision. *Journal of Educational Psychology, 74*(5), 533–548. doi:10.1037/0022-0663.74.5.733

Dunne, T., Bishop, L., Avery, S., & Darcy, S. (2016). A Review of Effective Youth Engagement Strategies for Mental Health and Substance Use Interventions. *The Journal of Adolescent Health, 60*(5), 487–512. doi:10.1016/j.jadohealth.2016.11.019 PMID:28087268

Duong, T. V., Aringazina, A., Baisunova, G., Nurjanah, Pham, T. V., Pham, K. M., ... Chang, P. W. (2017). Measuring health literacy in Asia: Validation of the HLS-EU-Q47 survey tool in six Asian countries. *Journal of Epidemiology, 27*(2), 80–86. doi:10.1016/j.je.2016.09.005 PMID:28142016

Durant, R. W., Wenzel, J. A., Scarinci, I. C., Paterniti, D. A., Fouad, M. N., Hurd, T. C., & Martin, M. Y. (2014). Perspectives on barriers and facilitators to minority recruitment for clinical trials among cancer center leaders, investigators, research staff, and referring clinicians: Enhancing minority participation in clinical trials EMPaCT). *Cancer, 120*(S7), 1097–1105. doi:10.1002/cncr.28574 PMID:24643647

Ebright, P. R., Urden, L., Patterson, E., & Chalko, B. (2004). Themes surrounding novice nurse near-miss and adverse-event situations. *The Journal of Nursing Administration, 34*(11), 531–538. doi:10.1097/00005110-200411000-00010 PMID:15586075

Eckman, M. H., Wise, R., Leonard, A. C., Dixon, E., Burrows, C., Khan, F., & Warm, E. (2012). Impact of health literacy on outcomes and effectiveness of an educational intervention in patients with chronic diseases. *Patient Education and Counseling, 87*(2), 143–151. doi:10.1016/j.pec.2011.07.020 PMID:21925823

Eggers, P. W. (1998). Effect of transplantation on the Medicare End Stage Renal Disease Program. *The New England Journal of Medicine, 38*, 223–229. PMID:3275896

Eichler, K., Wieser, S., & Brügger, U. (2009). The costs of limited health literacy: A systematic review. *International Journal of Public Health, 54*(5), 313–324. doi:10.100700038-009-0058-2 PMID:19644651

Eisenberg, A. (1992). Doctor-patient eye contact. *Dynamic Chiropractic, 10*(1). Retrieved June 10, 2017, from http://www.dynamicchiropractic.com/mpacms/dc/article.php?id=43000

Elbert, N. J., Os-Medendorp, H. V., Renselaar, W. V., Ekeland, A. G., Roijen, L. H., Raat, H., ... Pasmans, S. G. (2014). Effectiveness and cost-effectiveness of eHealth interventions in somatic diseases: A systematic review of systematic reviews and meta-analyses. *Journal of Medical Internet Research, 16*(4), e110. doi:10.2196/jmir.2790 PMID:24739471

Elbina, R., Kawasaki, F., Taniguchi, I., Togari, T., Yamasaki, Y., & Sparks, M. (2010). The effectiveness of Health Communication strategies in health education in Kushima, Japan. *Global Health Promotion, 17*(1), 5–15. doi:10.1177/1757975909356628 PMID:20357347

Elliott, C. (1995). Doing harm: Living organ donors, clinical research and The Tenth Man. *Journal of Medical Ethics, 21*(2), 91–96. doi:10.1136/jme.21.2.91 PMID:7608947

Ellison, M. D., McBride, M. A., Taranto, S. E., Delmonico, F. L., & Kauffman, H. M. (2002). Living kidney donors in need of kidney transplants: A report from the organ procurement and transplantation network. *Transplantation, 74*(9), 1349–1351. doi:10.1097/00007890-200211150-00025 PMID:12451277

Eng, T., Maxfield, A., Patrick, K., Deering, M. J., Ratzan, S. C., & Gustafson, D. H. (1998). Access to health information and support: A public highway or private road? *Journal of the American Medical Association, 280*(15), 1371–1375. doi:10.1001/jama.280.15.1371 PMID:9794322

Epstein, R. M., & Street, R. L., Jr. (2007). Patient-Centered Communication in Cancer Care: Promoting Healing and Reducing Suffering. National Cancer Institute, NIH Publication No. 07-6225.

Epstein, R. M., Fiscella, K., Lesser, C., & Stange, K. C. (2010). *Why the nation needs a policy push on patient-centered health care.* Retrieved on 11 June 2017 from http://content.healthaffairs.org/content/29/8/1489.short

Epstein, R. M., Alper, B. S., & Quill, T. E. (2004). Communicating evidence for participatory decision making. *Journal of the American Medical Association, 291*(19), 2359–2366. doi:10.1001/jama.291.19.2359 PMID:15150208

Epstein, R. M., & Street, R. L. Jr. (2011). The values and value of patient-centered care. *Annals of Family Medicine, 9*(2), 100–103. doi:10.1370/afm.1239 PMID:21403134

E-Source. (n.d.). *Behavioral and Social Science Research. Evaluating the Quality of Health Care.* Retrieved from: www.esourceresearch.org/Portals/0/Uploads/Documents/Public/Cleary_FullChapter.pdf

Espanha, R., Ávila, P., & Mendes, R. M. (2016). *A literacia em saúde em Portugal.* Lisboa: Fundação Calouste Gulbenkian.

Essman, C., & Thornton, J. (2006). Assessing medical student knowledge, attitudes, and behaviors regarding organ donation. *Transplantation Proceedings, 38*(9), 2745–2750. doi:10.1016/j.transproceed.2006.08.127 PMID:17112821

European Health Forum Gastein. (2005). *Gastein health declaration 2005.* Partnerships for Health. Retrieved from June 10, 2017, http://www.ehfg.org/

European Union. (2007). *Final Report Summary - IROHLA (Intervention Research on Health Literacy among Ageing population).* Retrieved from http://cordis.europa.eu/result/rcn/184975_en.html

European Union. (2014). *Journalist Workshop on Organ donation and transplantation.* Retrieved 24/06/17 from https://ec.europa.eu/health//sites/health/files/blood_tissues_organs/docs/ev_20141126_factsfigures_en.pdf

EuroQol-Group. (1990). EuroQol--a new facility for the measurement of health-related quality of life. *Health Policy (Amsterdam), 16*(3), 199–208. doi:10.1016/0168-8510(90)90421-9

Faber, M., Bosch, M., Wollersheim, H., Leatherman, S., & Grol, R. (2009). Public reporting in health care: How do consumers use quality-of-care information? A systematic review. *Medical Care, 47*(1), 1–8. doi:10.1097/MLR.0b013e3181808bb5 PMID:19106724

Faddoul, B. (2017). Gamification and health literacy. In I. Management Association (Ed.), Medical education and ethics: Concepts, methodologies, tools, and applications (pp. 51–62). Hershey, PA: IGI Global. doi:10.4018/978-1-5225-0978-3.ch003

Faden, R. R., & Beauchamp, T. L. (1986). *A history and theory of informed consent.* New York: Oxford University Press.

Fehrman-Ekuholm, I., Brink, B., Ericsson, C., Elinder, C. G., Dunér, F., & Lundgren, G. (2000). Kidney donors don't regret: Follow-up of 370 donors in Stockholm since 1964. *Transplantation, 69*, 2067–2071. PMID:10852598

Fellner, C. H., & Marshall, J. R. (1968). Twelve kidney donors. *Journal of the American Medical Association, 206*(12), 2703–2707. doi:10.1001/jama.1968.03150120037007 PMID:4880430

Fellner, C. H., & Marshall, J. R. (1970). Kidney donors: The myth of informed consent. *The American Journal of Psychiatry, 126*(9), 1245–1251. doi:10.1176/ajp.126.9.1245 PMID:4905016

Ferrari, P., Weimar, W., Johnson, R. J., Lim, W. H., & Tinckam, K. J. (2015). Kidney paired donation: Principles, protocols and programs. *Nephrology, Dialysis, Transplantation, 30*(8), 1276–1285. doi:10.1093/ndt/gfu309 PMID:25294848

Ford, J. G., Howerton, M. W., Lai, G. Y., Gary, T. L., Bolen, S., Gibbons, M. C., ... Bass, E. B. (2008). Barriers to recruiting underrepresented populations to cancer clinical trials: A systematic review. *Cancer, 112*(2), 228–242. doi:10.1002/cncr.23157 PMID:18008363

Fouad, M. N., Partridge, E., Green, B. L., Kohler, C., Wynn, T., Nagy, S., & Churchill, S. (2000). Minority recruitment in clinical trials: A conference at Tuskegee, researchers and the community. *Annals of Epidemiology, 10*(8), S35–S40. doi:10.1016/S1047-2797(00)00199-X PMID:11189091

Frampton, S., Guastello, S., Brady, C., Hale, M., Horowitz, S., Smith, S. B., & Stone, S. (2008). *The Patient-Centered Care Improvement Guide*. Derby, CT: The Planetree Association and The Picker Institute.

Fransen, M. P., von Wagner, C., & Essink-Bot, M. L. (2012). Diabetes self-management in patients with low health literacy: Ordering findings from literature in a health literacy framework. *Patient Education and Counseling, 88*(1), 44–53. doi:10.1016/j.pec.2011.11.015 PMID:22196986

Freedman, D. A., Bess, K., Tucker, H., Boyd, D., Tuchman, A., & Wallston, K. (2009). Public Health Literacy Defined. *American Journal of Preventive Medicine, 36*(5), 446–451. doi:10.1016/j.amepre.2009.02.001 PMID:19362698

Freid, V.M., Bernstein, A.B., & Bush, M.A. (2012 July). Multiple chronic conditions among adults aged 45 and over: trends over the past 10 years. *National Center for Health Statistics Data Brief, Number 100*, 1-8.

Freimuth, V. S., & Quinn, S. C. (2004). The contributions of health communication to eliminating health disparities. *American Journal of Public Health, 94*(12), 2053–2055. doi:10.2105/AJPH.94.12.2053 PMID:15569949

Fremgmen, B. (2010). *Medical Law and Ethics Prentice* (3rd ed.). Upper Saddle River, NJ: Prentice Hall.

Frömel, K., Svozil, Z., Chmelík, F., Jakubec, L., & Groffik, D. (2016). The Role of Physical Education Lessons and Recesses in School Lifestyle of Adolescents. *The Journal of School Health, 86*(2), 143–151. doi:10.1111/josh.12362 PMID:26762826

Frosch, D. L., Kaplan, R. M., & Felitti, V. J. (2003). A randomized controlled trial comparing Internet and video to facilitate patient education for men considering the prostate-specific antigen test. *Journal of General Internal Medicine, 18*(10), 781–787. doi:10.1046/j.1525-1497.2003.20911.x PMID:14521639

Furlong, W., Feeny, D., Torrance, G., & Barr, R. T. (2001). *The Health Utilities Index (HUI) System for Assessing Health-Related Quality of Life in Clinical Studies*. Academic Press.

Gabolde, M., Herve, C., & Moulin, A. M. (2001). Evaluation, selection, and follow-up of live kidney donors: A review of current practice in French renal transplant centers. *Nephrology, Dialysis, Transplantation, 16*(10), 2048–2052. doi:10.1093/ndt/16.10.2048 PMID:11572895

Galesic, M., Garcia-Retamero, R., & Gigerenzer, G. (2009). Using icon arrays to communicate medical risks: Overcoming low numeracy. *Health Psychology, 28*(2), 210–216. doi:10.1037/a0014474 PMID:19290713

Garcia-Retamero, R., & Galesic, M. (2010). Who profits from visual aids: Overcoming challenges in people's understanding of risks. *Social Science & Medicine*, *70*(7), 1019–1025. doi:10.1016/j.socscimed.2009.11.031 PMID:20116159

Gazmararian, J. A. (1999). Health literacy among Medicare enrollees in a managed care organization. *Journal of the American Medical Association*, *281*(6), 545–551. doi:10.1001/jama.281.6.545 PMID:10022111

Gazmararian, J. A., Williams, M. V., Peel, J., & Baker, D. W. (2002). Health literacy and knowledge of chronic disease. *Patient Education and Counseling*, *51*(3), 267–275. doi:10.1016/S0738-3991(02)00239-2 PMID:14630383

Gerteis, M., Edgman-Levitan, S., Daley, J., & Delblanco, T. L. (Eds.). (1993). *Through the patient's eyes. Understanding and promoting patient-centered care*. San Francisco, CA: Jossey-Bass.

Gevers, S., Janssen, A., & Friele, R. (2004). Consent systems for post mortem organ donation in europe. *European Journal of Health Law*, *11*(2), 175–186. doi:10.1163/1571809041457422 PMID:15387424

Ghanbari, S., Ramezankhani, A., Montazeri, A., & Mehrabi, Y. (2016). Health Literacy Measure for Adolescents (HELMA): Development and Psychometric Properties. *PLoS One*, *11*(2), e0149202. doi:10.1371/journal.pone.0149202 PMID:26881933

Ghods, A. J., & Nasrollahzadeh, D. (2005). Transplant tourism and the Iranian model of renal transplantation program: Ethical considerations. *Experimental and Clinical Transplantation*, *3*, 351. PMID:16417442

Gibbons, M. C. (2005). A historical overview of health disparities and the potential of eHealth solutions. *Journal of Medical Internet Research*, *7*(5), e50. doi:10.2196/jmir.7.5.e50 PMID:16403714

Gill, J. S., Delmonico, F. L., Klarenbach, S., & Capron, A. M. (2017). Providing coverage for the unique life-long health care needs of living kidney donors within the framework of financial neutrality. *American Journal of Transplantation*, *17*(5), 1176–1181. doi:10.1111/ajt.14147 PMID:27888569

Gkiourda, C. (2017). Αντιμετωπίζοντας τις χρόνιες παθήσεις στο φαρμακείο [Facing chronic diseases in the pharmacy]. Retrieved from http://www.y-o.gr/επικαιρότητα/634-αντιμετωπίζοντας-τις-χρόνιες-παθήσεις-στο-φαρμακείο

Glazier, A. K., Danovitch, G. M., & Delmonico, F. L. (2014). Organ transplantation for nonresidents of the United States: A policy for transparency. *American Journal of Transplantation*, *14*(8), 1740–1743. doi:10.1111/ajt.12770 PMID:24840545

Goguen, J. (2016). Health literacy and patient preparation in radiology. *Journal of Medical Imaging and Radiation Sciences*, *47*(3), 283–286. doi:10.1016/j.jmir.2016.06.002

Golbeck, A., Ahlers-Schmidt, C., Paschal, A., & Dismuke, S. (2005). A definition and operational framework for health numeracy. *American Journal of Preventative Medicine, 29*(4), 375-376. doi: .10.1016/j.amepre.2005.06.012

Gordon, E.J., & Wolf, M.S. (2009). Health literacy skills of kidney transplant recipients. *Progress in Transplantation, 19*(1), 25-34.

Gordon, C., Purciel-Hill, M., Ghai, N. R., Kaufman, L., Graham, R., & Van Wey, G. (2011). Measuring food deserts in New York City's low-income neighborhoods. *Health & Place*, *17*(2), 696–700. doi:10.1016/j.healthplace.2010.12.012 PMID:21256070

Gordon, E. J., & Wolf, M. S. (2009). Health literacy skills of kidney transplant recipients. *Progress in Transplantation (Aliso Viejo, Calif.)*, *19*(1), 25–34. doi:10.1177/152692480901900104 PMID:19341060

Gray, N. J., Klein, J. D., Noyce, P. R., Sesselberg, T. S., & Cantrill, J. A. (2005). The Internet: A window on adolescent health literacy. *The Journal of Adolescent Health*, *37*(3), 243.e1–243.e7. doi:10.1016/j.jadohealth.2004.08.023 PMID:16109345

Green, G., Jackisch, J., & Zamaro, G. (n.d.). *Healthy cities as catalysts for caring and supportive environments and 3 Friuli Venezia Giulia*. Regional Health Trust for Purchasing and Shared Services. 10.1093/heapro/dav037

Greenhalgh, T., & Heath, I. (2010). *Measuring quality in the therapeutic relationship: An inquiry into the quality of general practice in England*. London: The King's Fund.

Gregory, A. (2008). Competencies of senior communication practitioners in the UK: An initial study. *Public Relations Review*, *34*(3), 215–223. doi:10.1016/j.pubrev.2008.04.005

Gridelli, B., & Remuzzi, G. (2000). Strategies for making more organs available for transplantation. *The New England Journal of Medicine*, *343*(6), 404–410. doi:10.1056/NEJM200008103430606 PMID:10933740

Groene, O., & Rudd, R. E. (2011). Results of a feasibility study to assess the health literacy environment: Navigation, written and oral communication in ten hospitals in Catalonia, Spain. *Journal of Communication in Healthcare*, *4*(4), 227–237. doi:10.1179/1753807611Y.0000000005

Gruman, J. (2014). *Self-Monitoring Health IT Falls Short of Providing the Information We Need*. Available from: http://www.cfah.org/blog/2014/self-monitoring-health-it-falls-short-of-providing-the-information-we-need

Gunby, P. (1983). Media-abetted liver transplants raise questions of "equity and decency". *Journal of the American Medical Association*, *249*(15), 1973–1974. doi:10.1001/jama.249.15.1973 PMID:6339755

Hagell, A., Rigby, E., & Perrow, F. (2015). Promoting health literacy in secondary schools: A review. *British Journal of School Nursing*, *10*(2), 82–87. doi:10.12968/bjsn.2015.10.2.82

Haj, H., Lamrini, M., & Rais, N. (2013). Quality of Care Between Donabedian Model and ISO9001V2008. *International Journal of Quality Research*, *7*(1), 17–30.

Hall, S. (1973). *Encoding and decoding in the media discourse. Stencilled Paper 7*. Birmingham: CCCS.

Hall, S. (1980). Encoding/decoding. In D. Hobson, A. Lowe, & P. Willis (Eds.), *Culture, Media, Language* (pp. 128–138). London: Hutchinson.

Hall, S. (1996). Cultural studies and its theoretical legacies. In *D. Morley & K.-H. Chen, Critical dialogues in cultural studies* (pp. 261–274). London, New York: Routledge.

Halm, E. A., Mora, P., & Leventhal, H. (2006). No symptoms, no asthma: The acute episodic disease belief is associated with poor self-management among inner-city adults with persistent asthma. *Chest*, *129*(3), 573–580. doi:10.1378/chest.129.3.573 PMID:16537854

Hamburger, J., & Crosnier, J. (1968). Moral and ethical problems in transplantation. In F. Rapaport & J. Daussert (Eds.), *Human transplantation*. New York: Grunn and Stratton.

Hanson-Divers, E. C. (1997). Developing a medical achievement reading test to evaluate patient literacy skills: A preliminary study. *Journal of Health Care for the Poor and Underserved*, *8*(1), 56–69. doi:10.1353/hpu.2010.0304 PMID:9019026

Harbaugh, C., Afana, M., Burdick, S., East, J., Kodali, S., Lee, J., ... Mathur, A. K. (2011). Portrayal of organ donation and transplantation on american primetime television. *Clinical Transplantation*, *25*(4), 375–380. doi:10.1111/j.1399-0012.2011.01427.x PMID:21410759

Hargie, O., & Dickson, D. (2004). *Skilled interpersonal communication: Research, theory, and practice*. London: Routledge.

Hart, L. M., Mason, R. J., Kelly, C. M., Cvetkovski, S., & Jorm, A. F. (2016). "teen Mental Health First Aid": A description of the program and an initial evaluation. *International Journal of Mental Health Systems*, *10*(1), 3. doi:10.118613033-016-0034-1 PMID:26788123

Health Catalyst. (2014). *Late-Binding™ Data Warehouse Platform*. Retrieved from: https://www.healthcatalyst.com/late-binding-data-warehouse-platform

Health Industry Insights, an IDC Company. (2009). *The Future of Business and Clinical Intelligence in the U.S. Provider Market*. Retrieved from: http://www-07.ibm.com/solutions/au/healthcare/presentations/downloads/The_Future_of_Business_Clinical.pdf

Health Level 7. (2009). *What is HL7?* Retrieved from: www.hl7.org/about/hl7about.htm

Health Service Executive. (2009). *National Adult Literacy Agency*. Dublin: Literacy Audit for Healthcare Settings.

Healthcare, I. T. New. (2014). *Deaths by medical mistakes hit records: The way IT is designed remains part of the problem*. Retrieved from: http://www.healthcareitnews.com/news/deaths-by-medical-mistakes-hit-records

Healthcare, I. T. New. (2015). *American Recovery and Reinvestment Act (ARRA)*. Retrieved from: http://www.healthcareitnews.com/directory/american-recovery-and-reinvestment-act-arra

HealthCare.gov. (n.d.). *Essential Health Benefits*. Retrieved from: www.healthcare.gov/glossary/essential-health-benefits

HealthDay News. (2017, April 11). Is 'desktop medicine' chipping away at patient care? *MedlinePlus*. Retrieved June 10, 2017, from https://medlineplus.gov/news/fullstory_164571.html

Heinrich, C. (2012). Health literacy: The sixth vital sign. *Journal of the American Academy of Nurse Practitioners*, *24*(4), 218–223. doi:10.1111/j.1745-7599.2012.00698.x PMID:22486837

Hellenic American College. (n.d.). *About Hellenic American College*. Retrieved from http://haec.gr/en/aboutus/about-haec-college

Hellenic American University. (n.d.). *Vision and mission*. Retrieved from http://hauniv.edu/about/charter-mission

Hellenic Statistical Authority (ELSTAT). (2017). *Greece in Figures*. Retrieved from http://www.statistics.gr/documents/20181/1515741/GreeceInFigures_2017Q2_EN.pdf/adec1d58-1d39-43ca-b07c-72a8a3741cb2

Herrman, H., & Jané-llopis, E. (n.d.). The Status of Mental Health Promotion. *Public Health Reviews*, *34*(2), 1–21.

Hibbard, J. H., & Greene, J. (2013). What the evidence shows about patient activation: Better health outcomes and care experiences; fewer data on costs. *Health Affairs*, *32*(2), 207–214. doi:10.1377/hlthaff.2012.1061 PMID:23381511

Hibbard, J. H., Peters, E., Dixon, A., & Tusler, M. (2007). Consumer competencies and the use of comparative quality information: It isn't just about literacy. *Medical Care Research and Review: MCRR*, *64*(4), 379–394. doi:10.1177/1077558707301630 PMID:17684108

Higgins, J. P. T., & Green, S. (2011). *Cochrane handbook for systematic reviews of interventions Version 5.1.0*. Chichester, UK: Wiley-Blackwell.

Hinami, K., Whelan, C. T., Konetzka, R. T., & Meltzer, D. O. (2012). Provider expectations and experiences of comanagement. *Journal of Hospital Medicine*, *6*(7), 401–404. doi:10.1002/jhm.914 PMID:21916002

HLS-EU Consortium. (2012). *Comparative report of health literacy in eight EU member states. The European health literacy survey HLS-EU* (second revised and extended version, July 22th, 2014). Retrieved June 10, 2017, from HTTP://WWW.HEALTH-LITERACY.EU

HLS-EU consortium. (2012). *Comparative report of health literacy in eight EU member states*. The European health literacy survey HLS-EU. Retrieved from http://www.health-literacy.eu

HLS-EU Consortium. (2012). *Comparative report of health literacy in eight EU member states. The European health literacy survey HLS-EU.* Retrieved from http://www.health-literacy.eu

HLS-EU Consortium. (2012). *Comparative report of health literacy in eight European member states.* The European Health Literacy Survey-hls-eu. Retrieved April 26, 2017 from https://www.healthliteracyeurope.net/hls-eu

Holmes, L. (2016, May 16). What Happens When Major Companies Take Mental Health Seriously. *Huffington Post.* Retrieved from http://www.huffingtonpost.com/entry/mental-health-workplace_us_572b5a92e4b016f37894d142

Holmes, M. M., Lewith, G., Newell, D., Field, J., & Bishop, F. L. (2017). The impact of patient-reported outcome measures in clinical practice for pain: A systematic review. *Quality of Life Research: An International Journal of Quality of Life Aspects of Treatment, Care and Rehabilitation, 26*(2), 245–257. doi:10.100711136-016-1449-5 PMID:27815820

Holm, S. (2004). The child as organ and tissue donor: Discussions in the Danish council of ethics. *Cambridge Quarterly of Healthcare Ethics, 13*(02), 156–160. doi:10.1017/S0963180104132076 PMID:15124403

Hostetter, M. (2011, October/November). Health care quality improvement: There's an app for that. *Quality Matters.* Retrieved from http://www.commonwealthfund.org/publications/newsletters/quality-matters/2011/october-november-2011/in-focus

Hou, S. (2000). Expanding the kidney donor pool: Ethical and medical considerations. *Kidney International, 58*(4), 1820–1836. doi:10.1046/j.1523-1755.2000.00345.x PMID:11012922

Hovland, C. I., Janis, I. L., & Kelley, H. H. (1953). *Communication and Persuasion: Psychological studies of opinion change. Yale.* Yale University Press.

Howard, D. H., Gazmararian, J. A., & Parker, R. M. (2005). The impact of low health literacy on the medical costs of Medicare managed care enrollees. *The American Journal of Medicine, 118*(4), 371–377. doi:10.1016/j.amjmed.2005.01.010 PMID:15808134

Howard, D. H., Sentell, T., & Gazmararian, J. A. (2006). Impact of health literacy on socioeconomic and racial differences in health in an elderly population. *Journal of General Internal Medicine, 21*(8), 857–861. doi:10.1111/j.1525-1497.2006.00530.x PMID:16881947

Howard, T., Jacobson, K. L., & Kripalani, S. (2013). Doctor talk: Physicians' use of clear verbal communication. *Journal of Health Communication, 18*(8), 991–1001. doi:10.1080/10810730.2012.757398 PMID:23577746

How, C. H. (2011). A review of health literacy: Problem, tools and interventions. *Proceedings of Singapore Healthcare, 20*(2), 119–125. doi:10.1177/201010581102000209

Howerton, M. W., Gibbons, M. C., Baffi, C. R., Gary, T. L., Lai, G. Y., Bolen, S., ... Ford, J. G. (2007). Provider roles in the recruitment of underrepresented populations to cancer clinical trials. *Cancer, 109*(3), 465–476. doi:10.1002/cncr.22436 PMID:17200964

Hulme, W., Allen, J., Manara, A. R., Murphy, P. G., Gardiner, D., & Poppitt, E. (2016). Factors influencing the family consent rate for organ donation in the UK. *Anaesthesia, 71*(9), 1053–1063. doi:10.1111/anae.13535 PMID:27440055

Hunsicker, L. G. (1999). Survival advantage for renal transplantation. *The New England Journal of Medicine, 341*(23), 1762–1763. doi:10.1056/NEJM199912023412310 PMID:10580078

Hussain-Gambles, M., Atkin, K., & Leese, B. (2004). Why ethnic minority groups are under-represented in clinical trials: A review of the literature. *Health & Social Care in the Community, 12*(5), 382–388. doi:10.1111/j.1365-2524.2004.00507.x PMID:15373816

Ingelfinger, F. J. (1972). Informed (but uneducated) consent. *The New England Journal of Medicine*, *287*(9), 465–466. doi:10.1056/NEJM197208312870912 PMID:5044921

Institute for Quality and Efficiency in Health Care. (2004). *The Institute*. Retrieved from: https://www.iqwig.de/en/home.2724.html

Institute of Medicine. (2004). *Health literacy: A prescription to end confusion*. Washington, DC: Institute of Medicine.

International Development Finance Club. (2014). *Investing in Sustainable Cities: Challenges and Opportunities*. Author.

International Registry in Organ Donation and Transplantation (IRODAT). (2017). Retrieved from http://www.irodat.org/img/database/pdf/NEWSLETTER2017_firstedition.pdf

International Summit on Transplant Tourism and Organ Trafficking. (2008). The Declaration of Istanbul on organ trafficking and transplant tourism. *Kidney International*, *74*(7), 854–859. doi:10.1038/ki.2008.388 PMID:18810784

International Technology Education Association. (2007). *Standards for Technological Literacy: Content for the Study of Technology* (3rd ed.) Retrieved from https://www.iteea.org/39197.aspx

IOM (Institute of Medicine). (2004). *Health literacy: A prescription to end confusion*. Washington, DC: The National Academy Press. Retrieved from http:www.iom.edu/Reports/2004/Health-Literacy-A-Prescription-to-End-Confusion.aspx

IOM (Institute of Medicine). (2009). *Race, Ethnicity, and Language Data: Standardization for Health Care Quality Improvement*. Washington, DC: The National Academies Press.

Ishikawa, H., & Kiuchi, T. (2010). Health literacy and health communication. *BioPsychoSocial Medicine*, *4*(1), 1–5. doi:10.1186/1751-0759-4-18 PMID:21054840

Ishikawa, H., Takeuchi, T., & Yano, E. (2008). Measuring functional, communicative, and critical health literacy among diabetic patients. *Diabetes Care*, *31*(5), 874–879. doi:10.2337/dc07-1932 PMID:18299446

Ismail, S. Y., Luchtenburg, A. E., Timman, R., Zuidema, W. C., Boonstra, C., Weimar, W., . . . Massey, E. K. (2014). *Home-based family intervention increases knowledge, communication and living donation rates: a randomized controlled trial*. Retrieved on 11 June 2017 from http://onlinelibrary.wiley.com/doi/10.1111/ajt.12751/

Jackson, L. D. (1992). Information complexity and medical communication: The effects of technical language and amount of information in a medical message. *Health Communication*, *4*(3), 197–210. doi:10.120715327027hc0403_3

Jacobson, B., Aldana, S., Goetzel, R., Vardell, K., Adams, T., & Pietras, R. (1996). The relationship between perceived stress and self-reported illness-related absenteeism. *American Journal of Health Promotion*, *11*(1), 54–61. doi:10.4278/0890-1171-11.1.54 PMID:10163451

Jacobson, T. A., Thomas, D. M., Morton, F. J., Offutt, G., Shevlin, J., & Ray, S. (1999). Use of a low-literacy patient education tool to enhance pneumococcal vaccination rates: A randomized controlled trial. *Journal of the American Medical Association*, *282*(7), 646–650. doi:10.1001/jama.282.7.646 PMID:10517717

Jagdeo, A., Cox, B., Stein, M., & Sareen, J. (2009, November). Negative attitudes toward help seeking for mental illness in 2 population-based surveys from the United States and Canada. *Canadian Journal of Psychiatry*, *54*(11), 757–766. doi:10.1177/070674370905401106 PMID:19961664

Jakab, Z., Celarc, M., & Ossinovski, J. (2016). Introducing the 20th Ljubljana Charter Anniversary issue. *Eurohealth (London)*, *22*(2), 2.

James, B. (n.d.). *Quality Management for Health Care Delivery. The Hospital Research and Educational Trust of the American Hospital Association*. Retrieved from: www.ghdonline.org/uploads/QMMP.pdf

Jansen, L. A. (2004). Child organ donation, family autonomy, and intimate attachments. *Cambridge Quarterly of Healthcare Ethics*, *13*(02), 133–142. doi:10.1017/S0963180104132040 PMID:15124400

Jensen, J. D., King, A. J., Davis, L. A., & Guntzviller, L. M. (2010). Utilization of internet technology by low-income adults: The role of health literacy, health numeracy, and computer assistance. *Journal of Aging and Health*, *22*(6), 804–826. doi:10.1177/0898264310366161 PMID:20495159

Jha, V., Garcia-Garcia, G., Iseki, K., Li, Z., Naicker, S., Plattner, B., ... Yang, C. W. (2013). Chronic kidney disease: Global dimension and perspectives. *Lancet*, *382*(9888), 260–272. doi:10.1016/S0140-6736(13)60687-X PMID:23727169

Jiang, S., & Beaudoin, C. E. (2016). Health literacy and the Internet: An exploratory study on the 2013 HINTS survey. *Computers in Human Behavior*, *58*, 240–248. doi:10.1016/j.chb.2016.01.007

Johnson, A. (2014). Health literacy, does it make a difference? *The Australian Journal of Advanced Nursing*, *31*(3), 39–45.

Johnston, B. C., Patrick, D. L., Busse, J. W., Schünemann, H. J., Agarwal, A., & Guyatt, G. H. (2013). Patient-reported outcomes in meta-analyses – Part 1: Assessing risk of bias and combining outcomes. *Health and Quality of Life Outcomes*, *11*(1), 109–109. doi:10.1186/1477-7525-11-109 PMID:23815754

Jones, A. H., Dizon, Z. B., & October, T. W. (2018). Investigation of public perception of brain death, using the internet. *Chest*. doi:10.1016/j.chest.2018.01.021 PMID:29382473

Jones, J. A., Kreps, G. L., & Phillips, G. M. (1995). *Communicating with your doctor: getting the most out of health care*. Cresskill, NJ: Hampton Press.

Jones, J. A., Kreps, G. L., & Phillips, G. M. (1995). *Communicating with your doctor: Getting the most out of health care*. Cresskill, NJ: Hampton Press.

Joppa, M. C., Rizzo, C. J., Nieves, A. V., & Brown, L. K. (2016). Pilot Investigation of the Katie Brown Educational Program: A School-Community Partnership. *The Journal of School Health*, *86*(4), 288–297. doi:10.1111/josh.12378 PMID:26930241

Jorm, A. F. (2000). Mental Health Literacy: Public Knowledge and beliefs about mental disorders. *The British Journal of Psychiatry*, *177*(05), 396–401. doi:10.1192/bjp.177.5.396 PMID:11059991

Joseph, S. (Ed.). (2015). Positive psychology in practice: Promoting human flourishing in work, health, education, and everyday life. Hoboken, NJ: John Wiley & Sons.

JustiaU. S. Law. (1975). *In Re Guardianship of Pescinski*. Retrieved from https://law.justia.com/cases/wisconsin/supreme-court/1975/668-6.html

Kaas, J., Stasková, V., & Šulistová, R. (2016). The concept of health literacy in contemporary nursing. *Kontakt*, *18*(4), e219–e223. doi:10.1016/j.kontakt.2016.10.001

Kabir, R., & Khan, H. T. A. (2013). Utilization of antenatal care among pregnant women of urban slums of Dhaka City, Bangladesh. *IOSR Journal of Nursing and Health Science*, *2*(2), 55–59. doi:10.9790/1959-0221519

Kabir, R., Rahman, S., Monte-Serrat, D. M., & Arafat, S. M. Y. (2017). Exploring the decision-making power of Bangladeshi women of reproductive age: Results from a national survey. *South East Asia Journal of Medical Sciences*, *1*(1), 4–8.

Kahn, J., & Matas, A. J. (2002). What's special about the ethics of living donors? *Transplantation*, *74*(3), 421–422. doi:10.1097/00007890-200208150-00026

Kantar, T. N. S. (n.d.). *Who we are*. Retrieved from http://www.tnsglobal.com/who-we-are

Karczewski, S. A., Carter, J. S., & DeCator, D. D. (2016). The Role of Ethnicity in School-Based Obesity Intervention for School-Aged Children: A Pilot Evaluation. *The Journal of School Health*, *86*(11), 778–786. doi:10.1111/josh.12433 PMID:27714874

Karpati, A., Kerker, B., Mostashari, F., Singh, T., Hajat, A., Thorpe, L., ... Frieden, T. (2004). *Health Disparities in New York City*. New York: New York City Department of Health and Mental Hygiene. Retrieved from http://www.commonwealthfund.org/~/media/files/publications/other/2004/jul/health-disparities-in-new-york-city/karpati_disparities-pdf.pdf

Kasemsap, K. (2017a). The fundamentals of health literacy. In N. Wickramasinghe (Ed.), *Handbook of research on healthcare administration and management* (pp. 507–527). Hershey, PA: IGI Global. doi:10.4018/978-1-5225-0920-2.ch030

Kasemsap, K. (2017b). Promoting health literacy in global health care. In N. Wickramasinghe (Ed.), *Handbook of research on healthcare administration and management* (pp. 485–506). Hershey, PA: IGI Global. doi:10.4018/978-1-5225-0920-2.ch029

Kasemsap, K. (2017c). Telemedicine and electronic health: Issues and implications in developing countries. In K. Moahi, K. Bwalya, & P. Sebina (Eds.), *Health information systems and the advancement of medical practice in developing countries* (pp. 149–167). Hershey, PA: IGI Global. doi:10.4018/978-1-5225-2262-1.ch009

Kasemsap, K. (2017d). Digital storytelling and digital literacy: Advanced issues and prospects. In D. Loveless, P. Sullivan, K. Dredger, & J. Burns (Eds.), *Deconstructing the education-industrial complex in the digital age* (pp. 151–171). Hershey, PA: IGI Global. doi:10.4018/978-1-5225-2101-3.ch009

Kasemsap, K. (2017e). The perspectives of medical errors in the health care industry. In M. Riga (Ed.), *Impact of medical errors and malpractice on health economics, quality, and patient safety* (pp. 113–143). Hershey, PA: IGI Global. doi:10.4018/978-1-5225-2337-6.ch005

Kasemsap, K. (2018a). Challenges and implications of health literacy in global health care. In M. Khosrow-Pour (Ed.), *Encyclopedia of information science and technology* (4th ed.; pp. 3734–3744). Hershey, PA: IGI Global. doi:10.4018/978-1-5225-2255-3.ch324

Kasemsap, K. (2018b). Mobile health systems and electronic health record: Applications and implications. In J. Machado, A. Abelha, M. Santos, & F. Portela (Eds.), *Next-generation mobile and pervasive healthcare solutions* (pp. 67–85). Hershey, PA: IGI Global. doi:10.4018/978-1-5225-2851-7.ch005

Kasemsap, K. (2018c). Advanced issues of health informatics and clinical decision support system in global health care. In J. Machado, A. Abelha, M. Santos, & F. Portela (Eds.), *Next-generation mobile and pervasive healthcare solutions* (pp. 153–170). Hershey, PA: IGI Global. doi:10.4018/978-1-5225-2851-7.ch010

Kasemsap, K. (2018d). Encouraging digital literacy and ICT competency in the information age. In M. Khosrow-Pour (Ed.), *Encyclopedia of information science and technology* (4th ed.; pp. 2253–2263). Hershey, PA: IGI Global. doi:10.4018/978-1-5225-2255-3.ch196

Kasemsap, K. (2018e). Knowledge management: Applications and implications. In A. Gyamfi & I. Williams (Eds.), *Evaluating media richness in organizational learning* (pp. 232–261). Hershey, PA: IGI Global. doi:10.4018/978-1-5225-2956-9.ch012

Kasemsap, K. (2018f). The role of knowledge transfer in modern organizations. In F. Di Virgilio (Ed.), *Social media for knowledge management applications in modern organizations* (pp. 190–217). Hershey, PA: IGI Global. doi:10.4018/978-1-5225-2897-5.ch009

Kasiske, B., Ravenscraft, M., Ramos, E. L., Gaston, R. S., Bia, M. J., & Danovitch, G. M. (1996). The evaluation of living renal transplant donors: Clinical practice guidelines. *Journal of the American Society of Nephrology*, *7*, 2288–2313. PMID:8959619

Katz, M. G., Jacobson, T. A., Veledar, E., & Kripalani, S. (2007). Asking questions in the medical encounter. *General Internal Medicine*, *22*, 782–786. doi:10.100711606-007-0184-6

Kaufman, L., & Karpati, A. (2007). Understanding the sociocultural roots of childhood obesity: Food practices among Latino families of Bushwick, Brooklyn. *Social Science & Medicine*, *64*(11), 2177–2188. doi:10.1016/j.socscimed.2007.02.019 PMID:17383060

Kazley, A., Hund, J., Simpson, K., Chavin, K., & Baliga, P. (2015). Health literacy and kidney transplant outcomes. *Progress in Transplantation*, *25*(1), 85-90.

Keller, D. B., Sarkar, U., & Schillinger, D. (2014). Health literacy and information exchange in medical settings. In L. R. Martin & M. R. DiMatteo (Eds.), *The Oxford handbook of health communication, behavior change, and treatment adherence* (pp. 23–37). Oxford, UK: Oxford University Press.

Kentikelenis, A., Karanikolos, M., Papanicolas, I., Basu, S., McKee, M., & Stuckler, D. (2011). Health effects of financial crisis: Omens of a Greek tragedy. *Lancet*, *378*(9801), 1457–1458. doi:10.1016/S0140-6736(11)61556-0 PMID:21988763

Keown, P. (2001). Improving the quality of life: The new target for transplantation. *Transplantation*, *7*, S67–S74. PMID:11833144

Kerka, S. (2003). *Health Literacy Beyond Basic Skills*. ERIC Digest. ERIC Clearinghouse on Adult Career and Vocational Education Columbus.

Kessler, R., Aguilar-Gaxiola, S., Alonso, J., Chatterji, S., Lee, S., Ormel, J., ... Wang, P. (2009). The global burden of mental disorders: An update from the WHO World Mental Health (WMH) Surveys. *Epidemiologia e Psichiatria Sociale*, *18*(1), 23–33. doi:10.1017/S1121189X00001421 PMID:19378696

Khalil, G. E., & Rintamaki, L. S. (2014). A televised entertainment-education drama to promote positive discussion about organ donation. *Health Education Research*, *29*(2), 284–296. doi:10.1093/her/cyt106 PMID:24399264

Khanna, D., Furst, D. E., Wong, W. K., Tsevat, J., Clements, P. J., Park, G. S., ... Hays, R. D. (2007). Reliability, validity, and minimally important differences of the SF-6D in systemic sclerosis. *Quality of Life Research: An International Journal of Quality of Life Aspects of Treatment, Care and Rehabilitation*, *16*(6), 1083–1092. doi:10.100711136-007-9207-3 PMID:17404896

Kickbusch, I., Wait, S., & Maag, D. (2005). *Navigating health: The role of health literacy*. Retrieved from http://www.ilcuk.org.uk/index.php/publications/publication_details/ navigating_health_the_role_of_health_literacy

Kickbusch, I. (2001). Health literacy: Addressing the health and education divide. *Health Promotion International*, *16*(3), 289–297. doi:10.1093/heapro/16.3.289 PMID:11509466

Kickbusch, I. (2004). Health and citizenship: The characteristics of 21st century health. *World Hospitals and Health Services*, *40*(4), 12–14. PMID:15751547

Kickbusch, I., & Maag, D. (2008). Health literacy. In K. Heggenhougen & S. Quah (Eds.), *International Encyclopedia of Public Health* (Vol. 3, pp. 204–211). San Diego: Academic Press. doi:10.1016/B978-012373960-5.00584-0

Kickbusch, I., Pelikan, J. M., Apfel, F., & Tsouros, A. D. (Eds.). (2013). *Health literacy: The solid facts*. Copenhagen, Denmark: World Health Organization, Regional Office for Europe.

Kickbusch, I., Pelikan, J., Apfel, F., & Agis, T. (2013). *Health literacy: the solid facts*. Copenhagen: World Health Organisation Regional Office for Europe.

Kickbusch, I., Wait, S., & Maag, D. (2005). *Navigating health. The role of health literacy*. Alliance for Health and the Future, International Longevity Centre-UK.

Kickbush, I., Wait, S., & Maag, D. (2005). Navigating health: The role of health literacy. London: Alliance for Health and the Future. International Longevity Centre.

Kim, H., & Xie, B. (2017). Health literacy in the eHealth era: A systematic review of the literature. *Patient Education and Counseling*, *100*(6), 1073–1082. doi:10.1016/j.pec.2017.01.015 PMID:28174067

Kim, J. Y., Wineinger, N. E., Taitel, M., Radin, J. M., Akinbosoye, O., Jiang, J., ... Steinhubl, S. (2016). Self-Monitoring utilization patterns among individuals in an incentivized program for healthy behaviours. *Journal of Medical Internet Research*, *18*(11), e292. doi:10.2196/jmir.6371 PMID:27856407

Kim, S. H., & Kim, S. H. (2009). Health literacy and functional health status in Korean older adults. *Journal of Clinical Nursing*, *18*(16), 2337–2343. doi:10.1111/j.1365-2702.2008.02739.x PMID:19583664

King, M. T., Winters, Z. E., Olivotto, I. A., Spillane, A. J., Chua, B. H., Saunders, C., ... Rutherford, C. (2017). Patient-reported outcomes in ductal carcinoma in situ: A systematic review. *European Journal of Cancer (Oxford, England)*, *71*, 95–108. doi:10.1016/j.ejca.2016.09.035 PMID:27987454

Kintsch, W. (1994). Text comprehension, memory, and learning. *The American Psychologist*, *49*(4), 294–303. doi:10.1037/0003-066X.49.4.294 PMID:8203801

Kirk, S. M., & Kirk, E. P. (2016). Sixty Minutes of Physical Activity per Day Included Within Preschool Academic Lessons Improves Early Literacy. *The Journal of School Health*, *86*(3), 155–163. doi:10.1111/josh.12363 PMID:26830501

Kirsch, J. S., Junegeblut, A., Jenkins, L., & Kolstad, L. A. (1993). *Adult literacy in America: a first look at the results of the National Adult Literacy Survey (NALS)*. Washington, DC: Department of Education.

Kline R., (2015). *Beyond the snowy white peaks of the NHS?* Better Health. Retrieved on 31 May 2017 from Betterhealth.org.uk

Kline, R. (2014) *The snowy peaks of the NHS: a survey of discrimination in governance and leadership and the potential impact on patient care in London and England*. Retrieved on 15 June 2017 from https://www.england.nhs.uk/wp-content/uploads/2014/08/edc7-0514.pdf

Knight, G. D. (2017). Health literacy: An essential ingredient for better health outcomes –Overview of health literacy theoretical concepts. In I. Management Association (Ed.), Medical education and ethics: Concepts, methodologies, tools, and applications (pp. 22–50). Hershey, PA: IGI Global. doi:10.4018/978-1-5225-0978-3.ch002

Knowledge Network on Urban Settings. (2008). *Our cities, our health, our future Acting on social determinants for health equity in urban settings*. Kobe, Japan: Author.

Koh, H. K., Berwick, D. M., Clancy, C. M., Baur, C., Brach, C., Harris, L. M., & Zerhusen, E. G. (2012). New federal policy initiatives to boost health literacy can help the nation move beyond the cycle of costly 'crisis care'. *Health Affairs (Project Hope)*, *31*(2), 434–443. doi:10.1377/hlthaff.2011.1169 PMID:22262723

Koh, K. K., Brach, C., Harris, L. M., & Parchman, M. L. (2013). A proposed health literate care model would constitute a systems approach to improving patients' engagement in care. *Health Affairs*, *32*(2), 357–367. doi:10.1377/hlthaff.2012.1205 PMID:23381529

Kondilis, B. (2016, September). *Student Discourses of Civic Engagement and Global Citizenship in a Time of Crisis in Greece.* Paper presented at the "Europe in Discourse: Identity, Diversity, Borders" 1st International Conference, Hellenic American College, Athens, Greece. Retrieved from http://europeindiscourse.eu/2016-conference/conference-proceedings

Kondilis, B., Akrivos, P., Salloum, S., & Falagas, M. (2008, June). *Health literacy in Athens, Greece: Exploring sources of health information in adults.* EHMA Annual Conference, Athens, Greece. Retrieved from www.ehma.org/files/16.40%20B%20Kondilis.ppt

Kondilis, B., Magoulas, C., Ioannidi, E., & Agrafiotis, D. (2012, March). *The European Health Literacy Survey Greece.* Hellenic National School of Public Health. Retrieved from http://www.nsph.gr/files/006_Koinoniologias/HLSEU%20country%20report_Greece_2012_ENG.pdf

Kondilis, B., Akrivos, P., Soteriades, E., & Falagas, M. (2010). Readability Levels of Health Pamphlets distributed in Athens Hospitals & Health Centers. *Public Health, 124*(10), 547–552. doi:10.1016/j.puhe.2010.05.010 PMID:20832835

Kondilis, E., Giannakopoulos, S., Gavana, M., Ierodiakonou, I., Waitzkin, H., & Benos, A. (2013, April 18). Economic crisis, restrictive policies, and the population's health and healthcare: The Greek Case. *American Journal of Public Health*, e1–e8. doi:10.2105/AJPH.2012.301126 PMID:23597358

Kostagiolas, P. A., Samioti, F., Alexias, G., Korfiatis, N., & Niakas, D. (2012). Examining patterns of information behavior among healthcare professionals: A case study on health psychologists. *New Review of Information Networking, 17*(2), 108–119. doi:10.1080/13614576.2012.724300

Kranenburg, L. W., Visak, T., Weimar, W., Zuidema, W., de Klerk, M., Hilhorst, M., ... Busschbach, J. J. (2004). Starting a crossover kidney transplantation program in the Netherlands: Ethical and psychological considerations. *Transplantation, 78*(2), 194–197. doi:10.1097/01.TP.0000129259.02340.F7 PMID:15280677

Kreps, G. L. (1988a). The pervasive role of information in health and health care: Implications for health communication policy. In J. Anderson (Ed.), *Communication yearbook 11* (pp. 238–276). Newbury Park, CA: Sage.

Kreps, G. L. (1988b). Relational communication in health care. *Southern Speech Communication Journal, 53*(4), 344–359. doi:10.1080/10417948809372736

Kreps, G. L. (1996). Promoting a consumer orientation to health care and health promotion. *Journal of Health Psychology, 1*(1), 41–48. doi:10.1177/135910539600100104 PMID:22011519

Kreps, G. L., & O'Hair, D. (Eds.). (1995). *Communication and health outcomes.* Cresskill, New Jersey: Hampton Press.

Kreps, G. L., & Query, J. L. (1990). Health communication and interpersonal competence. In G. M. Phillips & J. T. Wood (Eds.), *Speech communication: Essays to commemorate the 75th anniversary of the Speech Communication Association* (pp. 292–323). Carbondale, IL: Southern Illinois University Press.

Kripalani, S., & Weiss, B. D. (2006). Teaching about health literacy and clear communication. *Journal of General Internal Medicine, 21*(8), 888–890. doi:10.1111/j.1525-1497.2006.00543.x PMID:16881953

Krish, S.R., Lawrence, R.H., & Aron, D.C. (2008). Tailoring an intervention to the context and system redesign related to the intervention: A case study of implementing shared medical appointments for diabetes. *Implementation Science*, 3-34. doi:10.1186/1748-5908-3-34

Krist, A. H., & Woolf, S. H. (2011). A vision for patient-centered health information systems. *Journal of the American Medical Association, 305*(3), 300–301. doi:10.1001/jama.2010.2011 PMID:21245186

Kumar, A., & Shim, S. J. (2005). Using computer simulation for surgical care process reengineering in hospitals. *Information Systems and Operational Research, 43*(4), 303–319. doi:10.1080/03155986.2005.11732732

Kummervold, P.E., & Wynn, R. (2012). Health information accessed on the internet: The development in 5 European countries. *International Journal of Telemedicine and Applications*, 1-3. doi:10.1155/2012/297416

Kutner, M., Greenberg, E., Jin, Y., & Paulson, C. (2003). The health literacy of America's adults: results from the 2003 National Assessment of Adult Literacy. Washington, DC: National Center for Educational Statistics; NCES publication no.2006-483.

Kutner, M., Greenburg, E., Jin, Y., & Paulsen, C. (2006). *The health literacy of America's adults: Results from the 2003 National Assessment of Adult Literacy. NCES 2006-483. U.S. Department of Education.* Washington, DC: National Center for Education Statistics.

Labrie, J., Berghmans, B. L. C. M., Fischer, K., Milani, A. L., van der Wijk, I., Smalbraak, D. J. C., ... van der Vaart, C. H. (2013). Surgery versus Physiotherapy for Stress Urinary Incontinence. *The New England Journal of Medicine, 369*(12), 1124–1133. doi:10.1056/NEJMoa1210627 PMID:24047061

Ladd, R. E. (2004). The child as living donor: Parental consent and child assent. *Cambridge Quarterly of Healthcare Ethics, 13*(02), 143–148. doi:10.1017/S0963180104132052 PMID:15124401

Lahana, E., Pappa, E., & Niakas, D. (2011). Do place of residence and ethnicity affect health services utilization? Evidence from Greece. *International Journal for Equity in Health, 10*(16), 1–9. PMID:21521512

Lara, P. N. Jr, Higdon, R., Lim, N., Kwan, K., Tanaka, M., Lau, D. H., ... Lam, K. S. (2001). Prospective evaluation of cancer clinical trial accrual patterns: Identifying potential barriers to enrollment. *Journal of Clinical Oncology, 19*(6), 1728–1733. doi:10.1200/JCO.2001.19.6.1728 PMID:11251003

Larsen, A. L., Liao, Y., Alberts, J., Huh, J., Robertson, T., & Dunton, G. F. (2017). RE-AIM Analysis of a School-Based Nutrition Education Intervention in Kindergarteners. *The Journal of School Health, 87*(1), 36–46. doi:10.1111/josh.12466 PMID:27917488

Lazar, J. (Ed.). (2007). *Universal usability: Designing computer interfaces for diverse user populations.* John Wiley & Sons.

Lazarus, A. A. (1971). *Behavior therapy and beyond.* New York: McGraw-Hill.

Lazarus, A. A. (1973). On assertive behavior: A brief note. *Behavior Therapy, 4*(5), 697–699. doi:10.1016/S0005-7894(73)80161-3

Lee, D., & Bauer, C. *(2013). Wayfinding elements in the environment of care.* Health Facilities Management. Retrieved May 14, 2017 from http://www.hfmmagazine.com/articles/284-signs-of-change

Lee, Y. J., Shin, S. J., Wang, R. H., Lin, K. D., Lee, Y. L., & Wang, Y. H. (2016). Pathways of empowerment perceptions, health literacy, self-efficacy, and self-care behaviors to glycemic control in patients with type 2 diabetes mellitus. *Patient Education and Counseling, 99*(2), 287–294. doi:10.1016/j.pec.2015.08.021 PMID:26341940

Lee, Y. M., Yu, H. Y., You, M. E., & Son, Y. J. (2017). Impact of health literacy on medication adherence in older people with chronic diseases. *Collegian (Royal College of Nursing, Australia), 24*(1), 11–18. doi:10.1016/j.colegn.2015.08.003 PMID:29218957

Leonard, K. (2004). The role of patients in designing health information systems: The case of applying simulation techniques to design an electronic patient record (EPR) interface. *Health Care Management Science, 7*(4), 275–284. doi:10.100710729-004-7536-0 PMID:15717812

Lesselroth, B., Felder, R., Adams, S., Cauthers, P., Dorr, D., Wong, G., & Douglas, D. (2009). Design and implementation of a medication reconciliation kiosk: The Automated Patient History Intake Device (APHID). *Journal of the American Medical Informatics Association, 16*(3), 300–304. doi:10.1197/jamia.M2642 PMID:19261949

Levinsky, N. (1984). The doctor's master. *The New England Journal of Medicine*, *311*(24), 1573–1575. doi:10.1056/NEJM198412133112412 PMID:6438510

Levy, E., Saenger, A. K., Steffes, M. W., & Delvin, E. (2017). Pediatric Obesity and Cardiometabolic Disorders: Risk Factors and Biomarkers. *EJIFCC*, *28*(1), 6–24. PMID:28439216

Lewenstein, B. V. (1992). The Meaning of 'Public Understanding of Science' in the United States after World War II. *Public Understanding of Science (Bristol, England)*, *1*(1), 45–68. doi:10.1088/0963-6625/1/1/009

Lewis, A., & Caplan, A. (2016). Brain death in the media. *Transplantation*, *100*(5), e24. doi:10.1097/TP.0000000000001147 PMID:27116579

Lewis, M. (1974). Kidney donation by a 7-year-old identical twin child: Psychological, legal, and ethical considerations. *Journal of the American Academy of Child and Adolescent Psychiatry*, *13*(2), 221–245. doi:10.1016/S0002-7138(09)61313-3 PMID:4596778

Lindley, C. M., Hirsch, J. D., O'Neill, C. V., Transau, M. C., Gilbert, C. S., & Osterhaus, J. T. (1992). Quality of life consequences of chemotherapy-induced emesis. *Quality of Life Research: An International Journal of Quality of Life Aspects of Treatment, Care and Rehabilitation*, *1*(5), 331–340. doi:10.1007/BF00434947 PMID:1299465

Lipkus, I., Samsa, G., & Rimer, B. (2001). General performance on a numeracy scale among highly educated samples. *Medical Decision Making*, *21*(1), 37–44. doi:10.1177/0272989X0102100105 PMID:11206945

Liu, Y. B., Liu, L., Li, Y. F., & Chen, Y. L. (2015). Relationship between Health Literacy, Health-Related Behaviors and Health Status: A Survey of Elderly Chinese. *International Journal of Environmental Research and Public Health*, *12*(8), 9714–9725. doi:10.3390/ijerph120809714 PMID:26295246

Living Kidney Donors Network. (2018). *Matching Recipient and Donors*. Retrieved from http://lkdn.org/matching_recip_donors.html

Locke, J., Kang-Yi, C. D., Pellecchia, M., Marcus, S., Hadley, T., & Mandell, D. S. (2017). Ethnic disparities in school-based behavioral health service use for children with psychiatric disorders. *The Journal of School Health*, *87*(1), 47–54. doi:10.1111/josh.12469 PMID:27917490

Logan, R. A., Wong, W. F., Villaire, M., Daus, G., Parnell, T. A., Willis, E., & Paasche-Orlow, M. (2015). *Health literacy: A necessary element for achieving health equity*. Discussion Paper. Institute of Medicine. Retrieved April 26, 2017 from http://www.nam.edu/perspectives/2015/Health-literacy-a-necessary-element-for-achieving-health-equity

Lohr, K. N., Aaronson, N. K., Alonso, J., Burnam, M. A., Patrick, D. L., Perrin, E. B., & Roberts, J. S. (1996). Evaluating quality-of-life and health status instruments: Development of scientific review criteria. *Clinical Therapeutics*, *18*(5), 979–992. doi:10.1016/S0149-2918(96)80054-3 PMID:8930436

Longo, D. R., & Patrick, T. B. (2001). Consumer reports and health care information: A call for research. *Journal of Health Care Finance*, *28*, 92–96. PMID:11669296

Loosier, P. S., Doll, S., Lepar, D., Ward, K., Gamble, G., & Dittus, P. J. (2016). Effectiveness of an Adaptation of the Project Connect Health Systems Intervention: Youth and Clinic-Level Findings. *The Journal of School Health*, *86*(8), 595–603. doi:10.1111/josh.12414 PMID:27374349

Lucena, A. de F., & de Góes, M. O. (1999). O processo de comunicação no cuidado do paciente submetido ao eco-stress: Algumas reflexões. *Revista Gaúcha de Enfermagem*, *20*, 37–48.

Lurio, J., Morrison, F. P., Pichardo, M., Berg, R., Buck, M. D., Wu, W., ... Calman, N. (2010). Using electronic health record alerts to provide public health situational awareness to clinicians. *Journal of the American Medical Informatics Association, 17*(2), 217–219. doi:10.1136/jamia.2009.000539 PMID:20190067

Lustria, M. L., Smith, S. A., & Hinnant, C. C. (2011). Exploring digital divides: An examination of eHealth technology use in health information seeking, communication and personal health information management in the USA. *Health Informatics Journal, 17*(3), 224–243. doi:10.1177/1460458211414843 PMID:21937464

Luthans, F., Youssef, C. M., & Avolio, B. J. (2007). *Psychological capital*. New York: Oxford University Press.

Maastricht University CAPHRI. (2012). *European health award for the HLS-EU project*. Retrieved from https://www.caphri.nl/european-health-award-hls-eu-project

Mackert, M., Ball, J., & Lopez, N. (2011). Health literacy awareness training for healthcare workers: Improving knowledge and intentions to use clear communication techniques. *Patient Education and Counseling, 85*(3), e225–e228. doi:10.1016/j.pec.2011.02.022 PMID:21474264

Ma, G. X., Tan, Y., Blakeney, N. C., Seals, B. F., Ma, X. S., Zhai, S., ... Michaels, M. (2014). The impact of a community-based clinical trial educational intervention among underrepresented Chinese Americans. *Cancer Epidemiology, Biomarkers & Prevention, 23*(3), 424–432. doi:10.1158/1055-9965.EPI-13-0773 PMID:24092627

Maisano, G. (2006). *Therapeutic education of patients with coronary heart disease: Training guide for general practitioners*. Udine, Italy: World Health Organization.

Majeske, R. A., Parker, L. S., & Frader, J. E. (1996). In search of an ethical framework for consideration of decisions regarding live donation. In B. Spielman (Ed.), *Organ and Tissue Donation: Ethical, Legal, and Policy Issues*. Carbondale, IL: Southern Illinois University Press.

Manara, A. R., Murphy, P. G., & O'Callaghan, G. (2012). Donation after circulatory death. *BJA: British Journal of Anaesthesia, 108*(suppl_1), i121. doi:10.1093/bja/aer357

Mancuso, J. M. (2008). Health literacy: A concept/dimensional analysis. *Nursing & Health Sciences, 10*(3), 248–255. doi:10.1111/j.1442-2018.2008.00394.x PMID:18786068

Mancuso, J. M. (2009). Assessment and measurement of health literacy: An integrative review of the literature. *Nursing & Health Sciences, 11*(1), 77–89. doi:10.1111/j.1442-2018.2008.00408.x PMID:19298313

Manganello, J. A. (2008). Health literacy and adolescents: A framework and agenda for future research. *Health Education Research, 23*(5), 840–847. doi:10.1093/her/cym069 PMID:18024979

Manning, D. I., & Dickens, C. (2006). Health literacy: More choice, but do cancer patients have the skills to decide? *European Journal of Cancer Care, 15*(5), 448–452. doi:10.1111/j.1365-2354.2006.00687.x PMID:17177901

Mantwill, S., & Schulz, P. J. (2015). Low health literacy associated with higher medication costs in patients with type 2 diabetes mellitus: Evidence from matched survey and health insurance data. *Patient Education and Counseling, 98*(12), 1625–1630. doi:10.1016/j.pec.2015.07.006 PMID:26198546

Marks, L., & Power, E. (2002). Using technology to address recruitment issues in the clinical trial process. *Trends in Biotechnology, 20*(3), 105–109. doi:10.1016/S0167-7799(02)01881-4 PMID:11841861

Marks, R. (2009). Schools and health education: What works, what is needed, and why? *Health Education, 109*(1), 4–8. doi:10.1108/09654280910923345

Marks, R. (2012). *Health literacy and School-based education*. New York: Emerald.

Marks, R. (2012). *Health literacy and school-based health education.* Emerald Group Publishing.

Marmot, M., Friel, S., Bell, R., Houweling, T. A., & Taylor, S. (2008). Closing the gap in a generation: Health equity through action on the social determinants of health. *Lancet, 372*(9650), 1661–1669. doi:10.1016/S0140-6736(08)61690-6 PMID:18994664

Martin, L. R., & Di Matteo, M. R. (Ed.). (2014). The Oxford handbook of Health Communication, behavieoural change and Treatment Adherence. New York: Oxford.

Martini, C. J., & McDowell, I. (1976). Health status: Patient and physician judgments. *Health Services Research, 11*(4), 508–515. PMID:1025054

Martin, L., Schonlau, M., Hass, A., Derose, K., Rosenfeld, L., Buka, S., & Rudd, R. (2011). Patient activation and advocacy: Which literacy skills mater most? *Journal of Health Communication, 16*(3), 177–190. doi:10.1080/10810730.2011.604705 PMID:21951251

Matas, A. J., Garvey, C. A., Jacobs, C. L., & Kahn, J. P. (2000). Nondirected donation of kidneys from living donors. *The New England Journal of Medicine, 343*(6), 433–436. doi:10.1056/NEJM200008103430611 PMID:10933745

Mathus-Vliegen, E. M., & de Wit, L. T. (2007). Health-related quality of life after gastric banding. *British Journal of Surgery, 94*(4), 457–465. doi:10.1002/bjs.5607 PMID:17310505

Matsumoto, M., & Nakayama, K. (2017). Development of the health literacy on social determinants of health questionnaire in Japanese adults. *BMC Public Health, 17*(1), 30. doi:10.118612889-016-3971-3 PMID:28056903

Matsuyama, R. K., Wilson-Genderson, M., Kuhn, L., Moghanaki, D., Vachhani, H., & Paasche-Orlow, M. (2011). Education level, not health literacy, associated with information needs for patients with cancer. *Patient Education and Counseling, 85*(3), e229–e236. doi:10.1016/j.pec.2011.03.022 PMID:21543182

Matthews, D. (2015). The impact of ethnicity on health inequalities. *Nursing Times, 111*(44), 18–20. PMID:26665383

Matthews, P. H., Darbisi, C., Sandmann, L., Galen, R., & Rubin, D. (2008). Disseminating health information and diabetes care for Latinos via electronic information kiosks. *Journal of Immigrant and Minority Health, 11*(6), 520–526. doi:10.100710903-008-9134-6 PMID:18392935

Mayeaux, E. J. Jr, Murphy, P. W., Arnold, C., Davis, T. C., Jackson, R. H., & Sentell, T. (1996). Improving patient education for patients with low literacy skills. *American Family Physician, 53*(1), 205–211. PMID:8546047

Mazaris, E., & Papalois, V. (2006). Ethical Issues in Living Donor Kidney Transplantation. *Experimental and Clinical Transplantation, 2*, 485–497. PMID:17238845

McCaffery, K. J., Holmes-Rovner, M., Smith, S. K., Rovner, D., Nutbeam, D., Clayman, M. L., ... Sheridan, S. L. (2013). Addressing health literacy in patient decision aids. *BMC Medical Informatics and Decision Making, 13*(Suppl 2), S10. doi:10.1186/1472-6947-13-S2-S10 PMID:24624970

McCauley, C. (2006). *Developmental Assignments: Creating Learning Experiences without Changing Jobs.* Retrieved from: www.worldcat.org/title/adaptability-responding-effectively-to-change/oclc

McCormack, L., Thomas, V., Lewis, M. A., & Rudd, R. (2017). Improving low health literacy and patient engagement: A social ecological approach. *Patient Education and Counseling, 100*(1), 8–13. doi:10.1016/j.pec.2016.07.007 PMID:27475265

McCray, A. T. (2005). Promoting health literacy. *Journal of the American Medical Informatics Association, 1*(2), 152–163. doi:10.1197/jamia.M1687 PMID:15561782

McCune, R. L., Lee, H., & Pohl, J. M. (2016). Assessing health literacy in safety net primary care practices. *Applied Nursing Research, 29*, 188–194. doi:10.1016/j.apnr.2015.04.004 PMID:26856512

McLellan, F. (2003). US surgeons do first "triple-swap" kidney transplantation. *Lancet, 362*(9382), 456. doi:10.1016/S0140-6736(03)14106-2 PMID:12931692

McLeod, L. D., Coon, C. D., Martin, S. A., Fehnel, S. E., & Hays, R. D. (2011). Interpreting patient-reported outcome results: US FDA guidance and emerging methods. *Expert Review of Pharmacoeconomics & Outcomes Research, 11*(2), 163–169. doi:10.1586/erp.11.12 PMID:21476818

Mcluckie, A., Kutcher, S., Wei, Y., & Weaver, C. (2014). Sustained improvements in students¿ mental health literacy with use of a mental health curriculum in Canadian schools. *BMC Psychiatry, 14*(1), 1694. doi:10.118612888-014-0379-4 PMID:25551789

McNamara, D. S., Kintsch, E., Butler-Songer, N., & Kintsch, W. (1996). Are good texts always better? Interactions of text coherence, background knowledge, and levels of understanding in learning from text. *Cognition and Instruction, 14*(1), 1–43. doi:10.12071532690xci1401_1

McNeil, A., & Arena, R. (2017). The evolution of health literacy and communication: Introducing health harmonics. *Progress in Cardiovascular Diseases, 59*(5), 463–470. doi:10.1016/j.pcad.2017.02.003 PMID:28216109

McPherson, W. (1999). *The Stephen Lawrence inquiry – report of an inquiry* retrieved on 14 June 2017 from https://www.gov.uk/government/uploads/system/uploads/attachment_data/file/277111/4262.pdf

Mead, G. H. (1934). *Mind, self, and society.* Chicago: University of Chicago Press.

Melvin, D. (2015, July 13). Between rock, hard place, Greece picks austerity. How did it get into this mess? *CNN.* Retrieved from http://www.cnn.com/2015/07/13/europe/how-greece-reached-this-point/

Mendoza, D. B., Williams, M. T., Chapman, L. K., & Powers, M. (2012). Minority inclusion in randomized clinical trials of panic disorder. *Journal of Anxiety Disorders, 26*(5), 574–582. doi:10.1016/j.janxdis.2012.02.011 PMID:22445317

Merai, R., Siegel, C., Rakotz, M., Basch, P., Wright, J., Wong, B., & Thorpe, P. (2016). CDC Grand Rounds: A Public Health Approach to Detect and Control Hypertension. *MMWR. Morbidity and Mortality Weekly Report, 65*(45), 1261–1264. doi:10.15585/mmwr.mm6545a3 PMID:27855138

Merga, M. K., & Hu, Q. M. (2016). Health education beyond the school gates: Use of school newsletters to communicate health messages to parents and their families. *Australian Journal of Education, 60*(1), 73–85. doi:10.1177/0004944115627567

Merrill, J. P., Murray, J. E., Harrison, J. H., & Guild, W. R. (1956). Successful homotransplantation of human kidneys between identical twins. *Journal of the American Medical Association, 160*(4), 277–282. doi:10.1001/jama.1956.02960390027008 PMID:13278189

Michielutte, R., Alciati, M. H., & El Arculli, R. (1999). Cancer control research and literacy. *Journal of Health Care for the Poor and Underserved, 10*(3), 281–297. doi:10.1353/hpu.2010.0585 PMID:10436728

Michie, S., & Williams, S. (2003). Reducing Work Related Psychological Ill Health and Sickness Absence: A Systematic Literature Review. *Occupational and Environmental Medicine, 60*(1), 3–9. doi:10.1136/oem.60.1.3 PMID:12499449

Middleton, P. F., Duffield, M., Lynch, S. V., Padbury, R. T., House, T., Stanton, P., ... Maddern, G. (2006). Living donor liver transplantation: Adult donor outcomes—a systematic review. *Liver Transplantation, 12*(1), 24–30. doi:10.1002/lt.20663 PMID:16498709

Miller, N. (2013). Apps for your smart phone. *Clinical Psychiatry News*. Retrieved from http://www.clinicalpsychiatrynews.com/views/blognosis/blog/apps-for-your-smartphone/ff1923da2e4f57803957dbbb7fca029f.html

Miller, J. D. (1983). Scientific literacy: A conceptual and empirical review. *Daedalus*, 29–48.

Miller, T. A. (2016). Health literacy and adherence to medical treatment in chronic and acute illness: A meta-analysis. *Patient Education and Counseling*, *99*(7), 1079–1086. doi:10.1016/j.pec.2016.01.020 PMID:26899632

Mills, H. (2017). *Health Literacy Training In Stoke-On-Trent An overview of 2 training courses on offer*. Retrieved June 15, 2017, from http://slideplayer.com/slide/8888367/

Mokkink, L. B., Terwee, C. B., Patrick, D. L., Alonso, J., Stratford, P. W., Knol, D. L., ... de Vet, H. C. (2010). The COSMIN checklist for assessing the methodological quality of studies on measurement properties of health status measurement instruments: An international Delphi study. *Quality of Life Research: An International Journal of Quality of Life Aspects of Treatment, Care and Rehabilitation*, *19*(4), 539–549. doi:10.100711136-010-9606-8 PMID:20169472

Montgomery, R. A., Gentry, S. E., Marks, W. H., Warren, D. S., Hiller, J., Houp, J., ... Segev, D. L. (2006). Domino paired kidney donation: A strategy to make best use of live non-directed donation. *Lancet*, *368*(9533), 419–421. doi:10.1016/S0140-6736(06)69115-0 PMID:16876670

Moonseong, H., Erica, I., Natania, O., Carmen, I., Shawn, H., & Judith, W.-R. (2016). Behaviors and Knowledge of HealthCorps New York City High School Students: Nutrition, Mental Health and Physical Activity. *The Journal of School Health*, *86*(2), 84–95. doi:10.1111/josh.12355 PMID:26762819

Morgan, S. E., Harrison, T. R., Long, S. D., Afifi, W. A., Stephenson, M. S., & Reichert, T. (2005). Family discussions about organ donation: How the media influences opinions about donation decisions. *Clinical Transplantation*, *19*(5), 674–682. doi:10.1111/j.1399-0012.2005.00407.x PMID:16146561

Morgan, S. E., Movius, L., & Cody, M. J. (2009). The power of narratives: The effect of entertainment television organ donation storylines on the attitudes, knowledge, and behaviors of donors and nondonors. *Journal of Communication*, *59*(1), 135–151. doi:10.1111/j.1460-2466.2008.01408.x

Morgan, S., & Miller, J. (2002). Communicating about gifts of life: The effect of knowledge, attitudes, and altruism on behavior and behavioral intentions regarding organ donation. *Journal of Applied Communication Research*, *30*(2), 163–178. doi:10.1080/00909880216580

Mosley, C. M., & Taylor, B. J. (2017). Integration of health literacy content into nursing curriculum utilizing the health literacy expanded model. *Teaching and Learning in Nursing*, *12*(2), 109–116. doi:10.1016/j.teln.2016.12.005

Mossialos, E., Costa-i-Font, J., & Rudisill, C. (2008). Does organ donation legislation affect individuals' willingness to donate their own or their relative's organs?: Evidence from European Union survey data. *BMC Health Services Research*, *8*(1), 48. doi:10.1186/1472-6963-8-48 PMID:18304341

Mougiakakou, S. G., Kyriacou, E., Perakis, K., Papadopoulos, H., Androulidakis, A., Konnis, G., ... Koutsouris, D. (2011). A feasibility study for the provision of electronic healthcare tools and services in areas of Greece, Cyprus and Italy. *Biomedical Engineering Online*, *10*(1), 49. doi:10.1186/1475-925X-10-49 PMID:21649924

Mukhopadhyay, S., & Postolache, O. (Ed.). (2013). *Pervasive and mobile sensing and computing for healthcare: technological and social issues*. Heidelberg, Germany: Springer.

Muller, E. (2016). Transplantation in Africa – an overview. *Clinical Nephrology*, *86*(13), 90-95.

Mullins, C. D., Blatt, L., Gbarayor, C. M., Yang, H. W., & Baquet, C. (2005). Health disparities: A barrier to high-quality care. *American Journal of Health-System Pharmacy*, *62*(18), 1873–1882. doi:10.2146/ajhp050064 PMID:16141106

Murff, H. J., Patel, V. L., Hripcsak, G., & Bateset, D. W. (2003). Detecting adverse events for patient safety research: A review of current methodologies. *Journal of Biomedical Informatics*, *36*(1), 131–143. doi:10.1016/j.jbi.2003.08.003 PMID:14552854

Murphy-Knoll, L. (2007). Low health literacy puts patients at risk: The Joint Commission proposes solutions to national problem. *Journal of Nursing Care Quality*, *22*(3), 205–209. doi:10.1097/01.NCQ.0000277775.89652.30 PMID:17563587

Muscat, D. M., Smith, S., Dhillon, H. M., Morony, S., Davis, E. L., Luxford, K., ... Buchbinder, R. (2016). Incorporating health literacy in education for socially disadvantaged adults: An Australian feasibility study. *International Journal for Equity in Health*, *15*(1), 84. doi:10.118612939-016-0373-1 PMID:27259476

Musil, C. M. (2006). *Assessing global leaning: Matching good intentions with good practice*. Washington, DC: Association of American Colleges and Universities.

Nair, S. C., Satish, K. P., Sreedharan, J., & Ibrahim, H. (2016). Assessing health literacy in the eastern and middle-eastern cultures. *BMC Public Health*, *16*(1), 831. doi:10.118612889-016-3488-9 PMID:27538529

Nanda, U., McLendon, P. M., Andresen, E. M., & Armbrecht, E. (2003). The SIP68: An abbreviated sickness impact profile for disability outcomes research. *Quality of Life Research: An International Journal of Quality of Life Aspects of Treatment, Care and Rehabilitation*, *12*(5), 583–595. doi:10.1023/A:1025036325886 PMID:13677503

National Centre for Social Research. (2014). *30 years of British social attitudes self-reported racial prejudice data*. Retrieved on 15 June 2017 from https://diversityuk.org/wp-content/uploads/2014/06/selfreported-racial-prejudice-datafinal.pdf

National Committee for Quality Assurance (NCQA). (2016). *Health Insurance Plan Rankings*. Retrieved from: http://www.ncqa.org/report-cards/health-plans/health-insurance-plan-rankings

National Heart, Lung, and Blood Institute (NHLBI). (2007). *Portion Distortion Interactive Quizzes Slides Sets*. Retrieved from https://www.nhlbi.nih.gov/health/educational/wecan/eat-right/portion-distortion.htm

National network of libraries of medicine. (2017). *Health literacy*. Retrieved June 16, 2017, from https://nnlm.gov/professional-development/topics/health-literacy

National Patient Safety Foundation. (n.d.). *Ask Me 3: Good questions for good health*. Retrieved May 11, 2017 from http://www.npsf.org/?page=askme3

National Research Council. (2013). *Core Measurement Needs for Better Care, Better Health, and Lower Costs: Counting What Counts: Workshop Summary*. Washington, DC: The National Academies Press.

National Science Foundation (NSF). (2003). *Science and engineering indicators*. National Science Board. Retrieved from www.nsf.gov/sbe/srs/seind93/chap7/doc/7d1a93.htm

Nelson, E. C., Eftimovska, E., Lind, C., Hager, A., Wasson, J. H., & Lindblad, S. (2015). Patient reported outcome measures in practice. *BMJ: British Medical Journal, 350*.

Nelson, D., Hesse, B., & Croyle, R. (2009). *Making data talk: Communicating public health data to the public, policy makers and the press*. New York, NY: Oxford University Press. doi:10.1093/acprof:oso/9780195381535.001.0001

Network. (n.d.). Retrieved July 13, 2017 from https://www.merriam-webster.com/dictionary/network

New York City Department of Health and Mental Hygiene, Bureau of Communications in cooperation with Bureau of Chronic Disease Prevention and Control. (2009). *Health Bulletin #51: How to Lose Weight*. Retrieved from http://www.nyc.gov/html/ doh/downloads/pdf/public/dohmhnews6-05.pdf

New York City Department of Health and Mental. (2012). *Reversing the Epidemic: The New York City Obesity Task Force Plan to Prevent and Control Obesity*. Retrieved from http://www.nyc.gov/html/om/pdf/2012/otf_report.pdf

Newby, M., & Christensen, H. (2016). NU SC. *Clinical Psychology Review*.

Newman, S., Steed, L., & Mulligan, K. (2004). Self-management interventions for chronic illness. *Lancet*, *364*(9444), 1523–1537. doi:10.1016/S0140-6736(04)17277-2 PMID:15500899

Newsweek. (2015). *Many Insured Americans Can't Afford Health Care*. Retrieved from http://www.newsweek.com/many-americans-insured-cant-afford-health-care-334624

NHS Blood and Transplant Organ Donation and Transplantation 2013-2014. (n.d.). Retrieved https://nhsbtmediaservices.blob.core.windows.net/organ-donation-assets/pdfs/activity_report_2013_14.pdf

NHS Blood and Transplant. (n.d.). *Living Donation Guidance and Resources on Living Donation and Trandplantation*. Retrieved from http://www.odt.nhs.uk/living-donation/

NHS Blood and Transplant. (n.d.a). *Donation After Brainstem Death*. Retrieved https://www.odt.nhs.uk/deceased-donation/best-practice-guidance/donation-after-brainstem-death/

NHS Blood and Transplant. (n.d.b). *Donation After Circulatory Death*. Retrieved https://www.odt.nhs.uk/deceased-donation/best-practice-guidance/donation-after-circulatory-death/

NICE. (2013). *Guide to the methods of technology appraisal 2013 (PMG9)*. Retrieved from nice.org.uk/process/pmg9

NICE. (2015). *NICE Clinical Knowledge Summary: Depression*. Retrieved from https://cks.nice.org.uk/depression

Nielsen-Bohlman, L., Panzer, A. M., & Kindig, D. A. (2004). Health Literacy: A Prescription to End Confusion. Washington, DC: The National Academy of Sciences.

Nielsen-Bohlman, L. T., Panzer, A. M., & Kindig, D. A. (2004). *Health Literacy: A Prescription to End Confusion. San Fransisco*: The National Academies Press.

Nielsen-Bohlman, L., Panzer, A. M., & Kindig, D. A. (2004). *Health Literacy, A Prescription to End Confusion*. Washington, DC: The National Academies Press.

Nielsen-Bohlman, L., Panzer, A. M., & Kindig, D. A. (Eds.). (2004). *Health literacy: a prescription to end confusion*. Washington, DC: Institute of Medicine, National Academies Press.

Nieto, T., Inston, N., & Cockwell, P. (2016). Renal transplantation in adults. *British Medical Journal*, *355*, i6158. doi:10.1136/bmj.i6158 PMID:27903494

Nijman, J., Hendriks, M., Brabers, A., de Jong, J., & Rademakers, J. (2014). Patient activation and health literacy as predictors of health information use in a general sample of Dutch health care consumers. *Journal of Health Communication: International Perspectives*, *19*(8), 955–969. doi:10.1080/10810730.2013.837561 PMID:24397280

Noar, S. M., Harrington, N. G., Van Stee, S. V., & Aldrich, R. S. (2011). Tailored health communication to change lifestyle behaviours. *American Journal of Lifestyle Medicine*, *5*(5), 112–122. doi:10.1177/1559827610387255

Nolte, S., Osborne, R. H., Dwinger, S., Elsworth, G. R., Conrad, M. L., Rose, M., ... Zill, J. M. (2017). German translation, cultural adaptation, and validation of the Health Literacy Questionnaire (HLQ). *PLoS One*, *12*(2), 12. doi:10.1371/journal.pone.0172340 PMID:28234987

Norman, C. D., & Skinner, H. A. (2006). eHealth Literacy: Essential Skills for Consumer Health in a Networked World. *Journal of Medical Internet Research*, *8*(2), e9. doi:10.2196/jmir.8.2.e9 PMID:16867972

Norman, C. D., & Skinner, H. A. (2006a). eHEALS: The eHealth Literacy Scale. *Journal of Medical Internet Research, 4*(4), e27. doi:10.2196/jmir.8.4.e27 PMID:17213046

Nuffield Council on Bioethics. (1995). *Human Tissue Ethical and Legal Issues.* London: Nuffield Council on Bioethics.

Nussbaum, M. C. (2000). *Women and Human Development. The Capabilities Approach.* Cambridge, UK: Press Syndicate of the University of Cambridge. doi:10.1017/CBO9780511841286

Nutbeam, D. (1998). Health Promotion Glossary. *Health Promotion International, 13*(4), 349–364. doi:10.1093/heapro/13.4.349

Nutbeam, D. (2000). Health literacy as a public health goal: A challenge for contemporary health education and communication strategies into the 21st century. *Health Promotion International, 15*(3), 259–267. doi:10.1093/heapro/15.3.259

Nutbeam, D. (2008). The evolving concept of health literacy. *Social Science & Medicine, 67*(12), 2072–2078. doi:10.1016/j.socscimed.2008.09.050 PMID:18952344

Nutbeam, D. (2009). Defining and measuring health literacy: What can we learn from literacy studies? *International Journal of Public Health, 54*(5), 303–305. doi:10.100700038-009-0050-x PMID:19641847

Nutbeam, D. (2017). *Discussion paper on promoting, measuring and implementing health literacy: Implications for policy and practice in non-communicable disease prevention and control (WHO GCM/NCD Working Group 3.3 2017).* University of Sydney.

Nutbeam, D., & Kickbusch, I. (2000). Advancing health literacy: A global challenge for the 21st century. *Health Promotion International, 15*(3), 183–184. doi:10.1093/heapro/15.3.183

O'Connor, A. M., & Jacobsen, M. J. (2006). *Decisional conflict: Supporting people experiencing uncertainty about options affecting their health.* Retrieved from http://careinaging.duke.edu/longtermcare/dynamic/resources/1027/Decisional_Conflict.pdf

Obamacare Facts. (n.d.). *Obamacare Bill: Full PPACA & Related Laws.* Retrieved from: http://obamacarefacts.com/obamacarebill

O'Donnell, J., Pham, S., Pashos, C., Miller, D., Smith, M. (2009). *Health Technology Assessment: Lessons Learned from Around the World—An Overview. Value In Health.* Wiley-Blackwell. doi:10.1111/j.1524-4733.2009.00550.x

Office for National Statistics. (2012). *Ethnicity and national identity in England and Wales: 2011.* Retrieved on 13 June 2017 from /www.ons.gov.uk/peoplepopulationandcommunity/culturalidentity/ethnicity/articles/ethnicityandnationalidentityinenglandandwales/2012-12-11

Office of Disease Prevention and Health Promotion. (2016). Heart disease and stroke. In *Healthy People 2020.* Retrieved May 14, 2017 from https://www.healthypeople.gov/2020/topics-objectives/topic/health-communication-and-health-information-technology/objectives

Ogden, C., Carroll, M., Fryar, C., & Flegal, K. (2015, November). *Prevalence of obesity among Adults and Youth: 2014-2015.* NCHS Data Brief, No. 219. Retrieved from https://www.cdc.gov/nchs/data/databriefs/db219.pdf

Ogden, C., Carroll, M., Curtin, L., Lamb, M., & Flegal, K. (2010). Prevalence of high body mass index in US children and adolescents, 2007–2008. *Journal of the American Medical Association, 303*(3), 242–249. doi:10.1001/jama.2009.2012 PMID:20071470

Ojio, Y. (2015). Development of a mental health literacy program for secondary school students and its effects: In-school mental health literacy education. *School Mental Health: Global Challenges and Opportunities*, (3).

Okello, E. S., Abbo, C., Muhwezi, W. W., Akello, G., & Ovuga, E. (2014). Mental health literacy among secondary school students in North and Central Uganda: A qualitative study. *World Cultural Psychiatry Research Review*, *9*(3), 70–80. PMID:26113883

Oliver, M., Ahmed, A., & Woywodt, A. (2012). Donating in good faith or getting into trouble? religion and organ donation revisited. *World Journal of Transplantation*, *2*(5), 69–73. doi:10.5500/wjt.v2.i5.69 PMID:24175198

Olsen, M. F., Bjerre, E., Hansen, M. D., Hilden, J., Landler, N. E., Tendal, B., & Hrobjartsson, A. (2017). Pain relief that matters to patients: Systematic review of empirical studies assessing the minimum clinically important difference in acute pain. *BMC Medicine*, *15*(1), 35. doi:10.118612916-016-0775-3 PMID:28215182

ONC Office of the National Coordinator. (2015, April). *ONC Data Brief No. 23 April 2015*. Author.

Onjefu, O., & Olalekan, A. G. (2016). Human communication as a correlate of the essence of Man: A Philosophical perspective. *Arts and Social Sciences Journal*, *7*(1), 1–4.

Operations Research. (2007). *The Science of Better*. Retrieved from: The Science of Better website: www.scienceofbetter.org

Organ Procurement and Transplantation Network (OPTN). (n.d.). Retrieved September, 2017, from https://optn.transplant.hrsa.gov/

Osborn, C. Y., Paasche-Orlow, M. K., Bailey, S. C., & Wolf, M. S. (2011). The mechanisms linking health literacy to behavior and health status. *American Journal of Health Behavior*, *35*(1), 118–128. doi:10.5993/AJHB.35.1.11 PMID:20950164

Osborn, C. Y., Paasche-Orlow, M. K., Davis, T. C., & Wolf, M. S. (2007). Health literacy: An overlooked factor in understanding HIV health disparities. *American Journal of Preventive Medicine*, *33*(5), 374–378. doi:10.1016/j.amepre.2007.07.022 PMID:17950402

Osborne, H. (2012). *Health Literacy from A to Z: Practical Ways to Communicate Your Health Message*. Jones & Bartlett Publishers.

Otani, K., Kurz, R. S., & Harris, L. E. (2005). Managing primary care using patient satisfaction measures. *Journal of Healthcare Management*, *50*(5), 311–325. doi:10.1097/00115514-200509000-00007 PMID:16268410

Oxley 101. (2014). *Confused by SOX Compliance?* Retrieved from: www.sarbanes-oxley-101.com

Paasche-Orlow, M. K., & Wolf, M. S. (2007). The causal pathways linking health literacy to health outcomes. *American Journal of Health Behavior*, *31*(Suppl 1), S19–S26. doi:10.5993/AJHB.31.s1.4 PMID:17931132

Palombo, R. (2016). Designing health-literate health care organization: A literature review. *Health Services Management Research*, *29*(3), 79–87. doi:10.1177/0951484816639741

Palumbo, R. (2015). Discussing the Effects of Poor Health Literacy on Patients Facing HIV: A Narrative Literature Review. *International Journal of Health Policy and Management*, *4*(7), 417–430. doi:10.15171/ijhpm.2015.95 PMID:26188806

Palumbo, R., & Annarumma, C. (2014, August). The importance of being health literate: An organizational health literacy approach. *17th Toulon-Verona International Conference Proceedings*.

Palumbo, R., Annarumma, C., Adinolfi, P., Musella, M., & Piscopo, G. (2016). The Italian health literacy project: Insights from the assessment of health literacy skills in Italy. *Health Policy (Amsterdam)*, *120*(9), 1087–1094. doi:10.1016/j.healthpol.2016.08.007 PMID:27593949

Pandey, A., Hasan, S., Dubey, D., & Sarangi, S. (2012). Smartphone apps as a source of cancer information: Changing trends in health information-seeking behavior. *Journal of Cancer Education*, *28*(1), 138–142. doi:10.100713187-012-0446-9 PMID:23275239

Parikh, N. S., Parker, R. M., Nurss, J. R., Baker, D. W., & Williams, M. V. (1996). Shame and health literacy: The unspoken connection. *Patient Education and Counseling*, *27*(1), 33–39. doi:10.1016/0738-3991(95)00787-3 PMID:8788747

Parisod, H., Axelin, A., Smed, J., & Salanterä, S. (2016). Determinants of tobacco-related health literacy: A qualitative study with early adolescents. *International Journal of Nursing Studies*, *62*, 71–80. doi:10.1016/j.ijnurstu.2016.07.012 PMID:27459318

Parker, I. (2004). The gift: Zell Kravinsky gave away millions: but somehow it wasn't enough. *The New Yorker*, *2*, 54-63.

Parker, R., & Ratzan, S. C. (2010). Health Literacy: A Second Decade of Distinction for Americans. *Journal of Health Communication*, *15*(sup2), 20–33.

Parker, R. M., Baker, D. W., Williams, M. V., & Nurss, J. R. (1995). The test of functional health literacy in adults: A new instrument for measuring patients' literacy skills. *Journal of General Internal Medicine*, *10*(10), 537–541. doi:10.1007/BF02640361 PMID:8576769

Parker, R., & Kreps, G. L. (2005). Library outreach: Overcoming health literacy challenges. *Journal of the Medical Library Association: JMLA*, *93*(4), S81–S85. PMID:16239962

Park, K., Moon, J. I., Kim, S. I., & Kim, Y. S. (1999). Exchange donor program in kidney transplantation. *Transplantation*, *67*(2), 336–338. doi:10.1097/00007890-199901270-00027 PMID:10075605

Parnell, T. A. (2014). Nurse leader strategies, health literacy, and patient outcomes. *Nurse Leader*, *12*(6), 49–52. doi:10.1016/j.mnl.2014.09.005

Parnell, T. A. (2015). *Health Literacy in Nursing: Providing Person-Centered Care*. New York, NY: Springer Publishing Company.

Partners in Prolepsis: Institute of Preventive Medicine Environmental and Occupational Health. (2013). *Diatrofi*. Retrieved from http://diatrofi.prolepsis.gr/en/

Partners in Prolepsis: Institute of Preventive Medicine Environmental and Occupational Health. (n.d.). *IROHLA – Intervention Research on Health Literacy among Ageing Population*. Retrieved from http://www.prolepsis.gr/new/en/Projects/39/IROHLA---Intervention-Research-on-Health-Literacy-among-Ageing.html

Partners in Prolepsis: Institute of Preventive Medicine Environmental and Occupational Health. (n.d.a). *Mig-HealthCare*. Retrieved from http://www.prolepsis.gr/new/en/Projects/50/Mig-HealthCare:-Strengthen-Community-Based-Care-to-minimize-health-inequalities.html

Partners in Prolepsis: Institute of Preventive Medicine Environmental and Occupational Health. (n.d.b). *Program on Food Aid and Nutrition Education – DIATROFI: Implemented in Remote and Rural Areas*. Retrieved from http://www.prolepsis.gr/new/en/Projects/44/Program-on-Food-Aid-and-Nutrition-Education---DIATROFI.html

Partners in Prolepsis: Institute of Preventive Medicine Environmental and Occupational Health. (n.d.c). *Who we are*. Retrieved from http://www.prolepsis.gr/new/en/Content/2/8/Who-we-are.html

Patrick, D. L., Burke, L. B., Gwaltney, C. J., Leidy, N. K., Martin, M. L., Molsen, E., & Ring, L. (2011). Content validity--establishing and reporting the evidence in newly developed patient-reported outcomes (PRO) instruments for medical product evaluation: ISPOR PRO Good Research Practices Task Force report: part 2--assessing respondent understanding. *Value in Health*, *14*(8), 978–988. doi:10.1016/j.jval.2011.06.013 PMID:22152166

Payer, L. (1996). *Medicine and Culture: Varieties of Treatment in the United States, England, West Germany, and France* (Rev. ed.). New York, NY: First Owl Books Edition.

Pbert, L., Druker, S., Barton, B., Schneider, K. L., Olendzki, B., Gapinski, M. A., ... Osganian, S. (2016). A School-Based Program for Overweight and Obese Adolescents: A Randomized Controlled Trial. *The Journal of School Health, 86*(10), 699–708. doi:10.1111/josh.12428 PMID:27619760

Peerson, A., & Saunders, M. (2009). Health literacy revisited: What do we mean and why does it matter? *Health Promotion International, 24*(3), 285–296. doi:10.1093/heapro/dap014 PMID:19372101

Peters, L., & Paulussen, T. (1994). *School Health: A Review of the Effectiveness of Health Education and Health Promotion.* Utrecht: Dutch Centre for Health Promotion.

Peterson, F. L., Cooper, R. J., & Laird, J. A. (2001). Enhancing Teacher Health Literacy in School Health Promotion A Vision for the New Millennium. *The Journal of School Health, 71*(4), 138–144. doi:10.1111/j.1746-1561.2001.tb01311.x PMID:11354982

Peterson, U., Demerouti, E., Bergström, G., Samuelsson, M., Åsberg, M., & Nygren, Å. (2008). Burnout and physical and mental health among Swedish healthcare workers. *Journal of Advanced Nursing, 62*(1), 84–95. doi:10.1111/j.1365-2648.2007.04580.x PMID:18352967

Petrie, N. (2015). *Future Trends in Leadership Development.* Retrieved from: http://www.ccl.org/wp-content/uploads/2015/04/futureTrends.pdf

Pickard, A. S., Neary, M. P., & Cella, D. (2007). Estimation of minimally important differences in EQ-5D utility and VAS scores in cancer. *Health and Quality of Life Outcomes, 5*(1), 70–70. doi:10.1186/1477-7525-5-70 PMID:18154669

Pickering, C. (2014). Ferguson to implement kidney transplant policy. *WiredJa Online News.* Retrieved from http://www.wiredja.com/sci-tech-health/health/kidney-transplant-policy-coming

Pierce, E. G., & Pierce, R. A. (1973). The agony and the ecstasy. *Transplantation Proceedings, 5*, 1067–1068. PMID:4579042

Pignone, M., DeWalt, D. A., Sheridan, S., Berkman, N., & Lohr, K. N. (2005). Interventions to improve health outcomes for patients with low literacy. *Journal of General Internal Medicine, 20*(2), 185–192. doi:10.1111/j.1525-1497.2005.40208.x PMID:15836553

Plain Language Association International (PLAIN). (2011). Retrieved May 10, 2017 from http://plainlanguagenetwork.org/plain-language/what-is-plain-language/

Plant, W. D., Akyol, M. A., & Rudge, C. J. (2002). *The ethical dimension to organ transplantation in transplantation surgery* (J. L. R. Forsythe, Ed.; 2nd ed.). WB Saunders London.

Pleasant, A., & Kuruvilla, S. (2008). A tale of two health literacies: Public health and clinical approaches to health literacy. *Health Promotion International, 23*(2), 152–159. doi:10.1093/heapro/dan001 PMID:18223203

Pleasant, A., Rudd, R. E., O'Leary, C., Paasche-Orlow, M. K., Allen, M. P., Alvarado-Little, W., ... Rosen, S. (2016). *Considerations for a new definition of health literacy. Discussion Paper.* Washington, DC: National Academy of Medicine. Retrieved from http://nam.edu/wp-content/uploads/2016/04/Considerations-for-a-New-Definition-ofHealth-Literacy.pdf

Porter, M. E., Larsson, S., & Lee, T. H. (2016). Standardizing Patient Outcomes Measurement. *The New England Journal of Medicine, 374*(6), 504–506. doi:10.1056/NEJMp1511701 PMID:26863351

Powell, C. K., Hill, E. G., & Clancy, D. E. (2007). The relationship between health literacy and diabetes knowledge and readiness to take health actions. *The Diabetes Educator, 33*(1), 144–151. doi:10.1177/0145721706297452 PMID:17272800

Pradel, F. G., Mullins, C. D., & Bartlett, S. T. (2003). Exploring donors' and recipients' attitudes about living donor kidney transplantation. *Progress in Transplantation (Aliso Viejo, Calif.)*, *13*(3), 203–210. doi:10.1177/152692480301300307 PMID:14558635

Praksis. (n.d.). *About Praksis*. Retrieved from https://www.praksis.gr/en/about-praksis

Pramana, G., Parmanto, B., Kendall, P. C., & Silk, J. S. (2014). The SmartCAT: An m-health platform for ecological momentary intervention in child anxiety treatment. *Telemedicine Journal and e-Health*, *20*(5), 419–427. doi:10.1089/tmj.2013.0214 PMID:24579913

Pratt, M., & Searles, G. E. (2017). Using visual aids to enhance physician-patient discussions and increase health literacy. *Journal of Cutaneous Medicine and Surgery*, *21*(6), 497–501. doi:10.1177/1203475417715208 PMID:28614954

Price, D. (2000a). *Legal and ethical aspects of organ transplantation*. Cambridge University Press.

Price, D. (2000b). Informed consent. In *Legal and Ethical Aspects of Organ Transplantation*. Cambridge, UK: Cambridge University Press.

Price, D. (2009). *Human tissue in transplantation and research: A model legal and ethical donation framework*. Cambridge University Press. doi:10.1017/CBO9781139195652

Prior, D. (2006). Efficiency and total quality management in health care organizations: A dynamic frontier approach. *Annals of Operations Research*, *145*(1), 281–299. doi:10.100710479-006-0035-6

Protheroe, J., Nutbeam, D., & Rowlands, G. (2009). Health literacy: A necessity for increasing participation in health care. *The British Journal of General Practice*, *59*(567), 721–723. doi:10.3399/bjgp09X472584 PMID:19843420

Pruett, T. L., Tibell, A., Alabdulkareem, A., Bhandari, M., Cronin, D. C., Dew, M. A., ... Delmonico, F. L. (2006). The ethics statement of the Vancouver Forum on the Live Lung, Liver, Pancreas, and Intestine Donor. *Transplantation*, *81*(10), 1386–1387. doi:10.1097/01.tp.0000214976.36526.e3 PMID:16732173

Public Broadcasting System (PBS). (2017). *Health crisis: the uninsured*. Retrieved from http://www.pbs.org/healthcarecrisis/uninsured.html

Public Health Association of British Columbia. (2012). An inter-sectoral approach for improving health literacy for Canadians. A discussion paper. Victoria: Author.

Public Law 111-148. (2010). *The American Recovery and Reinvestment Act (ARRA)*. Retrieved from: www.gpo.gov/fdsys/pkg/PLAW-111publ148/pdf/PLAW-111publ148.pdf

Public Law 111-5. Medicaid.gov. (n.d.). *Affordable Care Act*. Retrieved from: http://www.gpo.gov/fdsys/pkg/PLAW-111publ148/pdf/PLAW-111publ148.pdfPublic Law 111-5.

Query, J. L. Jr, & Kreps, G. L. (1996). Testing a relational model for health communication competence among caregivers for individuals with Alzheimer's disease. *Journal of Health Psychology*, *1*(3), 335–351. doi:10.1177/135910539600100307 PMID:22011996

Quick, B. L., Kim, D. K., & Meyer, K. (2009). A 15-year review of ABC, CBS, and NBC news coverage of organ donation: Implications for organ donation campaigns. *Health Communication*, *24*(2), 137–145. doi:10.1080/10410230802676516 PMID:19280457

Quinn, S., Bond, R., & Nugent, C. (2017). Quantifying health literacy and eHealth literacy using existing instruments and browser-based software for tracking online health information seeking behavior. *Computers in Human Behavior*, *69*, 256–267. doi:10.1016/j.chb.2016.12.032

Radcliffe-Richards, J., Daar, A. S., Guttmann, R. D., Hoffenberg, R., Kennedy, I., Lock, M., … Tilney, N. (1998). The case for allowing kidney sales. International Forum for Transplant Ethics. *Lancet*, *27*, 1950-2.

Ralph, A., Chapman, J. R., Gillis, J., Craig, J. C., Butow, P., Howard, K., ... Tong, A. (2014). Family perspectives on deceased organ donation: Thematic synthesis of qualitative studies. *American Journal of Transplantation*, *14*(4), 923–935. doi:10.1111/ajt.12660 PMID:24612855

Randhawa, G., & Neuberger, J. (2011). Role of religion in organ donation - development of the United Kingdom faith and organ donation action plan. *Transplantation Proceedings*, *48*(3), 689–694. doi:10.1016/j.transproceed.2015.10.074 PMID:27234715

Rapaport, F. T. (1986). The case for a living emotionally related international kidney donor exchange registry. *Transplantation Proceedings*, *18*, 5–9. PMID:11649919

Ratzan, S. C. (2001). Health literacy: Communication for the public good. *Health Promotion International*, *16*(2), 207–214. doi:10.1093/heapro/16.2.207 PMID:11356759

Ratzan, S. C. (2016). Effective decision-making: A negotiation perspective for Health Psychology and Health Communication. *Journal of Health Psychology*, *1*(3), 323–333. doi:10.1177/135910539600100306 PMID:22011995

Ratzan, S. C., & Parker, R. M. (2000). Introduction. In C. R. Selden, M. Zorn, S. C. Ratzan, & R. M. Parker (Eds.), *National Library of Medicine current bibliographies in medicine: Health literacy. NLM Pub. No. CBM 2000-1*. Bethesda, MD: National Institutes of Health, U.S. Department of Health and Human Services.

Raynor, D. K., (2012). Health literacy – Is it time to shift our focus from patient to provider? *British Medical Journal*. doi:102236/bmj.e2188

Ready, R., Nath, J., Milford, D., Adu, D., & Jewitt-Harris, J. (2016). Establishing sustainable kidney transplantation programmes in developing world countries: A 10-year experience. *Kidney International*, *90*(5), 916–920. doi:10.1016/j.kint.2016.08.024 PMID:27742191

Reed, G. E. (2006). *Leadership and Systems Thinking*. Defense AT&L. Retrieved from: www.au.af.mil/au/awc/awcgate/dau/ree_mj06.pdf

Reese, P. P., Caplan, A. L., Kesselheim, A. S., & Bloom, R. D. (2006). Creating a medical, ethical, and legal framework for complex living kidney donors. *Clinical Journal of the American Society of Nephrology; CJASN*, *1*(6), 1148–1153. doi:10.2215/CJN.02180606 PMID:17699340

Rees, M. A., Kopke, J. E., Pelletier, R. P., Segev, D. L., Rutter, M. E., Fabrega, A. J., ... Montgomery, R. A. (2009). A nonsimultaneous, extended, altruistic-donor chain. *The New England Journal of Medicine*, *360*(11), 1096–1101. doi:10.1056/NEJMoa0803645 PMID:19279341

Reeve, C. L., & Basalik, D. (2014). Is health literacy an example of construct proliferation? A conceptual and empirical evaluation of its redundancy with general cognitive ability. *Intelligence*, *44*(1), 93–102. doi:10.1016/j.intell.2014.03.004

References for Business. (n.d.). *Electronic Data Interchange (EDI) eCommerce Fulfillment*. Retrieved from: http://www.referenceforbusiness.com/encyclopedia/Eco-Ent/Electronic-Data-Interchange-EDI.html

Regional Office for Europe, World Health Organization. (2014). WHO European Healthy Cities Network Phase VI 2018) of the WHO European Healthy Cities Network: Goals and requirements. Copenhagen: Author.

Rego, A. (2016). *Comunicação pessoal e organizacional*. Lisboa: Sílabo.

Revicki, D., Hays, R. D., Cella, D., & Sloan, J. (2008). Recommended methods for determining responsiveness and minimally important differences for patient-reported outcomes. *Journal of Clinical Epidemiology*, *61*(2), 102–109. doi:10.1016/j.jclinepi.2007.03.012 PMID:18177782

Revolvy. (2017). *Urbanization*. Retrieved June 17, 2017, from https://www.revolvy.com/main/index.php?s=Urbanization

Reychav, I., & Azuri, J. (2016). Including elderly patients in decision making via electronic health literacy. In M. Cruz-Cunha, I. Miranda, R. Martinho, & R. Rijo (Eds.), *Encyclopedia of e-health and telemedicine* (pp. 241–249). Hershey, PA: IGI Global. doi:10.4018/978-1-4666-9978-6.ch020

Reynolds, L. T., & Herman-Kinney, N. J. (2003). *Handbook of symbolic interactionism*. Walnut Creek, CA: AltaMira.

Roberson, N. L. (1994). Clinical trial participation: Viewpoints from racial/ethnic groups. *Cancer*, *74*(S9), 2687–2691. doi:10.1002/1097-0142(19941101)74:9+<2687::AID-CNCR28207418173.0.CO;2-B PMID:7954287

Rodrigue, J. R., Paek, M. J., Egbuna, O., Waterman, A. D., Schold, J. D., Pavlakis, M., & Mandelbrot, D. A. (n.d.). *Making house calls increases living donor inquiries and evaluations for blacks on the kidney transplant waiting list*. Retrieved on 24 May 2017 from https://www.ncbi.nlm.nih.gov/pmc/articles/PMC4218873/

Rogers, R., & Ellen, J. (n.d.). *Mining your Data for Health Care Quality Improvement*. Retrieved from: http://www2.sas.com/proceedings/sugi22/EMERGING/PAPER139.PDF

Roh, Y. H., Lee, B. K., Park, M. H., Noh, J. H., Gong, H. S., & Baek, G. H. (2016). Effects of health literacy on treatment outcome and satisfaction in patients with mallet finger injury. *Journal of Hand Therapy*, *29*(4), 459–464. doi:10.1016/j.jht.2016.06.004 PMID:27765527

Roodnat, J. I., Zuidema, W., van de Wetering, J., de Klerk, M., Erdman, R. A., Massey, E. K., ... Weimar, W. (2010). Altruistic donor triggered domino-paired kidney donation for unsuccessful couples from the kidney-exchange program. *American Journal of Transplantation*, *10*(4), 821–827. doi:10.1111/j.1600-6143.2010.03034.x PMID:20199504

Root, J., & Stablefod, S. (1998). Easy-to-read consumer communications: A missing link in Medicaid managed care. *Journal of Health Politics, Policy and Law*, *24*(1), 1–26. doi:10.1215/03616878-24-1-1 PMID:10342253

Rootman, I. (2002). *Health literacy and health promotion*. Ontario: Ontario Health Promotion E-Bulletin.

Rootman, I. (2003). Literacy and health in Canada: Is it really a problem? *Canadian Journal of Public Health*, *94*(6), 405–406. PMID:14700236

Rose, I. D., & Friedman, D. B. (2017). Schools. *The Journal of School Nursing*, *33*(2), 109–115. doi:10.1177/1059840516678910 PMID:28288553

Rosenbach, M., Lake, T., Williams, S. R., & Buck, J. (2009). Implementation of mental health parity: Lessons from California. *Psychiatric Services (Washington, D.C.)*, *60*(12), 1589–1594. doi:10.1176/ps.2009.60.12.1589 PMID:19952147

Rosenbaum, S. (2011). The Patient Protection and Affordable Care Act: Implications for Public Health Policy and Practice. *Public Health Reports*, *126*(1), 130–135. doi:10.1177/003335491112600118 PMID:21337939

Rosenblum, A. M., Horvat, L. D., Siminoff, L. A., Prakash, V., Beitel, J., & Garg, A. X. (2012). The authority of next-of-kin in explicit and presumed consent systems for deceased organ donation: An analysis of 54 nations. *Nephrology, Dialysis, Transplantation*, *27*(6), 2533–2546. doi:10.1093/ndt/gfr619 PMID:22121233

Ross, L. F. (2000). Donating a second kidney: A tale of family and ethics. *Seminars in Dialysis*, *13*(3), 201–203. doi:10.1046/j.1525-139x.2000.00054.x PMID:10833782

Ross, L. F., Glannon, W., & Josephson, M. A. (2002). Should all living donors be treated equally? *Transplantation, 74*(3), 418–421. doi:10.1097/00007890-200208150-00025 PMID:12177627

Ross, L. F., Rubin, D. T., Siegler, M., Josephson, M. A., Thistlethwaite, J. R. Jr, & Woodle, E. S. (1997). Ethics of a paired-kidney-exchange program. *The New England Journal of Medicine, 336*(24), 1752–1755. doi:10.1056/NEJM199706123362412 PMID:9180096

Ross, L. F., Siegler, M., & Thistlethwaite, J. R. Jr. (2007). We need a registry of living kidney donors. *The Hastings Center Report, 7*, 1. PMID:18179104

Ross, L. F., & Thistlethwaite, J. R. Jr. (2008a). Minors as Living Solid-Organ Donors. *Pediatrics, 122*(2), 454–461. doi:10.1542/peds.2008-1525 PMID:18676567

Rowlands, G., Protheroe, J., Price, H., & Rafi, I. (2014). *Health literacy report from an RCGP-led health literacy workshop*. London: Royal College of General Practitioners.

Rowlands, G., Protheroe, J., Winkley, J., Richardson, M., Seed, P., & Rudd, R. (2015). A mismatch between population health literacy and the complexity of health information: An observational study. *The British Journal of General Practice, 65*(635), 296–297. doi:10.3399/bjgp15X685285 PMID:26009533

Royal College of Physicians. (2015 March). *Work and wellbeing in the NHS: why staff health matters to patient care.* Retrieved from https://www.rcplondon.ac.uk/guidelines-policy/work-and-wellbeing-nhs-why-staff-health-matters-patient-care

Rudd, R. E., & Anderson, J. E. (2006). *The health literacy environment of hospitals and health centers*. Harvard School of Public Health. Retrieved May 11, 2017 from https://cdn1.sph.harvard.edu/wp-content/uploads/sites/135/2012/09/healthliteracyenvironment.pdf

Rudd, R. (2010). Improving Americans' health literacy. *The New England Journal of Medicine, 363*(24), 2283–2285. doi:10.1056/NEJMp1008755 PMID:21142532

Rudd, R. E. (2002). A maturing partnership. *Focus on Basics, 5*(c), 1–8.

Ruffin, T. R. (2015). Health Information Technology and Business Process Reengineering. In M. Khosrow-Pour (Ed.), Encyclopedia of Information Science and Technology (3rd ed.; pp. 3355–3365). Hershey, PA: IGI Global. doi:10.4018/978-1-4666-5888-2.ch329

Rungapadiachy, D. M. (1999). *Interpersonal communication and psychology for health care professionals: Theory and practice*. Edinburgh, UK: Butterworth-Heinemann.

Russell, C., & Kuhnert, K. (1992). Integrating skill acquisition and perspective-taking capacity in the development of leaders. *The Leadership Quarterly, 3*, 109–135. doi:10.1016/1048-9843(92)90029-F

Ryan, P., & Morgan, S. (2004). *Assertive outreach: A strengths approach to policy and practice*. London: Churchill Livingstone.

Ryan, R. R., & Deci, E. L. (2000). Intrinsic and extrinsic motivations: Classic definitions and new directions. *Contemporary Educational Psychology, 25*(1), 54–67. doi:10.1006/ceps.1999.1020 PMID:10620381

Ryan, R., Prictor, M., McLaughlin, K. J., & Hill, S. (2008). Audio-visual presentation of information for informed consent for participation in clinical trials. *The Cochrane Library*, 1. PMID:18254029

Rykhoff, M. E., Coupland, C., Dionne, J., Fudge, B., Gayle, C., Ortner, T. L., ... Wrobleska, M. (2010). A clinical group's attempt to raise awareness of organ and tissue donation. *Progress in Transplantation (Aliso Viejo, Calif.)*, *20*(1), 33–39. doi:10.1177/152692481002000106 PMID:20397344

Saboga-Nunes, L., Sørensen, K., & Pelikan, J. M. (2014). *Hermenêutica da literacia em saúde e sua avaliação em Portugal (HLS-EU-PT)*. Paper presented at the VIII Congresso Português de Sociologia, Évora, Portugal. Retrieved June 10, 2017, from http://www.aps.pt/viii_congresso/VIII_ACTAS/VIII_COM0526.pdf

Safeer, R. S., & Keenan, J. (2005). Health literacy: The gap between physicians and patients. *American Family Physician*, *72*(3), 463–468. PMID:16100861

Salomon, D. R., Langnas, A. N., Reed, A. I., Bloom, R. D., Magee, J. C., & Gaston, R. S(2015). AST/ASTS workshop on increasing organ donation in the United States: Creating an "arc of change" from removing disincentives to testing incentives. *American Journal of Transplantation*, *15*(5), 1173–1179. doi:10.1111/ajt.13233 PMID:25833653

Salter, A. (1949). *Conditioned reflex theory*. New York: Creative Age Press.

Salter, A. (2002). *Conditioned reflex therapy: The classic book on assertiveness that began behavior therapy*. Gretna, LA: Wellness Institute.

Salvatierra, O. Jr. (2001). Transplant physicians bear full responsibility for the consequences of kidney donation by a minor. *American Journal of Transplantation*, *2*(4), 297–298. doi:10.1034/j.1600-6143.2002.20402.x PMID:12118849

Samsa, G., Edelman, D., Rothman, M. L., Williams, G. R., Lipscomb, J., & Matchar, D. (1999). Determining clinically important differences in health status measures: A general approach with illustration to the Health Utilities Index Mark II. *PharmacoEconomics*, *15*(2), 141–155. doi:10.2165/00019053-199915020-00003 PMID:10351188

Sandiford, P. J., Cassel, M., & Sanchez, G. (1995). The impact of women's literacy on child health and its interaction with access to health services. *Population Studies*, *49*(1), 5–17. doi:10.1080/0032472031000148216

Sarkar, U., Karter, A. J., Liu, J. Y., Adler, N. E., Nguyen, R., López, A., & Schillinger, D. (2011). Social disparities in internet patient portal use in diabetes: evidence that the digital divide extends beyond access. *Journal of the American Medical Informatics Association, 18*(3), 318-321. doi:.10.1136/jamia.2010.006015

Sarkar, U., Karter, A. J., Liu, J. Y., Moffet, H. H., Adler, N. E., & Schillinger, D. (2010). Hypoglycemia is more common among type 2 diabetes patients with limited health literacy: The Diabetes Study of Northern California (DISTANCE). *Journal of General Internal Medicine*, *25*(9), 962–967. doi:10.100711606-010-1389-7 PMID:20480249

Save the Children. (2000). *State of the World's Mothers*. Westport, CT: Save the Children.

Sawyerr, A., & Bagley, C. (2017). Child Sexual Abuse and Adolescent and Adult Adjustment : A Review of British and World Evidence, with Implications for Social Work, and Mental Health and School Counselling. *Advances in Applied Sociology*, *7*(01), 15. doi:10.4236/aasoci.2017.71001

Sayah, F. A., & Williams, B. (2012). An integrated model of health literacy using diabetes as an exemplar. *Canadian Journal of Diabetes*, *36*(1), 27–31. doi:10.1016/j.jcjd.2011.08.001

Schachter, H. M., Girardi, A., Ly, M., Lacroix, D., Lumb, A. B., van Berkom, J., & Gill, R. (2008). Effects of school-based interventions on mental health stigmatization: A systematic review. *Child and Adolescent Psychiatry and Mental Health*, *2*(1), 18. doi:10.1186/1753-2000-2-18 PMID:18644150

Schillinger, D., Bindman, A., Wang, F., Stewart, A., & Piette, J. (2004). Functional health literacy and the quality of physician-patient communication among diabetes patients. *Patient Education and Counseling*, *52*(3), 315–323. doi:10.1016/S0738-3991(03)00107-1 PMID:14998602

Schillinger, D., Grumbach, K., Piette, J., Wang, F., Osmond, D., Daher, C., ... Bindman, A. B. (2002). Association of health literacy with diabetes outcomes. *Journal of the American Medical Association*, *288*(4), 475–482. doi:10.1001/jama.288.4.475 PMID:12132978

Schillinger, D., & Keller, D. (2013). The other side of the coin: Attributes of a health literate health care organization. In L. M. Hernandez (Ed.), *How can health care organizations become more health literate? workshop summary* (pp. 69–96). Washington, DC: National Academy Press.

Schillinger, D., Piette, J., Grumbach, K., Wang, F., Wilson, C., Daher, C., ... Bindman, A. B. (2003). Closing the Loop: Physician Communication With Diabetic Patients Who Have Low Health Literacy. *Archives of Internal Medicine*, *163*(1), 83–90. doi:10.1001/archinte.163.1.83 PMID:12523921

Schirmer, M., Mauksch, L., Lang, F., Marvel, K., Zoppi, K., Epstein, R. M., ... Pryzbylski, M. (2005). Assessing communication competence: A review of current tools. *Family Medicine*, *37*(3), 184–192. PMID:15739134

Schroen, A. T., Petroni, G. R., Wang, H., Gray, R., Wang, X. F., Cronin, W., & ... . (2010). Preliminary evaluation of factors associated with premature trial closure and feasibility of accrual benchmarks in phase III oncology trials. *Clinical Trials*, *7*(4), 312–321. doi:10.1177/1740774510374973 PMID:20595245

Schulz, P. J., & Nakamoto, K. (2013). Patient behavior and the benefits of artificial intelligence: The perils of "dangerous" literacy and illusory patient empowerment. *Patient Education and Counseling*, *92*(2), 223–228. doi:10.1016/j.pec.2013.05.002 PMID:23743214

Schwartzberg, J. G., VanGeest, J., & Wang, C. (2005). *Understanding health literacy: Implications for medicine and public health.* American Medical Association.

Schwartz, L. M., Woloshin, S., Black, W. C., & Welch, H. G. (1997). The role of numeracy in understanding the benefit of screening mammography. *Annals of Internal Medicine*, *127*(11), 966–972. doi:10.7326/0003-4819-127-11-199712010-00003 PMID:9412301

Scott, T. L., Gazmararian, J. A., Williams, M. V., & Baker, D. W. (2002). Health literacy and preventive health care use among Medicare enrollees in a managed care organization. *Medical Care*, *40*(5), 395–404. doi:10.1097/00005650-200205000-00005 PMID:11961474

Selden, C. R., Zorn, M., Ratzan, S., & Parker, R. M. (2000). *National Library of Medicine current bibliographies in medicine: Health literacy.* Retrieved from https://www.researchgate.net/profile/Marcia_Zorn/publication/230877250_National_Library_of_Medicine_Current_Bibliographies_in_Medicine_Health_Literacy/links/56794b7408ae6041cb49f348/National-Library-of-Medicine-Current-Bibliographies-in-Medicine-Health-Literacy.pdf

Sen, A. (1999). *Development as Freedom.* Oxford, UK: Oxford University Press.

Serper, M., Patzer, R. E., Curtis, L. M., Smith, S. G., O'Conor, R., Baker, D. W., & Wolf, M. S. (2014). Health literacy, cognitive ability, and functional health status among older adults. *Health Services Research*, *49*(4), 1249–1267. doi:10.1111/1475-6773.12154 PMID:24476068

Seymour, M. (Presenter). (2002). *The Method and the Magic: Ethics and Information Management.* CASE District VII Conference, Anaheim, CA. Retrieved from: http://www.usc.edu/dept/source/HIPPA.html

Sharma, S. V., Chow, J., Pomeroy, M., Raber, M., Salako, D., & Markham, C. (2017). Lessons Learned From the Implementation of Brighter Bites: A Food Co-op to Increase Access to Fruits and Vegetables and Nutrition Education Among Low-Income Children and Their Families. *The Journal of School Health*, *87*(4), 286–295. doi:10.1111/josh.12497 PMID:28260244

Shaw, D., Georgieva, D., Haase, B., Gardiner, D., Lewis, P., Jansen, N., ... Ploeg, R. (2017). Family over rules? an ethical analysis of allowing families to overrule donation intentions. *Transplantation*, *101*(3), 482–487. doi:10.1097/TP.0000000000001536 PMID:27764030

Shen, B.S.P. (1975). Science Literacy and the Public Understanding of Science. *Communication of Scientific Information*. 45-52. 10.1159/000398072

Shimazono, Y. (2007). *The state of the international organ trade: a provisional picture based on integration of available information.* Retrieved from http://www.who.int/bulletin/volumes/85/12/06-039370/en/

Silverman, J., Krutz, S., & Draper, J. (2013). *Skills for communicating with patients.* Boca Raton, FL: Taylor & Francis Group.

Siminoff, L. A., Zhang, A., Colabianchi, N., Sturm, C. M. S., & Shen, Q. (2000). Factors that predict the referral of breast cancer patients onto clinical trials by their surgeons and medical oncologists. *Journal of Clinical Oncology*, *18*(6), 1203–1211. doi:10.1200/JCO.2000.18.6.1203 PMID:10715289

Simmons, R. G., Marine, S. K., & Simmons, R. L. (1987). *Gift of Life. The Effect of Organ Transplantation on Individual, Family, and Societal Dynamics*. New Brunswick, NJ: Transaction Books.

Simmons, R. G., Marine, S. K., & Simmons, R. L. (1987). *Gift of life: the effect of organ transplantation on individual, family, and societal dynamics* (2nd ed.). New Brunswick, NJ: Transaction Publishers.

Simou, E., & Koutsogeorgou, E. (2014). Effects of the economic crisis on health and healthcare in Greece in the literature from 2009 to 2013: A systematic review. *Health Policy (Amsterdam)*, *115*(2-3), 111–119. doi:10.1016/j.healthpol.2014.02.002 PMID:24589039

Sinclair, S., Hayes-Reams, P., Myers, H. F., Allen, W., Hawes-Dawson, J., & Kington, R. (2000). Recruitment African Americans for health studies: Lessons From the Drew-Rand Center on Health and Aging. *Journal of Mental Health and Aging*, *6*(1), 39.

Sixsmith, J., & O'Shea, G. (2016). Health Literacy for Healthy Cities (HL4HC). Galway, Ireland: Academic Press.

Sixsmith, J., Doyle, P., D'Eath, M., & Barry, M.M. (2014). *Health communication and its role in the prevention and control of communicable diseases in Europe: Current evidence, practices and future developments.* European Centre for Disease Prevention and Control (ECDC Technical Report).

Skills for Life. (2003). *The Skills for Life survey: A national needs and impact survey of literacy, numeracy and ICT skills.* Author.

Skinner, H. A. (2002). What motivates people to change? In H. A. Skinner (Ed.), *Promoting health through organizational change* (pp. 113–146). San Francisco, CA: Benjamin Cummings.

Smith, J. L., & Haggerty, J. (2003). Literacy in primary care: Is it a problem? *Canadian Journal of Public Health*, *94*(6), 408–412. PMID:14700237

Smith, M. D., Kappell, D. F., Province, M. A., Hong, B. A., Robson, A. M., Dutton, S., ... Cameron, E. (1986). Living-related kidney donors: A multicenter study of donor education, socioeconomic adjustment, and rehabilitation. *American Journal of Kidney Diseases*, *8*(4), 223–233. doi:10.1016/S0272-6386(86)80030-0 PMID:3532770

Smith, M. J. (1985). *When I say no, I feel guilty*. New York: Bantam Books.

Smith, S. G., Curtis, L. M., Wardle, J., von Wagner, C., & Wolf, M. S. (2013). Skill Set or Mind Set? Associations between Health Literacy, Patient Activation and Health. *PLoS One*, *8*(9), e74373. doi:10.1371/journal.pone.0074373 PMID:24023942

Snowdown, A. (2015). Enhancing patient experience through personalization of health services. *Healthcare Management Forum*, *28*(5), 182–185. doi:10.1177/0840470415588656 PMID:26135292

Society for Human Resource Management (SHRM). (2015). *Leadership Competencies*. Retrieved from: http://www.shrm.org/research/articles/articles/pages/leadershipcompetencies.aspx

Somerville, M. (1979). *The duty to inform the patient or research subject for the purpose of obtaining "informed" consent. Consent to medical care*. Ottawa, Canada: Law Reform Commission of Canada.

Sorensen, K. (2013). *Health literacy: a neglected European public health disparity*. Maastricht: Universitaire Pers Maastricht.

Sørensen, K., & Brand, H. (2011). Health literacy: The essential catalyst for the responsible and effective translation of genome-based information for the benefit of population health. *Public Health Genomics*, *14*(4–5), 195–200. doi:10.1159/000324241 PMID:21734433

Sørensen, K., Pelikan, J. M., Röthlin, F., Ganahl, K., Slonska, Z., Doyle, G., ... Schyve, P. (2015). Health literacy in Europe: Comparative results of the European health literacy survey (HLS-EU). *European Journal of Public Health*, *25*(6), 1053–1058. doi:10.1093/eurpub/ckv043 PMID:25843827

Sorensen, K., Van den Broucke, S., Fullam, J., Doyle, G., Pelikan, J., Slonska, Z., & Brand, H. (2012). Health literacy and public health: A systematic review and integration of definitions and models. *BMC Public Health*, *12*(1), 80. doi:10.1186/1471-2458-12-80 PMID:22276600

Sørensen, K., Van den Broucke, S., Pelikan, J. M., Fullam, J., Doyle, G., Slonska, Z., ... Brand, H. (2013). Measuring health literacy in populations: Illuminating the design and the development process of the European Health Literacy Survey Questionnaire (HLS-EU-Q). *BMC Public Health*, *13*(1), 1–22. doi:10.1186/1471-2458-13-948 PMID:24112855

Spital, A. (1997). Should children ever donate kidneys? Views of U.S. transplant centers. *Transplantation*, *64*(2), 232–236. doi:10.1097/00007890-199707270-00009 PMID:9256179

Spital, A. (1998). When a stranger offers a kidney: Ethical issues in living organ donation. *American Journal of Kidney Diseases*, *32*(4), 676–691. doi:10.1016/S0272-6386(98)70037-X PMID:9774135

Spital, A. (2001). Ethical Issues in Living Organ Donation: Donor Autonomy and Beyond. *American Journal of Kidney Diseases*, *38*(1), 189–195. doi:10.1053/ajkd.2001.25213 PMID:11431202

Spital, A. (2001). Ethical issues in living related donors. In W. Shelton & J. Balint (Eds.), *The Ethics of Organ Transplantation*. New York, NY: Elsvier Science. doi:10.1016/S1479-3709(01)80008-X

Spital, A. (2004). Donor benefit is the key to justified living organ donation. *Cambridge Quarterly of Healthcare Ethics*, *13*(01), 105–109. doi:10.1017/S0963180104131174 PMID:15045922

Spivack, J. G., Swietlik, M., Alessandrini, E., & Faith, M. S. (2010). Primary care providers' knowledge, practices, and perceived barriers to the treatment and prevention of childhood obesity. *Obesity (Silver Spring, Md.)*, *18*(7), 1341–1347. doi:10.1038/oby.2009.410 PMID:19910934

St. Leger, L. (2001). Schools, health literacy and public health: Possibilities and challenges. *Health Promotion International*, *16*(2), 197–205. doi:10.1093/heapro/16.2.197 PMID:11356758

St. Leger, L., & Nutbeam, D. (2000). A model for mapping linkages between health and education agencies to improve school health. *The Journal of School Health*, *70*(2), 45–50. doi:10.1111/j.1746-1561.2000.tb07239.x PMID:10715824

Stableford, S., & Mettger, W. (2007). Plain Language: A Strategic Response to the Health Literacy Challenge. *Journal of Public Health Policy*, *28*(1), 71–93. doi:10.1057/palgrave.jphp.3200102 PMID:17363939

Stansfield, M. P. (1979). Malpractice: Toward a viable disclosure standard for informed consent. *Oklahoma Law Review*, *32*, 868–890. PMID:11665171

Steering Committee of the Istanbul Summit. (2008). Organ trafficking and transplant tourism and commercialism: The Declaration of Istanbul. *Lancet*, *372*(9632), 5–6. doi:10.1016/S0140-6736(08)60967-8 PMID:18603141

Steiner, R. W., & Gert, B. (2000). Ethical selection of living kidney donors. *American Journal of Kidney Diseases*, *36*(4), 677–686. doi:10.1053/ajkd.2000.17611 PMID:11007668

Stein, S., & Book, H. (2006). *The EQ edge: Emotional intelligence and your success.* Toronto: Jossey-Bass.

Steinwachs, D. M., & Hughes, R. G. (2008). Health Services Research: Scope and Significance. In *Patient Safety and Quality: An Evidence-Based Handbook for Nurses.* Rockville, MD: Agency for Healthcare Research and Quality (US). Retrieved from: http://www.ncbi.nlm.nih.gov/books/NBK2660

Stemple, J. C., & Hapner, E. R. (2014). *Voice therapy: Clinical case studies.* San Diego, CA: Plural Publishing.

Stewart, W., Ricci, J., Chee, E., Hahn, S., & Morganstein, D. (2003). Cost of Lost Worker Productive Work Time Among US Workers with Depression. *Journal of the American Medical Association*, *289*(23), 3135–3144. doi:10.1001/jama.289.23.3135 PMID:12813119

Stoke on Trent City Council. (2017). *Stoke on Trent City Council - Health Literacy on Vimeo.* Retrieved June 15, 2017, from https://vimeopro.com/inspiredfilm/stoke-on-trent-city-council-health-literacy

Stonbraker, S., Schnall, R., & Larson, E. (2015). Tools to measure health literacy among Spanish speakers: An integrative review of the literature. *Patient Education and Counseling*, *98*(12), 1513–1523. doi:10.1016/j.pec.2015.07.012 PMID:26227578

Stothers, L., Gourlay, W. A., & Liu, L. (2005). Attitudes and predictive factors for live kidney donation: A comparison of live kidney donors versus nondonors. *Kidney International*, *67*(3), 1105–1111. doi:10.1111/j.1523-1755.2005.00176.x PMID:15698451

Stott, D. J., Rodondi, N., Kearney, P. M., Ford, I., Westendorp, R. G., Mooijaart, S. P., ... Bauer, D. C. (2017). Thyroid hormone therapy for older adults with subclinical hypothyroidism. *The New England Journal of Medicine*, *376*(26), 2534–2544. doi:10.1056/NEJMoa1603825

Street, B. V. (Ed.). (1993). *Cross-cultural approaches to literacy.* Cambridge, UK: Cambridge University Press.

Sudore, R. L., & Schillinger, D. (2009). Interventions to improve care for patients with limited health literacy. *Journal of Clinical Outcomes Management: Journal of Clinical Outcomes*, *16*(1), 20. PMID:20046798

Sun, C. Y., Lee, C. C., Chang, C. T., Hung, C. C., & Wu, M. S. (2006). Commercial cadaveric renal transplant: An ethical rather than medical issue. *Clinical Transplantation*, *20*(3), 340–345. doi:10.1111/j.1399-0012.2006.00491.x PMID:16824152

Suri, V. R., Majid, S., Chang, Y. K., & Foo, S. (2016). Assessing the influence of health literacy on health information behaviors: A multi-domain skills-based approach. *Patient Education and Counseling*, *99*(6), 1038–1045. doi:10.1016/j.pec.2015.12.017 PMID:26794667

Tarlov, A. R., Ware, J. E. Jr, Greenfield, S., Nelson, E. C., Perrin, E., & Zubkoff, M. (1989). The Medical Outcomes Study. An application of methods for monitoring the results of medical care. *Journal of the American Medical Association, 262*(7), 925–930. doi:10.1001/jama.1989.03430070073033 PMID:2754793

Teixeira, J. A. C. (2004). *Comunicação em saúde: Relação técnicos de saúde – utentes*. Lisboa: Instituto Superior de Psicologia Aplicada.

Tench, R., & Konczos, M. (2013). Mapping European communication practitioners competencies: A review of the European communication professionals skills and innovation programme. *ECOPSI*, 35-64.

Terwee, C. B., Bot, S. D. M., de Boer, M. R., van der Windt, D. A. W. M., Knol, D. L., Dekker, J., ... de Vet, H. C. W. (2007). Quality criteria were proposed for measurement properties of health status questionnaires. *Journal of Clinical Epidemiology, 60*(1), 34–42. doi:10.1016/j.jclinepi.2006.03.012 PMID:17161752

The Declaration of Istanbul on organ trafficking and transplant tourism. (2008a). *Transplantation, 86*(8), 1013-1018. Retrieved from https://journals.lww.com/transplantjournal/Fulltext/2008/10270/The_Declaration_of_Istanbul_on_Organ_Trafficking.1.aspx

The Declaration of Istanbul on Organ Trafficking and Transplant Tourism. (2008b). Istanbul Summit April 30-May 2. *Nephrology, Dialysis, Transplantation, 23*, 3375. PMID:18922861

The Declaration of Istanbul on Organ Trafficking and Transplant Tourism. (2018). Retrieved from http://www.declarationofistanbul.org/

The Department of Health. (2013). Healthy Ireland. A framework for improved health and wellbeing 2013-2025. Dublin, Ireland: Author.

The European Network Against Racism. (2014). *Invisible visible minority – confronting Afrophobia and advancing equality for people of African descent and black Europeans in Europe*. Brussels: European Network Against Racism.

The Joint Commission, Division of Health Care Improvement (2016, November). Advancing patient-provider communication and activating patients. *Quick Safety,* (29).

The Joint Commission. (2010). *Advancing Effective Communication, Cultural Competence, and Patient- and Family-Centered Care: A Roadmap for Hospitals*. Oakbrook Terrace, IL: The Joint Commission.

The Joint Commission. (2010). *Frequently Asked Questions about Accrediting Hospitals in Accordance with their CMS' Certification Number (CCN).* Retrieved from: www.jointcommission.org/faqs_ccn/default.aspx

The Ohio State University-Office of Outreach & Engagement. (2008). *Health Literacy: It's Time To Take It Seriously!* AHEC Clear Health Communication Program.

The Sullivan Commission on Diversity in the Healthcare Workforce. (2004). *Missing persons: Minorities in the health professions*. Retrieved from http://www.aacn.nche.edu/Media/pdf/SullivanReport.pdf

Things Are Looking App. (2016, March 10). *The Economist.* Retrieved from https://www.economist.com/news/business/21694523-mobile-health-apps-are-becoming-more-capable-and-potentially-rather-useful-things-are-looking

Threlfall, J. M., Auslander, W., Gerke, D., Mcginnis, H., & Myers, S. (2017). Mental Health and School Functioning for Girls in the Child Welfare System : The Mediating Role of Future Orientation and School Engagement. *School Mental Health, 9*(2), 194–204. doi:10.100712310-017-9207-6 PMID:28572859

Thuong, M., Ruiz, A., Evrard, P., Kuiper, M., Boffa, C., Akhtar, M. Z., ... Ploeg, R. (2016). New classification of donation after circulatory death donors definitions and terminology. *Transplant International*, *29*(7), 749–759. doi:10.1111/tri.12776 PMID:26991858

Tieu, L. (2017). Online patient websites for electronic health record access among vulnerable populations: Portals to nowhere? *Journal of the American Medical Informatics Association*, *24*(e1), e47–e54. doi:10.1093/jamia/ocw098 PMID:27402138

Tones, K. (2002). Health literacy: New wine in old bottles? *Health Education Research*, *17*(3), 287–290. doi:10.1093/her/17.3.287 PMID:12120844

Transplant Links Community. (2017). Retrieved from http://www.transplantlinks.org

Trevena, L. J., Davey, H. M., Barratt, A., Butow, P., & Caldwell, P. (2006). A systematic review on communicating with patients about evidence. *Journal of Evaluation in Clinical Practice*, *12*(1), 13–23. doi:10.1111/j.1365-2753.2005.00596.x PMID:16422776

Truog, R. D. (2005). The ethics of organ donation by living donors. *The New England Journal of Medicine*, *353*(5), 444–446. doi:10.1056/NEJMp058155 PMID:16079366

Tsouros, A. (n.d.). City Leadership for Health and Well-being: Back to the Future. *Journal of Urban Health: Bulletin of the New York Academy of Medicine, 90*. 10.1007/s11524-013-9825-8

Tsouros, A. (2009). City leadership for health and sustainable development: The World Health Organization European Healthy Cities Network. *Health Promotion International*, *24*(Suppl 1), i4–i10. doi:10.1093/heapro/dap050 PMID:19914987

Tu, H. T., & Hargraves, J. L. (2003). Seeking health care information: Most consumers still on the sidelines. *Center for Studying Health System Change,* (61). Retrieved June 10, 2017, from http://www.hschange.org/CONTENT/537/?words=Tu%20&%20Hargraves%20200344

U. S. Department of Health and Human Services. (2010). *National Action Plan to Improve Health Literacy*. U.S. Department of Health and Human Services, Office of Disease Prevention and Promotion. Retrieved from http://www.health.gov/communication/HLActionPlan/

U.S. Census Bureau. (2012). *U.S. Census Bureau Projections Show a Slower Growing, Older, More Diverse Nation a Half Century from Now*. Retrieved from https://www.census.gov/newsroom/releases/archives/population/cb12-243.html

U.S. Department of Health and Human Services, Office of Disease Prevention and Health Promotion. (2010). *National Action Plan to Improve Health Literacy*. Washington, DC: Author.

U.S. Department of Health and Human Services. (2000). *Healthy People 2010*. Washington, DC: U.S. Government Printing Office.

U.S. Department of Health and Human Services. (2001). *Mental health: Culture, race, and ethnicity—A supplement to mental health: A report of the Surgeon General*. Author.

U.S. National Library of Medicine. (2017). *Urbanization*. Retrieved June 17, 2017, from https://meshb.nlm.nih.gov/record/ui?ui=D014507

Ubel, P. A., & Mahowald, M. B. (1995). Ethical and legal issues regarding living donors. In W. T. Reich (Ed.), *Encyclopedia of Bioethics*. New York: Simon Schuster Macmillan.

Ueno, M., Takayama, A., Adiatman, M., Ohnuki, M., Zaitsu, T., & Kawaguchi, Y. (2014). Application of visual oral health literacy instrument in health education for senior high school students. *International Journal of Health Promotion and Education*, *52*(1), 38–46. doi:10.1080/14635240.2013.845412

United Nations Economic and Social Council (ECOSOC). (2011). Health literacy and the Millennium Development Goals: United Nations Economic and Social Council (ECOSOC) regional meeting background paper (Abstracted). *Journal of Health Communication, 15*(Suppl. 2), 211–223. doi:10.1080/10810730.2010.499996 PMID:20845205

United Nations Educational Scientific and Cultural Organization. (1997). *The Hamburg Declaration on Adult Learning (CONFINTEA V)*. Author.

United Nations Educational Scientific and Cultural Organization. (2014). Adult and Youth Literacy. Institute for Statistics, (32), 1–4.

United Nations Educational Scientific and Cultural Organization. (2015). *Education For All 2000-2015: Achievements and Challenges. EFA Global Monitoring Report.* Author.

United Nations General Assembly. (2015). *Transforming our world: The 2030 agenda for sustainable development.* Author.

United Nations Office on Drugs and Crime. (2015). *Trafficking in Persons for the Purpose of Organ Removal.* Retrieved from https://www.unodc.org/documents/human-trafficking/2015/UNODC_Assessment_Toolkit_TIP_for_the_Purpose_of_Organ_Removal.pdf

United States Congress House of Representatives. (1967). *Committee on Science and Astronautics. Technology assessment.* Statement of Emilio QDaddario, chair, Subcommittee on Science, Research, and Development. Washington: 90th Congress, 1st session; 1967. pp. 9–13.

United States Department of Health & Human Services (HHS). (n.d.). *Privacy.* Retrieved from: http://www.hhs.gov/foia/privacy

United States Department of Health and Human Services Health Resources and Service Administration (HRSA). (2011). *Quality Improvement. Part 1: Quality Improvement (QI) and the Importance of QI.* Retrieved from: www.hrsa.gov/quality/toolbox/methodology/qualityimprovement

University Mental Health Research Institute (UMHRI) Ε.Π.Ι.Ψ.Υ. (n.d.). *About us.* Retrieved from http://www.epipsi.gr/index%20eng.htm

UNOS. (2016). *Increasing the number of Transplants in the United States: 2016 in review.* Retrieved from https://unos.org/about/annual-report/2016-annual-report/

Unrelated Live Transplant Regulatory Authority (ULTRA). (1998). Retrieved from http://www.advisorybodies.doh.gov.uk/ultra/index.htm

Val Derde Regional Medical Center. (2015). *Health Insurance Portability and Accountability Act (HIPAA).* Retrieved from: http://www.vvrmc.org/hipaa.html

Valapour, M. (2008). The live organ donor's consent: Is it informed and voluntary? *Transplantation Reviews*, *22*(3), 196–199. doi:10.1016/j.trre.2008.02.004 PMID:18631878

Valderas, J. M., Ferrer, M., Mendivil, J., Garin, O., Rajmil, L., Herdman, M., & Alonso, J. (2008). Development of EMPRO: A tool for the standardized assessment of patient-reported outcome measures. *Value in Health*, *11*(4), 700–708. doi:10.1111/j.1524-4733.2007.00309.x PMID:18194398

Valois, R. F., & Hoyle, T. B. (2005). Health in Education: The Challenge Continues. *American Journal of Health Education, 36*(1), 43–47. doi:10.1080/19325037.2005.10608156

van der Heide, I., Heijmans, M., Schuit, A. J., Uiters, E., & Rademakers, J. (2015). Functional, interactive and critical health literacy: Varying relationships with control over care and number of GP visits. *Patient Education and Counseling, 98*(8), 998–1004. doi:10.1016/j.pec.2015.04.006 PMID:25956070

van Jagt, R. K., Hoeks, J. C. J., Duizer, E., Baron, M., Molina, G. B., Unger, J. B., & Jansen, C. J. M. (2017). Sweet temptations: How does reading a fotonovela about diabetes affect Dutch adults with different levels of literacy? *Health Communication*, 284–290. Retrieved online http://www.tandfonline.com/doi/full/10.1080/10410236.2016.1258617 PMID:28094559

Van Wert, R. (2017, June 8). Dichotomous endings: A physician's personal reflection [Blog Post]. Retrieved from http://healthaffairs.org/blog/2017/06/08/dichotomous-endings-a-physicians-personal-reflection/

Van't Jagt, K., de Winter, A. F., Reijneveld, S. A., Hoeks, J. C., & Jansen, C. J. (2016). Development of a communication intervention for older adults with limited health literacy: Photo stories to support doctor-patient communication. *Journal of Health Communication, 21*(sup2), 69–82. doi:10.1080/10810730.2016.1193918 PMID:27662265

Vardavas, C., Kondilis, B., Patelarou, E., Akrivos, P., & Falagas, M. (2009). Health literacy and sources of health education among adolescents in Greece. *International Journal of Adolescent Medicine and Health, 21*(2), 179–186. doi:10.1515/IJAMH.2009.21.2.179 PMID:19702197

Vaz de Almeida, C. (2011). Communication and Literacy in e-Health. In *V SEMiME Exclusão Digital na Sociedade da Informação*. FMH-Universidade Técnica de Lisboa.

Veale, J., & Hil, G. (2011). The National Kidney registry: 175 transplants in 1 year. *Clinical Transplantation*, 255–278. PMID:22755419

Veatch, R. M., & Ross, L. F. (2015). *Transplantation ethics* (2nd ed.). Washington, DC: Georgetown University Press.

Veenhof, B., Clermont, Y., & Sciadis, G. (2005). *Literacy and digital technologies: Linkages and outcomes*. Ottawa, Canada: Statistics Canada.

Vernon, J. A., Trujillo, A., Rosenbaum, S. J., & Pfizer, B. D. (2007). *Low Health Literacy: Implications for National Health Policy*. Academic Press.

Vernon, J., Trujillo, A., Rosenbaum, S., & DeBuono, B. (2007). *Low health literacy: Implications for national policy*. Academic Press.

Vida Estacio, Saidy-Khan, Karic, McKinley, Sargeant, Murray, … Wydell. (2012). Action on health literacy in Stoke-on-Trent: Engaging South Asian men and Young men with Diabetes. Stoke-on-Trent, UK: Academic Press.

Visiomed Group. (2017). Bewell Connect Products. Products Exhibited at Consumer Electronics Show 2017 (CES 2017), Las Vegas, NV.

Vozikis, A., Drivas, K., & Milioris, K. (2014). Health literacy among university students in Greece: Determinants and association with self-perceived health, health behaviours and health risks. *Archives of Public Health, 72*(1), 15. doi:10.1186/2049-3258-72-15 PMID:24987522

Wagner, E. H. (1998). Chronic disease management: What will it take to improve care for chronic illness? *Effective Clinical Practice, 1*(1), 2–4. PMID:10345255

Wang, N. (2015, March 13). Mental Health: A New Priority in Corporate America. *US News & World Report*. Retrieved from https://www.usnews.com/news/articles/2015/03/13/mental-health-a-new-priority-in-corporate-america

Wang, H., Li, T., Siahpush, M., Chen, L.-W., & Huberty, J. (2017). Cost-Effectiveness of Ready for Recess to Promote Physical Activity in Children. *The Journal of School Health*, *87*(4), 278–285. doi:10.1111/josh.12495 PMID:28260240

Ware, J. E., & Sherbourne, C. D. (1992). The MOS 36-Item Short-Form Health Survey (SF-36): I. Conceptual Framework and Item Selection. *Medical Care*, *30*(6), 473–483. doi:10.1097/00005650-199206000-00002 PMID:1593914

Waterman, A. D., Morgievich, M., Cohen, D. J., Butt, Z., Chakkera, H. A., Lindower, C., … LaPoint Rudow, D. (2015). Living donor kidney transplantation: improving education outside of transplant centers about live donor transplantation – recommendations from a concensus conference. *Clinical Journal of the American Society of Nephrology*. Retrieved 17 May 2017, from https://www.ncbi.nlm.nih.gov/pmc/articles/PMC4559502/

Watson, B., Gallois, C., Hewett, D., & Jones, L. (2014). Culture and healthcare: intergroup communication and its consequences. Academic Press.

Watson, R. (2011). Europeans with poor" health literacy" are heavy users of health services. *British Medical Journal*, 343. PMID:22127773

Watzlawick, P., Beavin, J. H., & Jackson, D. D. (1967). *Pragmática da comunicação humana: Um estudo dos padrões, patologias e paradoxo da interação* (S. Paulo, Ed.). Cultrix.

Webb, G., Phillips, N., Reddiford, S., & Neuberger, J. (2015). Factors affecting the decision to grant consent for organ donation: A survey of adults in England. *Transplantation*, *99*(7), 1396–1402. doi:10.1097/TP.0000000000000504 PMID:25675195

Weisman, H. L., Kia-Keating, M., Lippincott, A., Taylor, Z., & Zheng, J. (2016). Mental Health Stigma Prevention: Pilot Testing a Novel, Language Arts Curriculum-Based Approach for Youth. *The Journal of School Health*, *86*(10), 709–716. doi:10.1111/josh.12427 PMID:27619761

Weiss, B. D., Blanchard, J. S., McGee, D. L., Hart, G., Warren, B., Burgoon, M., & Smith, K. J. (1994). Illiteracy among Medicaid recipients and its relationship to health care costs. *Journal of Health Care for the Poor and Underserved*, *5*(2), 99–111. doi:10.1353/hpu.2010.0272 PMID:8043732

Weiss, B. D., & Palmer, R. (2004). Relationship between health care costs and very low literacy skills in a medically needy and indigent Medicaid population. *The Journal of the American Board of Family Practice*, *17*(1), 44–47. doi:10.3122/jabfm.17.1.44 PMID:15014052

Wei, Y., Hayden, J. A., Kutcher, S., Zygmunt, A., & McGrath, P. (2013). The effectiveness of school mental health literacy programs to address knowledge, attitudes and help seeking among youth. *Early Intervention in Psychiatry*, *7*(2), 109–121. doi:10.1111/eip.12010 PMID:23343220

Wei, Y., McGrath, P. J., Hayden, J., & Kutcher, S. (2016). Measurement properties of tools measuring mental health knowledge: A systematic review. *BMC Psychiatry*, *16*(1), 297. doi:10.118612888-016-1012-5 PMID:27553955

Westin, A. (2012). *National Partnership for Women & Families. Making IT Meaningful: How Consumers Value and Trust Health IT*. Retrieved from http://go.nationalpartnership.org/site/DocServer/HIT_Making_IT_Meaningful_National_Partnership_February_2.pdf

WHO Regional Office for Europe. (1999). *Health 21. The health for all policy framework for the WHO European region*. Copenhagen: WHO Regional Office for Europe.

WHO Regional Office for Europe. (2013). *WHO European Ministerial Conference on the Prevention and Control of Noncommunicable Diseases in the Context of Health 2020 Ashgabat Declaration on the Prevention and Control of Noncommunicable Diseases in the Context of Health 2020*. Ashgabat: Author.

WHOQOL-Group. (1998a). Development of the World Health Organization WHOQOL-BREF quality of life assessment. The WHOQOL Group. *Psychological Medicine*, *28*(3), 551–558. doi:10.1017/S0033291798006667 PMID:9626712

WHOQOL-Group. (1998b). The World Health Organization quality of life assessment (WHOQOL): Development and general psychometric properties1. *Social Science & Medicine*, *46*(12), 1569–1585. doi:10.1016/S0277-9536(98)00009-4 PMID:9672396

Wickramasinghe, N. (2017). *Handbook of research on healthcare administration and management*. Hershey, PA: IGI Global. doi:10.4018/978-1-5225-0920-2

Wieclaw, J., Agerbo, E., Mortensen, P., & Bonde, J. (2006). Risk of affective and stress related disorders among employees in human service professions. *Occupational and Environmental Medicine*, *6*(5), 314–319. doi:10.1136/oem.2004.019398 PMID:16621851

Wilkinson, R., & Marmot, M. (Eds.). (2003). *Social Determinants of Health. The solid facts*. Geneva: WHO Europe International Centre for Health and Society.

Williams, M. V., Baker, D. W., Parker, R. M., & Nurss, J. R. (1998). Relationship of functional health literacy to patients' knowledge of their chronic disease. *Archives of Internal Medicine*, *158*(2), 166–172. doi:10.1001/archinte.158.2.166 PMID:9448555

Williams, M. V., Davis, T., Parker, R. M., & Weiss, B. D. (2002). The role of health literacy in patient-physician communication. *Family Medicine*, *34*(5), 383–389. PMID:12038721

Williams, M. V., Davis, T., Parker, R. M., & Weiss, B. D. (2002). The role of health literacy in patient-physician communication. *Family Medicine-Kansas City*, *34*(5), 383–389. PMID:12038721

Williams, M., Parker, R., Baker, D., Parikh, K., Coates, W., & Nurss, J. (1995). Inadequate functional health literacy among patients at two public health hospitals. *Journal of the American Medical Association*, *2714*, 1677–1682.

Willis, E., Wang, Y., & Rodgers, S. (2013). Online health communities and health literacy: Applying a framework for understanding domains of health literacy. In I. Management Association (Ed.), User-driven healthcare: Concepts, methodologies, tools, and applications (pp. 180–196). Hershey, PA: IGI Global. doi:10.4018/978-1-4666-2770-3.ch010

Wilson, C., & Peterson, A. (2010). *Managing Personal Health Information: An Action Agenda*. AHRQ Publication No. 10-0048-EF. Rockville, MD: Agency for Healthcare Research and Quality, U.S. Department of Health and Human Services.

Winkelman, W., Leonard, K., & Rossos, P. (2005). Patient-perceived usefulness of online electronic medical records: employing grounded theory in the development of information and communication technologies for use by patients living with chronic illness. *Journal of the American Medical Informatics Association, 12*(3), 306-314. doi:.10.1197/jamia.M1712

Wittenberg, E., Goldsmith, J., Ferrell, B., & Platt, C. S. (2015). Enhancing communication related to symptom management through plain language: A brief report. *Journal of Pain and Symptom Management*, *50*(5), 707–711. doi:10.1016/j.jpainsymman.2015.06.007 PMID:26162506

Wodchis, W., Dixon, A., & Anderson, G. (2015). Integrating care to older people and those with complex needs: Examining the lessons from international case studies. *International Journal of Integrated Care*, *15*(1), 1–15.

Wolf, M. S., Gazmararian, J. A., & Baker, D. W. (2005). Health literacy and functional health status among older adults. *Archives of Internal Medicine*, *165*(17), 1946–1952. doi:10.1001/archinte.165.17.1946 PMID:16186463

Wolf, M. S., Knight, S. J., Lyons, E. A., Durazo-Arvizu, R., Pickard, S. A., Arseven, A., ... Bennett, C. L. (2006). Literacy, race, and PSA level among low-income men newly diagnosed with prostate cancer. *Urology, 68*(1), 89–93. doi:10.1016/j.urology.2006.01.064 PMID:16844451

Wolf, M. S., Williams, M. V., Parker, R. M., Parikh, N. S., Nowlan, A. W., & Baker, D. W. (2007). Patients' shame and attitudes toward discussing the results of literacy screening. *Journal of Health Communication, 12*(8), 721–732. doi:10.1080/10810730701672173 PMID:18030638

Wolpe, J. (1968). Psychotherapy by Reciprocal Inhibition. *Conditional Reflex: A Pavlovian Journal of Research & Therapy, 3*(4), 234-240.

Wolpe, J. (1990). *The practice of behavior therapy.* New York: Pergamon.

Wolters, H. H., Heidenreich, S., & Senninger, N. (2003). Living donor kidney transplantation: Chance for the recipient--financial risk for the donor? *Transplantation Proceedings, 35*(6), 2091–2092. doi:10.1016/S0041-1345(03)00675-4 PMID:14529850

Wood, R. Y., & Duffy, M. E. (2004). Video breast health kits: Testing a cancer education innovation in older high-risk populations. *Journal of Cancer Education, 19*(2), 98–104. doi:10.120715430154jce1902_10 PMID:15456666

World Bank. (1993). *World Development Report 1993. Investing in Health.* Oxford, UK: Oxford University Press.

World Health Organisation. (2013). *Health literacy the solid facts.* Retrieved on 14 May 2017 from http://www.euro.who.int/__data/assets/pdf_file/0008/190655/e96854.pdf

World Health Organization (WHO). (2009). *The Financial Crisis and Global Health.* Retrieved from http://www.who.int/topics/financial_crisis/financialcrisis_report_200902.pdf

World Health Organization WHO. (2009). *Guiding principles on human cell, tissue and organ transplantation.* World Health Organization.

World Health Organization. (1986). *The Ottawa Charter for health promotion.* Geneva: WHO.

World Health Organization. (1996). *The Status of School Health.* Geneva: WHO.

World Health Organization. (1998). *Health Promotion Glossary.* Geneva: WHO.

World Health Organization. (2009). *Nairobi Call To Action.* Geneva: WHO.

World Health Organization. (2016). Global report on urban health: equitable, healthier cities for sustainable development. Kobe, Japan: WHO.

World Health Organization. (2016). Health as the pulse of the new urban agenda: United Nations conference on housing and sustainable urban development, Quito, October 2016. Geneva: WHO.

World Health Organization. (2016). *Policy brief 4: Health literacy.* Retrieved from http://www.who.int/healthpromotion/conferences/9gchp/policy-brief4-health-literacy.pdf?ua=1

World Health Organization. (2016). Shanghai Declaration on Health Promotion in the 2030 Agenda for Sustainable Development. Geneva: WHO.

World Health Organization. (2017). *Chronic Diseases and Health Promotion.* Retrieved from: http://www.who.int/chp/en/

Wu, E. (2015). *SB853 Bill Health Care language assistance.* Retrieved from http://cpehn.org/policy-center/cultural-and-linguistic-competency/sb-853-health-care-language-assistance-act

Wynia, M. K., & Osborn, C. Y. (2010). Health Literacy and Communication Quality in Health Care Organizations. *Journal of Health Communication*, *15*(2), 102–115. doi:10.1080/10810730.2010.499981 PMID:20845197

Yamin, C., Emani, S., Williams, D. H., Lipsitz, S. R., Karson, A. S., Wald, J. S., & Bates, D. W. (2011). The digital divide in adoption and use of a personal health record. *Archives of Internal Medicine*, *171*(6), 568–574. doi:10.1001/archinternmed.2011.34 PMID:21444847

Yang, R. C., Thiessen-Philbrook, H., Klarenbach, S., Vlaicu, S., & Garg, A. X. (2007). Insurability of living organ donors: A systematic review. *American Journal of Transplantation*, *7*(6), 1542–1551. doi:10.1111/j.1600-6143.2007.01793.x PMID:17430400

Yassi, A., Pawson, D., Leary, T., Sikorski, J., Parent, D., & Gilbert, M. (2004). *Trends in workplace injuries, illness, and policies in healthcare across Canada: workers' compensation patterns and policy changes in healthcare organizations. Report for Health Canada Ottawa*. Ontario: Health Canada.

Yen, H. (2000). PA plans financial aid for organ donors. *Philadelphia Inquirer*.

Yildirim, F., & Çakir, M. (2017). Are adult women or men who use the Internet as a health information resource more health literate? In I. Management Association (Ed.), Medical education and ethics: Concepts, methodologies, tools, and applications (pp. 1208–1234). Hershey, PA: IGI Global. doi:10.4018/978-1-5225-0978-3.ch055

Zandieh, S. O., Yoon-Flannery, G. J., Kuperman, D., Langsam, D. J., Hyman, D., & Kaushal, R. (2008). Challenges to EHR implementation in electronic- versus paper-based office practices. *Journal of General Internal Medicine*, *23*(6), 755–761. doi:10.100711606-008-0573-5 PMID:18369679

Zarcadoolas, C. (2010). The simplicity complex: Exploring simplified health messages in a complex world. *Health Promotion International*. doi:10.1093/heapro/daq075 PMID:21149317

Zarcadoolas, C., & Pleasant, A. (2008). Increasing Health Literacy. In J. C. Parker & E. Thorson (Eds.), *Healthcare Communication in the New Media Landscape*. New York, NY: Springer.

Zarcadoolas, C., Pleasant, A., & Greer, D. (2005). Understanding health literacy: An expanded model. *Health Promotion International*, *20*(2), 195–203. doi:10.1093/heapro/dah609 PMID:15788526

Zarcadoolas, C., Pleasant, A., & Greer, D. S. (2006). *Advancing Health Literacy: a framework for understanding and action*. San Francisco, CA: Jossey-Bass.

Zarcadoolas, C., Sealy, Y., Levy, J., Dresser, M., Ponieman, D., Young, S. M., ... Silver, L. (2011). Health literacy at work to address overweight and obesity in adults: The development of the obesity action kit. *Journal of Communication in Healthcare*, *4*(2), 88–101. doi:10.1179/175380611X13082296179316

Zelmer, J., & Hagens, S. (2014). Understanding the gap between the desire for and use of consumer health solutions. *Healthcare Papers*, *13*(4), 9–21. doi:10.12927/hcpap.2014.23871 PMID:25148119

Zhang, Q., Huang, F., Liu, Z., Zhang, N., Mahapatra, T., Tang, W., ... Zhang, J. (2016). Cross-Cultural Validation of the High Blood Pressure Health Literacy Scale in a Chinese Community. *PLoS One*, *11*(4), 12. doi:10.1371/journal.pone.0152182 PMID:27116336

Zhao, J., Freeman, B., & Li, M. (2016). Can mobile apps influence people's health behavior change? An evidence review. *Journal of Medical Internet Research*, *18*(11), e287. doi:10.2196/jmir.5692 PMID:27806926

Zuercher, E., Diatta, I. D., Burnand, B., & Peytremann-Bridevaux, I. (2017). Health literacy and quality of care of patients with diabetes: A cross-sectional analysis. *Primary Care Diabetes*, *11*(3), 233–240. doi:10.1016/j.pcd.2017.02.003 PMID:28292571

About the Contributors

Vassilios Papalois, MD, PhD, FICS, FRCS, FEBS, is Professor of Transplantation Surgery and Consultant Transplant and General Surgeon at the Hammersmith Hospital, Imperial College, London, UK. He leads a Transplant Centre of Excellence focusing on high risk and extended criteria kidney and pancreas transplantation. He has been active in surgical research for more than 20 years and has published 190 papers in peer review journals, 15 book chapters and 6 books. His research focuses on pre-transplant assessment and reconditioning of marginal kidney and pancreas grafts, use of stem cells for treatment of chronically scarred allografts, clinical ethics and health policy. He has been awarded, through competitive processes, more than £1,000,000 in research grants. Professor Papalois has extensive experience in the NHS in Clinical Governance and Medico-Legal issues, is NIHR NW London Subspecialty Lead for Transplantation, Chairs the Ethics Committee of the Avon and Somerset Constabulary and he is a member of the Research Ethics Committee of the UK Ministry of Defence. He is the President Elect of the European Society of Organ Transplantation (ESOT), the Secretary General of the European Union of Medical Specialists (UEMS), Member of the Executive Board of the Association of Surgeons of Great Britain and Ireland (ASGBI), Member of Council of the European Society of Surgery (ESS) and Member of the Council of the British Journal of Surgery Society (BJS). Professor Papalois organises annually a series of advanced international courses on transplant training, clinical ethics and health policy and has given more than 120 lectures in international forums as an invited speaker. He has been awarded a Bronze National Award for Clinical Excellence by the UK Department of the Health, a Senior Clinical Investigator Award by the European Society for Organ Transplantation and a Teaching Excellence Award by Imperial College.

Maria Theodosopoulou has studied Philosophy, Education and Psychology, has a Master's degree in Career Counselling, and a PhD in Lifelong Learning. Currently, she is finishing her second PhD, which focuses on Health Literacy at Imperial College London. She has worked for more than ten years in the fields of lifelong learning and adult education. Her work supports the idea that health literacy skills are part of a lifelong learning journey that first starts in families and schools.

***

Saliha Akhtar has held various positions in the pharmaceutical industry including Clinical Trial Manager and Strategic Development Manager. She has experience in the start-up through close-out phases of clinical trials. Saliha earned her PhD in Health Sciences from Seton Hall University, Master of Business Administration in Pharmaceutical Management from Fairleigh Dickinson University, Master of Science in Health Sciences from Rutgers University, and a Bachelor of Science in Biology from Montclair State University. Her research interests include understanding the factors that prevent clinical trials from recruiting on time and the reasons for low retention rates.

Lizette Alvarez is a graduate from two of the topped ranked women's universities and colleges in the United States. She holds an MBA from Mills College in the San Francisco Bay Area with a concentration in Socially Responsible Business. Her undergraduate degrees are in Psychology/Biology from Mount St. Mary's University, Los Angeles, California, USA. Her multifaceted work is that of a multilingual, ethical, and socially responsible organizational leader who delivers strong financial, cost effective performance while creating a positive societal impact on the communities and organizations she serves.

S. M. Yasir Arafat holds MBBS, MBA, MPH. Currently he is enrolled as MD Phase B Resident, Department of Psychiatry at Bangabandhu Sheikh Mujib Medical University. He is also affiliated as Adjunct Faculty at MPH Program, ASA University Bangladesh & School of Public Health, Independent University, Bangladesh.

Georgios Baskozos is a bioinformatician working as a postdoctoral research scientist at the University of Oxford. He did his Ph.D. in Bioinformatics at the University College in London, UK. He has studied computer science at the National and Kapodistrian University of Athens in Greece and then acquired his MSc degree in Bioinformatics from King's College London, UK.

Célia Belim is an Assistant Professor in the School of Social and Political Sciences, University of Lisbon (ISCSP-ULisboa) (Courses: e.g. Political Agenda; Agenda and Political Communication, Image Theory; Communication Theories; Press Techniques; Semiology; Social Psychology), and has a Ph.D in Communication Studies. She is co-editor of the book "Image of U.S. Presidential Administrations: The Cases of George W. Bush and Barack Obama" (Lexington Books, Rowman & Littlefiled). She also has a Master in Political Science. Her Master thesis is about Political Propaganda after the 11/9, focusing on analysis content of George W. Bush's and Al-Qaeda leaders' speeches. She had the best classification on Communication Studies Bachelor Degree in 2000 and received a Portuguese Ministry of Higher Education Science and Technology Doctorate scholarship. She has experience on Media Relations Management. Belim has been publishing and participating in conferences on her areas of interest, such as: Midwest Political Science Association (MPSA), the International Political Science Association (IPSA), the European Consortium for Political Research (ECPR), the Spanish Association of Political Science and Administration (AECPA), the Latin American Association of Political Science (ALACIP), the I Congress Of Semiotics of Culture in the Complutense University of Madrid (GESC), the International Association for Media and Communication Research (IAMCR). She has been interested on the contribution of communication competences to the effectiveness of communication, and recently on the communication competencies in the field of health.

Maria Irene Bellini has graduated from the Tor Vergata Medical School in Rome where she also qualified in General Surgery and HPB Surgery. She was a Transplant Fellow at Churchill Hospital in Oxford and has received her Ph. D. from Tor Vergata Medical School. Currently, she is a Senior Transplant Fellow in Renal and Transplant Surgery, at Hammersmith Hospital in London. She has received grants and awards, among others from British Transplantation Society and the European Society of Organ Transplantation.

Daniel Casanova is Professor of Surgery at the University of Cantabria in Spain and Head of Transplantation Surgery at the University Hospital Marqués de Valdecilla in Santander, Spain. Professor Casanova is also Chairman of the Board of Transplantation of the European Union of Medical Specialists (UEMS).

Mei Chen is an applied cognitive scientist specializing in educational technology, health education, and consumer eHealth innovation. Dr. Chen obtained her Ph. D. from McGill University in 2001.

Pierpaolo Di Cocco, MD, PhD, is a clinical fellow in Transplantation at the West London Renal and Transplant Centre, Imperial College NHS Healthcare. Clinical and scientific activities have been focused in solid organ transplantation, particularly in kidney and pancreas transplantation. Participation to multicenter research studies on clinical utility of machine perfusion as a preservation method in kidney transplantation. Memberships: Italian Society of Organ Transplantation (SITO), British Transplantation Society (BTS) and European Society for Organ Transplantation (ESOT).

Frank J. M. F. Dor, MD, PhD, FEBS, FRCS, is Consultant Transplant Surgeon and Head of Transplantation at Imperial College Renal and Transplant Centre, London, UK. Before moving to the UK in 2016, he was Consultant Transplant Surgeon and Surgical Director of the kidney transplant programme at Erasmus MC, Rotterdam, The Netherlands. He attended medical school in Antwerp and Rotterdam (MD 2001, cum laude), and conducted his PhD research in Transplant Immunology at Harvard Medical School, Boston, USA (PhD 2006, cum laude). He is an active clinical and translational scientist, and a passionate educationalist. He has been involved in ESOT since 2010 as ELPAT Board Member and co-chair of the Living Organ Donation Working Group. He has been the driving force behind the redesign of the ESOT educational landscape, as chair of the Hesperis Course and founder/chair of the LIDO Course (Living Donor Nephrectomy Course, since 2009). In 2012, he became Vice-Chair of the ESOT Education Committee, and Chair in 2015 and has since then served as Council Member. He was an active contributor to the organization of the 2015 ESOT Congress, and Scientific Programme Committee Member of the 2017 ESOT Congress. Frank has been Board Member and former president-elect of the Dutch Transplant Society, and Secretary General of the European Society for Surgical Research, and is currently Senior Secretary of the UEMS Division of Transplantation. He serves as Associate Editor and Social Media editor of Transplantation, Associate Editor of European Surgical Research, Advisor to the Peter Morris Centre of Evidence in Transplantation, and Member of the European Surgical Association. He is Chair of the European Chapter of the Peritoneal Dialysis University for Surgeons, and chair of the ISPD Guideline committee for PD catheter insertion. He has published and lectured widely on live kidney donation and transplantation.

Dela Idowu is the Executive Director and Founder of Gift of Living Donation (GOLD) an organisation set up to raise awareness, educate and engage the black population on living kidney donation after she came forward as a potential living kidney donor for her brother who had kidney failure. She is the author of 'More Than a Match', a book that gives a compelling personal account of her family's struggle to come to terms with kidney failure, dialysis and transplantation, she is the co writer and producer of 'We Are Family" a educational film on living kidney donation from a black family's perspective, both these resources are used at transplant centres to better engage black renal patients. She is a member of the Living Donor Kidney Transplantation 2020 Strategy Implementation Group, a member of Guy's & St Thomas's Organ Donation Committee and Kidney Patient's Association. Dela was the 2014 Pride of Brent Award Winner for her outstanding contribution to the London borough of Brent in the area of organ donation.

Jennie Jewitt-Harris is Founder and Chief Executive of Transplant Links Community (TLC), a UK registered charity dedicated to facilitating kidney transplantation in low and middle income countries across the world. She obtained her medical degree from King's College, London and has worked for many years in transplantation, in the pharmaceutical industry and other healthcare organisations. In pharmaceuticals, she was previously Head of Immunology Research, and Director of Corporate Communications and Government Affairs.

Russell Kabir is currently working as a Senior Lecturer in Research Methods in Department of Medical Science and Public Health at Anglia Ruskin University. Dr. Kabir obtained his BDS (Bachelor of Dentistry) degree from the University of Dhaka in 2004 and MPH (Masters of Public Health) degree from North South University in 2007. He completed his PhD degree from Middlesex University. Apart from his academic responsibilities, he is conducting research in different public health issues. He is a Fellow of Higher Education Academy and Royal Statistical Society. He is serving the role of an Editor in Chief for International Journal of Perceptions in Public Health and Associate Editor role for South East Asia Journal of Public Health.

Kijpokin Kasemsap received his BEng degree in Mechanical Engineering from King Mongkut's University of Technology, Thonburi, his MBA degree from Ramkhamhaeng University, and his DBA degree in Human Resource Management from Suan Sunandha Rajabhat University. Dr. Kasemsap is a Special Lecturer in the Faculty of Management Sciences, Suan Sunandha Rajabhat University, based in Bangkok, Thailand. Dr. Kasemsap is a Member of the International Economics Development and Research Center (IEDRC), the International Foundation for Research and Development (IFRD), and the International Innovative Scientific and Research Organization (IISRO). Dr. Kasemsap also serves on the International Advisory Committee (IAC) for the International Association of Academicians and Researchers (INAAR). Dr. Kasemsap is the sole author of over 250 peer-reviewed international publications and book chapters on business, education, and information technology. Dr. Kasemsap is included in the TOP 100 Professionals–2016 and in the 10th edition of 2000 Outstanding Intellectuals of the 21st Century by the International Biographical Centre, Cambridge, England.

Gillian King trained as a barrister and is the Project Administrator for the home-based education project currently run by Gift of Living Donation (GOLD) to increase access to living kidney donor transplantation for patients from the black population with End Stage Renal Disease. As a renal patient and Peer Volunteer at the Royal Free Hospital she uses her knowledge and experience as a peer volunteer at Guy's and St Thomas' NHS Trust to improve health outcomes for Black Minority Ethnic (BME) patients with Chronic Kidney Disease. She is very interested in how the Black British population in the UK identify themselves and is currently writing her first book on the subject. Her book on Black British Identity explores how people who are not white and British self-identify and how they are identified by the rest of the population and to what extent their ethnic origin affects their life as a British person."

Barbara Kondilis is Assistant Professor & Adjunct Faculty at Hellenic American University/ Hellenic American College, where she mainly teaches in the undergraduate psychology program, Psychology and General Education classes. She also teaches health communication and healthcare management classes in the M.B.A. program. She has extensive experience in public health, clinical social work, having worked with diverse populations as a health educator, counselor, and consultant, developing programs, health communication efforts, and creating relevant procedures/policies. Her most notable work involved working for the U.S. Centers for Disease Control & Prevention, as part of the Public Health Prevention Service, and for the Rhode Island Department of Health as the Coordinator of the Chronic Care Collaborative, Division of Diabetes Prevention & Control. She has done collaborative research with various private and public institutions including the National School of Public Health (Greece), on projects relating to tobacco control, bullying, and health literacy, among others. A Marie Curie Fellowship recipient (2006-2008), she collaborated with representatives from several EU-member states on national research on measuring health literacy (see HLS-EU project). Ms Kondilis is a Ph.D. student in Applied Linguistics (A.B.D.) at Hellenic American University, holds a Master's of Public Health and a Master's of Social Work from Boston University, and a B.A. in Psychology from Simmons College, Boston, Massachusetts.

Andre Kubler is a trainee physician with an interest in translational research, pre-clinical modelling and patient-centred, evidence-based clinical practice. He was awarded a Ph.D in Infectious Diseases and Immunology for research undertaken at Imperial College London, UK and Johns Hopkins Medical Institutes, Baltimore, USA, graduating from the Imperial College London MD PhD program.

Md Anwarul Azim Majumder is currently working as the Director of Medical Education in the Faculty of Medical Sciences, Cave Hill Campus, University of the West Indies, Barbados. Previously, he worked as a Lecturer at the Clinical Sciences Department, School of Medical Sciences, University of Bradford, UK (2004-16) and was actively involved in widening participation of medicine programme and problem-based learning. He also worked in the Centre for Medical Education, Bangladesh (1992-2001), and the Department of Medical Education of the School of Medical Sciences, Universiti Sains Malaysia (2001-04) and was actively involved with innovation and experimentation of medical curricula. Dr Majumder was the Founding General Secretary of the National Association of Medical Education, Bangladesh and the President of the Union of Risk Management for Preventive Medicine (URMPM), Bangladesh Society. He is also the Editor-in-Chief of the Advances in Medical Education and Practice and the Executive Editor of the South East Asia Journal of Public Health (published by the Public Health Foundation Bangladesh). He has published a number of peer reviewed papers on medical education and health care.

Konstantinos Papadopoulos has a background in physiotherapy, exercise rehabilitation and health-care sciences and has taught a variety of subjects in physiotherapy and allied health professions since 2010. He has always been interested in sports injuries, thus, he decided to expand his knowledge by studying an MSc course in Exercise Rehabilitation. During this course he contacted his first clinical study on knee pain. On successful completion of his MSc course he applied for a PhD Studentship in Healthcare Sciences and aimed to evaluate applied physiotherapy practice in NHS physiotherapy departments. Konstantinos is currently the programme leader of the MSc Sport Rehabilitation programme at Middlesex University, London.

Terri Ann Parnell, DNP, MA, RN, FAAN, is a nurse, an internationally recognized health literacy expert, and an award-winning author. She is a Clinical Associate Professor at Stony Brook University in the Graduate Program in Health Administration. Dr. Parnell is also Principal and Founder of Health Literacy Partners LLC, a corporation that specializes in providing a tapestry of solutions to promote health equity by enhancing person-centered care, effective communication, and the patient experience. Previously, Dr. Parnell was Vice President for Health Literacy and Patient Education for the Northwell Health System where she was responsible for the health literacy strategic plan and integrating concepts of health literacy, language access services, and cultural awareness into core activities across the system. She is a graduate of St. Vincent's Hospital School of Nursing in New York City. She earned a Bachelor of Science degree in Nursing from Adelphi University, a Masters Degree in Health Administration from Hofstra University and a Doctor of Nursing Practice degree from Case Western Reserve University. Dr. Parnell is a member of the Roundtable on Health Literacy of the National Academies of Sciences, Engineering, and Medicine. She is a Fellow in the American Academy of Nursing and the New York Academy of Medicine. In 2016, Dr. Parnell joined TVR Communications Advisory Board as their Chief Nursing Officer (CNO). Her second book, Health Literacy in Nursing: Providing Person-Centered Care received an American Journal of Nursing 2015 Book of the Year Award in the category of Nursing Management and Leadership.

Reshma Prashad is a PhD Candidate in the School of Health Policy and Management at York University in Toronto, Canada. She has completed an honours Bachelor of Health Studies Degree majoring in Health Informatics in 2009 at York University, followed by the completion of a Masters of Health Informatics Degree at the University of Toronto in 2011. Reshma's doctoral work focuses on the use of digital health technologies to engage and empower patients to self-manage their chronic conditions and prevent avoidable complications. Additionally she has a keen interest in how organizations can be designed to effectively support care providers in proactively managing their patients with chronic conditions. In addition to her academic background, Reshma has over 10 years of professional Project Management experience in information systems implementation at various levels of the health system in Canada.

Andrew Ready is Senior Consultant Renal Transplant Surgeon at the University Hospital Birmingham, UK. He is also an Honorary Senior Clinical Lecturer in Surgery at the University of Birmingham from where obtained his medical degree. During his postgraduate training gained Masters and Doctorate degrees for research into aspects of transplant immunology before undertaking a period as a postdoctoral research fellow at Stanford University, CA. He is Medical Director of Transplant Links Community (TLC) - an organisation dedicated to facilitating renal transplantation in LMICs.

T. Ray Ruffin's educational background has spawned and spanned a Bachelor of Business Administration from Northwood University. The completion of four graduate degrees, Master of Arts in Organizational Leadership, Master of Science in Human Resources, Master of Health Administration all from Chapman University, and Doctorate of Business Administration with a concentration in Information Systems from Argosy University. Additionally, Dr. Ruffin completed Post Doctorate Certificate in Health Care Management and Leadership from Colorado Technical University. Member of University of Phoenix Research Center for Workplace Diversity focusing on the different dimensions of diversity and their impact on the Workforce and successful management and leadership. Affiliated colleges and universities include: Faculty Member and Dissertation Chair for the University of Phoenix, focus on the

Doctoral Proposal for approval. Dr. Ruffin has received 10 Honorarium Awards and 6 Excellence in Publishing Awards. Colorado Technical University since 2103, were Dr. Ruffin received 9 Adjunct Faculty Funding Awards. Grand Canyon University since 2017, where Dr. Ruffin is a Dissertation Chairperson. Ashford University 2017, where Dr. Ruffin facilitates Masters of Health Administration for adult learners North Carolina Wesleyan College since in 2017, were Dr. Ruffin facilitates business and computer courses for adult learners. Dr. Ruffin is past member and officer of North Carolina Community College Faculty Association (NCCCFA), where he served as Vice President of Communications. North Carolina Computer Instruction Association (NCCIA), aiding the Leadership Team. Dr. Ruffin has over twenty years of management (including financial management), and information technology experience. Sponsors the Jack and Argavick Scarboro (grandparents) Memorial Scholarship through the North Carolina Computer Instruction Association (NCCIA) for students majoring in Health Information Technology (HIT); Health Care Management (HMT); Health Care Technology (HCT): Health Care Interpreting HCI); and Business Health Informatics (HBI). Sponsor for the Dr. T. Ray Ruffin Scholarship through Wake Technical Community College Foundation for students with financial need in Networking and Computer Technology Degree Programs. Creator and founder of the Dr. T. Ray Ruffin Scholarship in partnership with Everlasting Life Christian Church (ELCC) of Apex North Carolina, Pastor Stephen Lyons, for students attending trade schools, colleges, and universities.

Kristine Sørensen, PhD, MScPH, is a thought leader committed to advance the global scale and scope of health literacy to improve health and quality of life for all. She is the founding director of the Global Health Literacy Academy. Her primary focus is to manifest health literacy in Europe and on the global agenda. Her educational background is in medicine, public health and global health diplomacy. She has acted as advisor for McKinsey, EU, WHO, ECDC, the European Parliament and Council of Europe. Kristine Sørensen has received the European Health Award 2012 and the International Health Literacy Award 2017. She is the first president of the International Health Literacy Association and focal point for Health Literacy Europe - a network for advancing European health literacy.

Md Saleh Uddin completed graduation (MBBS) from Chittagong Medical College, Bangladesh and did post-graduation (MD-Psychiatry) from Bangabandhu Sheikh Mujib Medical University (BSMMU), Dhaka, Bangladesh. Currently Mr Uddin working as psychiatrist in the department of psychiatry, Chittagong Medical College Hospital under Ministry of Health and Family Welfare, Government Republic of Bangladesh. His research area of interest is Child Adolescent Mental Health (CAMH) and was awarded "Donald J Cohen Fellowship" by International Association of Child Adolescent Psychiatry and Allied Professions (IACAPAP) on 2014 for the first time from Bangladesh. He authored number of local and international original articles, review articles and scientific publications relevant to mental health issues. He is now acting as an associate editor of the Medical Journal of Clinical Trials and Case Studies (MJCCS), USA. Mr Uddin introduced school mental health research in Bangladesh and now conducting a relevant research collaboratively with Prof Stan Kutcher, Psychiatrist, Dalhousie University, Canada.

Cristina Vaz de Almeida is a PhD student on Communication Studies. She has a vast experience in Santa Casa da Misericórdia, in Lisboa. She is an experienced trainer on health literacy and on communication competences, having many health professionals, such as medical doctors and nurses, as her trainees. She has been publishing in the subject and has been participating in conferences and summer schools on health literacy.

Christina Zarcadoolas is a sociolinguist and internationally recognized expert in health literacy and public understanding of health and science. She focuses on analyzing and closing the gaps between expert & lay knowledge and understanding, paying particular attention to how people make meaning out of complex things. The New England J of Medicine called her critically acclaimed book, Advancing Health Literacy: A Framework for Understanding and Action, "required reading" for public health communication professionals. Dr. Zarcadoolas is a Professor at Hunter College, Department of Anthropology. Prior to this she was Professor at the CUNY School of Public Health and prior to that she was at Mount Sinai School of Medicine. She has a long tenure on the faculty at Brown University Center for Environmental Studies. She is the Founder and Director of the New York Roundtable on Public Health Literacy and founder of healthliteracylab.com which is an ever-expanding free library of communication and design lessons for health and safety communicators. Dr. Zarcadoolas is currently writing a book, "The Simplicity Complex", about the limits of simplifying complex information for the public.

Index

www.ingramcontent.com/pod-product-compliance
Lightning Source LLC
LaVergne TN
LVHW062137300926
849161LV00010B/2556